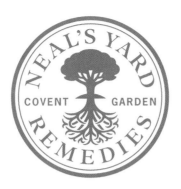

COMPLETE
HEALTH &
HEALING

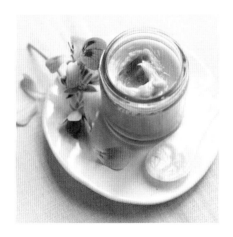

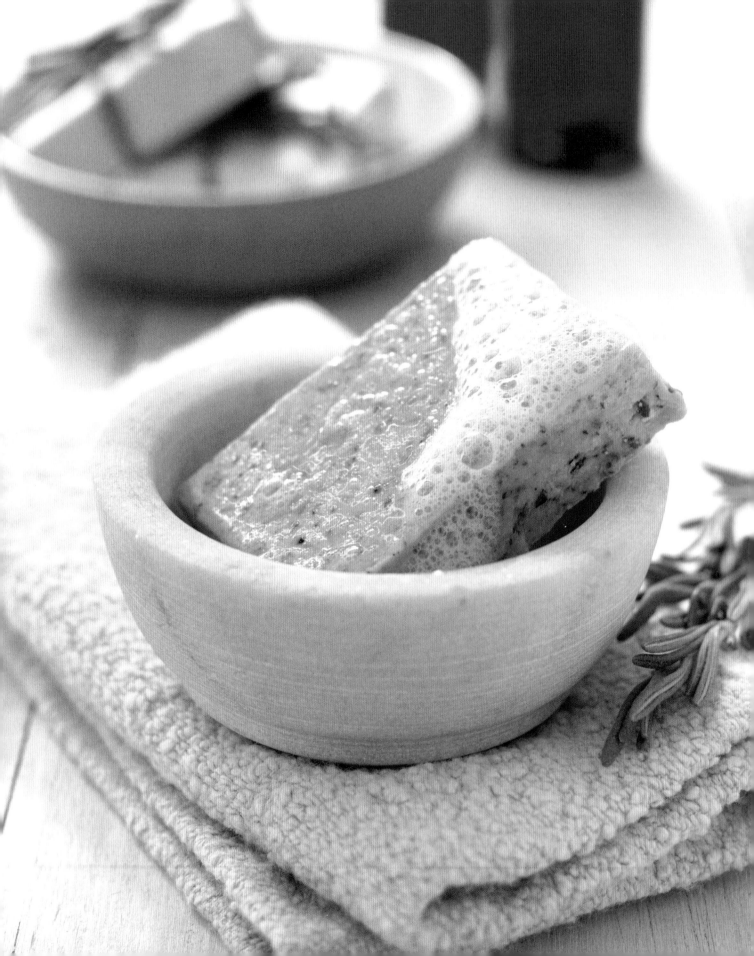

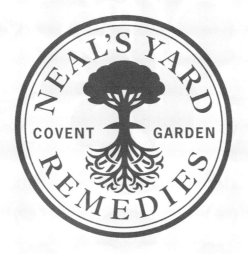

COMPLETE HEALTH & HEALING

**Natural ways to heal your body
and nourish your mind**

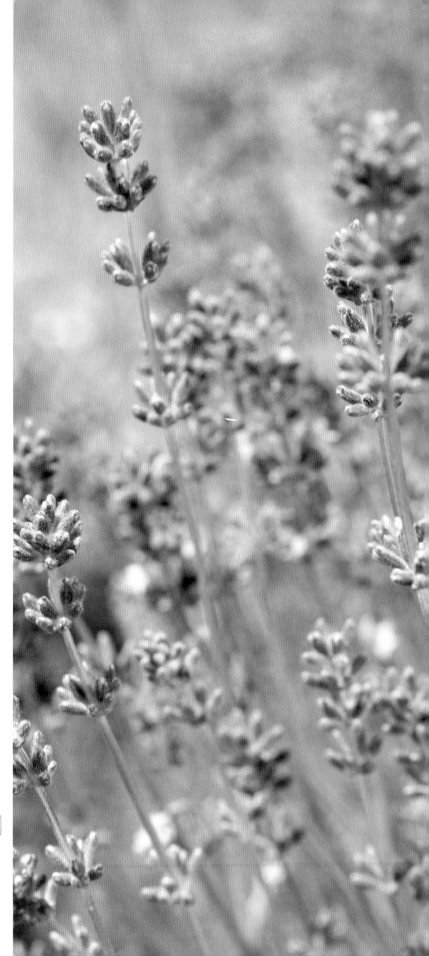

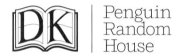
Penguin
Random
House

Editors Susannah Steel, Claire Cross, Libby Brown
Designers Colette Sadler, Kathryn Wilding,
Catherine Williams, Alison Gardner
Jacket Designer Vanessa Hamilton
Producer, Pre-Production Rebecca Fallowfield
Senior Production Controller Charlotte Oliver
Special Sales Creative Project Manager
Alison Donovan

Content previously published in *Neal's Yard
Essential Oils* (2016) and *Neal's Yard Remedies* (2011)
by Dorling Kindersley Limited
80 Strand, London, WC2R 0RL

2 4 6 8 10 9 7 5 3 1
001 – 309582 – Nov/2017

Copyright © 2011, 2016, 2017
Dorling Kindersley Limited
A Penguin Random House Company

A CIP catalogue record for this book is available
from the British Library.

ISBN 978-0-2413-3268-9

Printed and bound in China

A WORLD OF IDEAS
SEE ALL THERE IS TO KNOW
www.dk.com

DISCLAIMER: See page 398

Contents

Introduction *8*

A-Z OF HERBS *10*

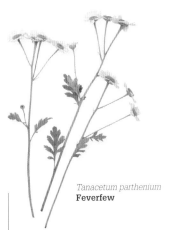

Tanacetum parthenium
Feverfew

USE HERBS

SOURCE HERBS

ESSENTIAL OILS

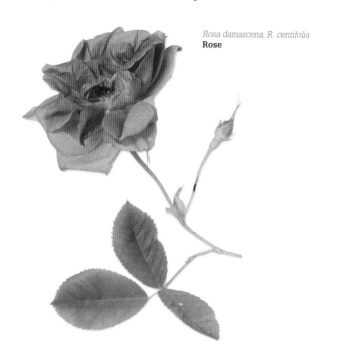

Rosa damascena, R. centifolia
Rose

A-Z ESSENTIAL OILS

Acacia dealbata
Mimosa

Achillea millefolium
Yarrow

Agathosma betulina
Buchu

Agonis fragrans
Fragonia

Aloysia triphylla
Lemon Verbena

Alpinia officinarum
Galangal

Anethum graveolens
Dill

Angelica archangelica
Angelica

Aniba rosaeodora
Rosewood

Artemisia dracunculus
Tarragon

Artemisia vulgaris
Mugwort

Betula alba
Birch (leaf)

Boswellia carterii, B. sacra, B. frereana, et al
Frankincense (Olibanum)

Cananga odorata
Ylang ylang

Canarium luzonicum
Elemi

Carum carui
Caraway

Cedrus atlantica
Cedarwood

Cinnamon camphora
Camphor

Cinnamon zeylanicum
Cinnamon

Cistus ladaniferus
Cistus

Citrus aurantifolia
Lime

Citrus aurantium
Neroli

Citrus aurantium amara
Petitgrain

Citrus aurantium bergamia
Bergamot

Citrus limonum
Lemon

Citrus paradisi
Grapefruit

Citrus reticulata, Citrus nobilis
Mandarin

Citrus sinensis
Orange

Commiphora myrrha, C. molmol
Myrrh

Coriandum saturum
Coriander

Cuminum cyminum
Cumin

Cupressus sempervirens
Cypress

Cymbopogon citratus, C. flexuosus
Lemongrass

Cymbopogon martinii
Palmarosa

Cymbopogon nardus
Citronella

Daucus carota
Carrot seed

Elettaria cardamomum
Cardamom

Eucalyptus globulus
Eucalyptus

Foeniculum vulgare
Fennel (sweet)

Gaultheria procumbens, G. fragrantissima
Wintergreen

Helichrysum italicum
Helichrysum (Immortelle)

Illicium verum
Star anise

Jasminum officinale
Jasmine

Juniperus communis
Juniper

Laurus nobilis
Bay laurel

Lavandula angustifolia
Lavender

Leptospermum scoparium
Manuka

Litsea cubeba
Litsea

Matricaria recutita
Chamomile (blue)

Melaleuca alternifolia
Tea tree

Melaleuca cajuputi
Cajuput

Melaleuca viridiflora, M. guinguenervia
Niaouli

Melissa officinalis
Lemon balm

Mentha piperita
Peppermint

Myristica fragrans
Nutmeg

Myrtus communis
Myrtle

Ocimum basilicum
Basil

Origanum majorana
Marjoram

Origanum vulgare
Oregano

Pelargonium graveolens
Geranium

Petroselinum crispum
Parsley seed

Pimenta dioica
Allspice

Pinus sylvestris
Pine

Piper nigrum
Black pepper

Pogostemon cablin
Patchouli

Polianthus tuberosa
Tuberose

*Ravensara aromatica,
Cinnamomum camphora*
Ravensara, Ravintsara

Rosa damascena, R. centifolia
Rose

Rosmarinus officinalis
Rosemary

Salvia officinalis
Sage (Dalmatian)

Salvia sclarea
Clary sage

Santalum album
Sandalwood

Satureja hortensis
Summer savory

Styrax benzoin
Benzoin

Syzygium aromaticum, Eugenia caryophyllata
Clove

Tagetes erecta
Tagetes

Thymus vulgaris
Thyme

Trigonella foenumgraecum
Fenugreek

Valeriana officinalis
Valerian

Vanilla planifolia
Vanilla

Vetiveria zizanioides
Vetiver

Viola odorata
Violet

Zingiber cassumunar, Z. montanum
Plai

Zingiber officinale
Ginger

THE AUTHORS

Susan Curtis
Susan runs a busy practice as a homeopath and naturopath and is the Director of Natural Health for Neal's Yard Remedies. She is the author of several books, including *Essential Oils*, and co-author of *Natural Healing for Women*. Susan has two children and is passionate about helping people to live a more natural and healthy lifestyle.

Louise Green
An avid supporter of the organic movement and eco-living, Louise has spent 15 years at Neal's Yard Remedies in a variety of roles ranging from buying to product development, and most recently as Head of Sustainability. Louise lives in London and is expecting her first child.

Penelope Ody MNIMH
Penelope qualified as a medical herbalist in the 1980s and practised as a consultant herbalist for 12 years. Since then she has written more than 20 books on both Western and Chinese herbalism and runs workshops on traditional uses of culinary and medicinal herbs at her home in Hampshire.

Dragana Vilinac
A fourth-generation herbalist widely respected for her vast knowledge and expertise, Dragana's passion for herbal medicine has taken her around the world, and has led her to train in disciplines including Western Herbal Medicine and Traditional Chinese Medicine. Dragana is Head Herbalist for Neal's Yard Remedies.

Pat Thomas
Pat is a journalist, campaigner, and broadcaster. Her previous books include *Cleaning Yourself to Death*, *What's in this Stuff?*, and *Skin Deep*. Through her work she has led the way in exposing harmful chemicals in many everyday products, as well as promoting natural alternatives that work. She is a former editor of *The Ecologist* magazine and is a trustee of the Organic Research Centre and editor of Neal's Yard Remedies' natural health website, *NYR Natural News*.

Fran Johnson
Fran is a passionate cosmetic scientist and aromatherapist, and has been part of the Product Development team at Neal's Yard Remedies since 2006, formulating therapeutic products for healing and wellbeing. She has written and teaches a number of Neal's Yard Remedies courses that cover aromatherapy, natural perfumery, and making cosmetic products.

Introduction

According to the World Health Organization, herbal remedies are the most widespread system of medicine used in the world. In recent years, an increased emphasis on holistic healing has also led to a resurgence of interest in the traditional use of essential oils in the practice of aromatherapy to enhance health and wellbeing. More and more people are recognizing the many benefits of using natural remedies to treat themselves and their family.

Author's **note**

Used appropriately, herbs can be a satisfying part of a more holistic lifestyle, and many herbs are of course the starting point of much of the modern medicine used today. When used with common sense, herbal remedies are a safe and effective form of home help. If we can treat colds, flu, or minor injuries in the early stages we can often prevent the development of something more serious and avoid using conventional drugs with their risk of side-effects.

Learning which herbs work for us enables us to learn more about the plants that surround us, as well as our own healing processes. However, some herbs are not suitable for everyone or at every stage of life (during pregnancy, for example); if in any doubt you should always consult a medical practitioner.

Pleasurable and extremely versatile, essential oils can be used as remedies for ailments and incorporated into cosmetics. The growth of interest in essential oils also coincides with a rise in stress-related conditions associated with hectic modern-day living. With their ability to soothe body and mind, essential oils are especially helpful for combatting the effects of chronic stress.

We have "tried and tested" all the recipes in this book. We are excited to have the opportunity to familairize you with the world of essential oils and introduce you to some more unusual plants so you can be more adventurous while trusting that your health and wellbeing will benefit.

Neal's Yard Remedies has over thirty years of expertise and passion in creating wonderful, natural products and remedies, and we are delighted to share some of our favourite ways of using herbs and oils to heal and nurture body and mind. Enjoy creating and using your own natural remedies!

Susan Curtis, Director of Natural Health, Neal's Yard Remedies

Consultant's **note**

Hippocrates, the father of medicine, wrote: "Let food be thy medicine, and medicine be thy food". Many herbs described in this book are used both as tasty foods and as medicines. Although the herbal medicines and essential oil remedies have not yet all been researched by modern science, most have stood the test of time. You should always see your doctor for serious health problems, but I hope this book will help readers to treat and prevent minor illnesses, and to understand treatments prescribed by their herbalist or aromatherapist.

Dr Merlin Willcox MRCGP MCPP

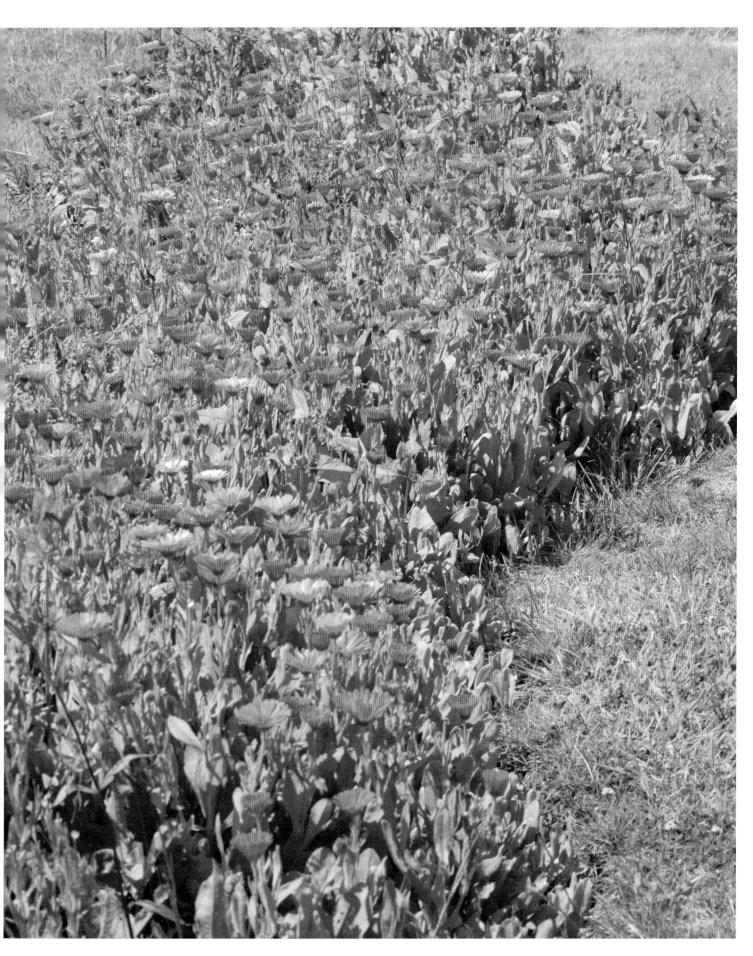

A–Z of Herbs

Discover 100 of the most useful medicinal herbs for natural health and well-being; find out how to use each herb to cure common ailments at home, as well as how to grow, forage, and harvest the herbs for yourself.

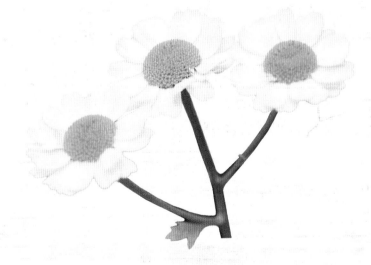

Achillea millefolium **Yarrow**

Native to Europe and western Asia, yarrow was traditionally used to treat wounds, although it was also once used in Germany and the Nordic countries as an alternative to hops in beer-making. Today it is valued for its astringent and anticatarrhal properties, and is used in remedies for colds and urinary disorders. It is widely naturalized in North America, New Zealand, and Australia.

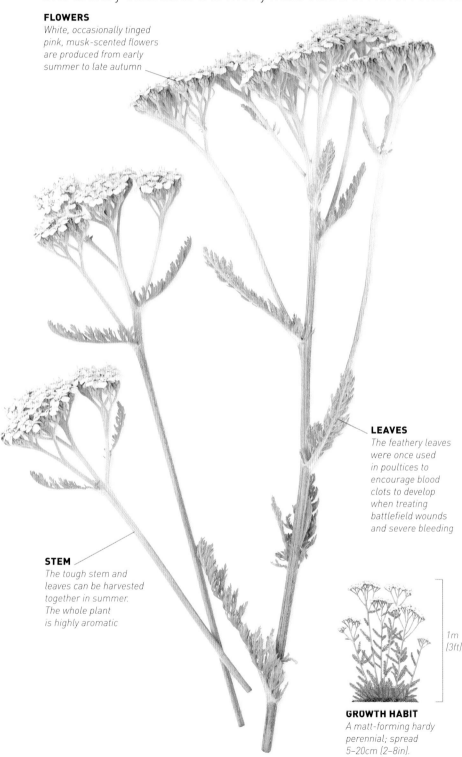

FLOWERS
White, occasionally tinged pink, musk-scented flowers are produced from early summer to late autumn

LEAVES
The feathery leaves were once used in poultices to encourage blood clots to develop when treating battlefield wounds and severe bleeding

STEM
The tough stem and leaves can be harvested together in summer. The whole plant is highly aromatic

1m (3ft)

GROWTH HABIT
A matt-forming hardy perennial; spread 5–20cm (2–8in).

PARTS USED Leaves, flowers, essential oil
MAIN CONSTITUENTS Volatile oil, isovalerianic acid, asparagine, salicylic acid, sterols, flavonoids
ACTIONS Astringent, diaphoretic, peripheral vasodilator, digestive stimulant, restorative for menstrual system, febrifuge Essential oil: anti-inflammatory, anti-allergenic

HOW TO USE

INFUSION Take 1 cup of a standard infusion (p.168) 3 times a day to encourage sweating and reduce fevers; combines well with elderflower and peppermint for common colds. One cup stimulates the appetite.
TINCTURE Use 1–2ml (20–40 drops) 3 times daily, usually with herbs such as couchgrass or buchu, for urinary disorders.
FRESH LEAVES A single leaf inserted in the nostril will rapidly stop a nosebleed.
OINTMENT Apply to minor cuts and grazes.
MASSAGE OIL Add 10 drops of yarrow essential oil to 25ml (5 tsp) of infused St John's wort oil to make a rub for hot, inflamed joints.
STEAM INHALATION Use 1 tbsp fresh flowers in boiling water to ease hayfever symptoms. Inhale the steam for at least 2–3 minutes.

HOW TO SOURCE

GROW Prefers a well-drained position in full sun, but is tolerant of a wide range of conditions. Sow seeds in spring. Propagation by root division is best in spring or autumn. It can easily become invasive.
FORAGE Generally found in pasture, hedgerows, or among grass in meadows throughout Europe.
HARVEST Gather leaves and aerial parts in summer, and flowers when they appear.

CAUTION In rare cases yarrow can cause skin rashes, and prolonged use can increase skin photosensitivity. Avoid during pregnancy. Essential oils should not be taken internally without professional advice.

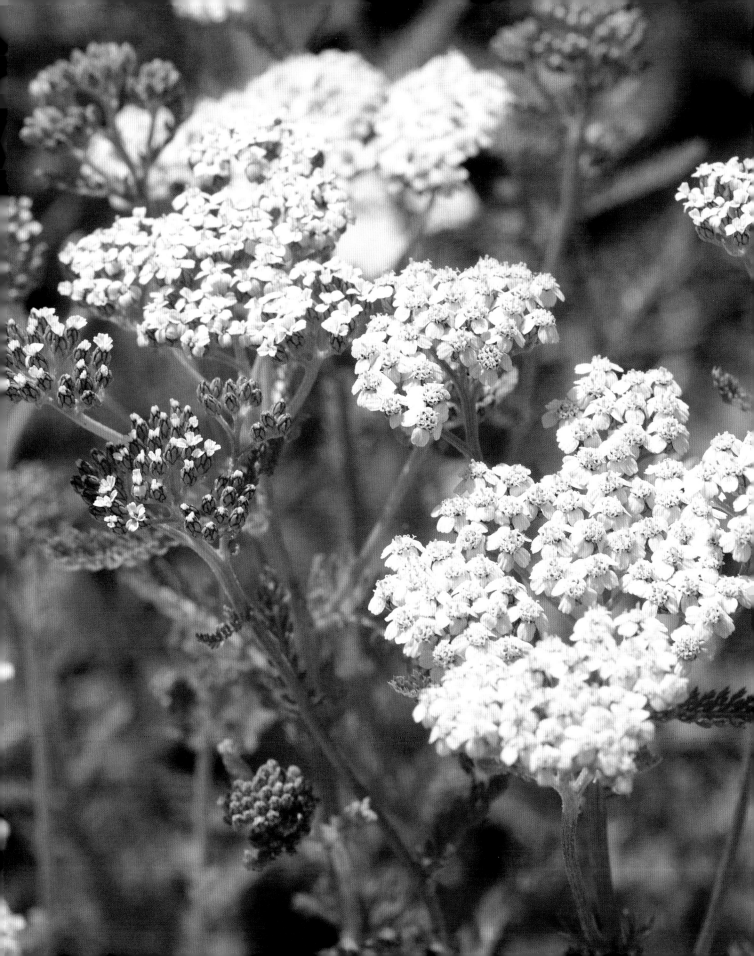

Actaea racemosa **Black cohosh**

Originally found in Canada and the eastern parts of the USA, black cohosh was a favourite remedy with Native Americans. It was used for a range of gynaecological disorders, snakebites, fevers, and rheumatism. It has been used in Europe since the 19th century, and is also known as *Cimicifuga racemosa*. Some cases of liver damage have been reported, and it is restricted in some countries.

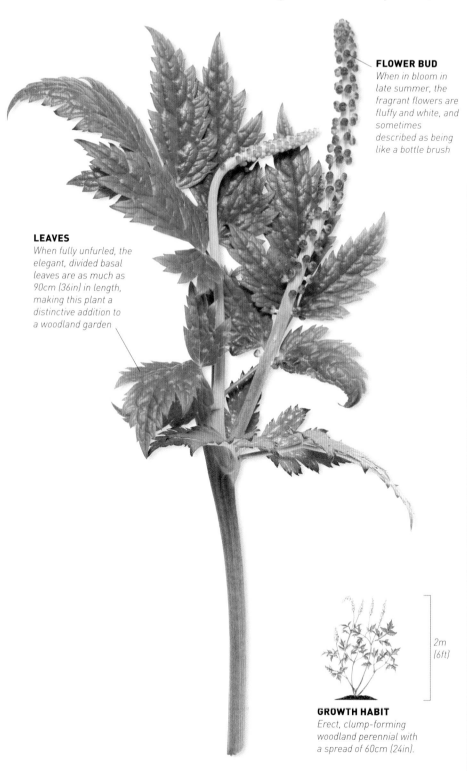

FLOWER BUD
When in bloom in late summer, the fragrant flowers are fluffy and white, and sometimes described as being like a bottle brush

LEAVES
When fully unfurled, the elegant, divided basal leaves are as much as 90cm (36in) in length, making this plant a distinctive addition to a woodland garden

GROWTH HABIT
Erect, clump-forming woodland perennial with a spread of 60cm (24in).

2m (6ft)

PARTS USED Root and rhizome
MAIN CONSTITUENTS Cinnamic acid derivatives, chromone, isoflavones, tannins, triterpene glycosides, salicylic acid
ACTIONS Antispasmodic, anti-arthritic, anti-inflammatory, antirheumatic, mild analgesic, relaxing nervine, relaxes blood vessels, emmenagogue, diuretic, sedative, antitussive, hypotensive, hypoglycaemic

HOW TO USE

TINCTURE Take 20–40 drops in a little water 3 times daily for period pain; combine with an equal amount of motherwort tincture and take 3 times daily for hot flushes, night sweats, and emotional upsets associated with the menopause. Take 20 drops 3 times daily with an equal amount of valerian to support treatments for high blood pressure.
DECOCTION Use 15g (½oz) of the root in 900ml (1½ pints) of water simmered for 15 minutes – twice daily for rheumatic pains, lumbago, facial neuralgia, sciatica, or tendonitis.
TABLETS/CAPSULES Use for menopausal problems or rheumatic disorders; follow dosage directions on the pack. It is best not to take more than 40–80mg daily.
SYRUP Combine 300ml (10fl oz) of a decoction (made as above) with 225g (8oz) of sugar or honey, bring to the boil, and simmer gently for 5–10 minutes to make a syrup. Take in 5ml (1 tsp) doses every 2–3 hours for whooping cough and bronchitis.

HOW TO SOURCE

GROW Prefers moist, fertile soil in dappled or partial shade. Sow ripe seeds in a cold frame and transplant to 7cm (3.5in) pots; plant in final positions in late spring.
FORAGE Found in woodland areas in North America and some parts of Europe.
HARVEST Dig mature roots in autumn.

CAUTION Do not exceed recommended dosage. May rarely cause liver problems. Do not use if you have a history of liver disease; if in doubt, consult your GP. Avoid during pregnancy.

Agastache rugosa **Purple giant hyssop**

Native to eastern Asia, including parts of India, China, and Japan, purple giant hyssop is also known as Korean mint. It is one of two species that are known as *huo xiang* in Chinese medicine, and which have been used for at least 1,500 years. *Huo xiang* is largely taken for digestive problems associated with nausea, vomiting, and poor appetite.

PARTS USED Aerial parts, essential oil
MAIN CONSTITUENTS Volatile oil (incl. methyl chavicol, anethole, anisaldehyde, limonene, pinene, linalool)
ACTIONS Antibacterial, antifungal, febrifuge, carminative, diaphoretic

HOW TO USE

INFUSION Take 1 cup of a standard infusion (p.168) of the aerial parts 1–2 times a day for abdominal bloating and indigestion.
LOTION/OINTMENT Use 1 cup of infusion to bathe ringworm patches, or make into an ointment and apply 2–3 times daily. Alternatively, add 10 drops of the essential oil to 15ml (1 tbsp) of almond oil.
TINCTURE Take 10–40 drops in a little water to relieve nausea.
DECOCTION In traditional Chinese medicine it is combined in decoctions with such herbs as *huang qin* (baikal skullcap, *Scutellaria baicalensis*) and *lian qiao* (forsythia fruits, *Forsythia suspensa*) for acute diarrhoea.
PATENT REMEDIES Included in various Chinese patent formulae, such as *huo xiang zheng qi san* (powder for dispelling turbidity with giant hyssop) which is used to clear "dampness". Follow the dosage directions on the pack.

HOW TO SOURCE

GROW Prefers well-drained, fertile soil with well-rotted organic matter in full sun. Can be grown from seeds planted in 7cm (3in) pots and transplanted to their final growing position when large enough to handle.
FORAGE Unlikely to be found growing wild beyond its native habitat, although cultivated plants that then self-seed are possible. Collect leaves throughout the growing season and use in any recipe that requires mint. They can also be infused to make a refreshing tea.
HARVEST Gather aerial parts in summer before flowering.

CAUTION In Chinese medicine it should be avoided in cases of fever. Avoid therapeutic doses in pregnancy.

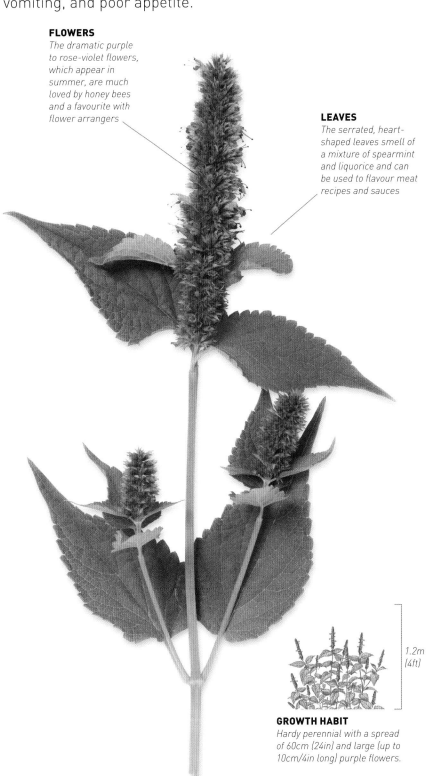

FLOWERS
The dramatic purple to rose-violet flowers, which appear in summer, are much loved by honey bees and a favourite with flower arrangers

LEAVES
The serrated, heart-shaped leaves smell of a mixture of spearmint and liquorice and can be used to flavour meat recipes and sauces

1.2m
(4ft)

GROWTH HABIT
Hardy perennial with a spread of 60cm (24in) and large (up to 10cm/4in long) purple flowers.

Agrimonia eupatoria **Agrimony**

Widely found in Europe, western Asia, and northern Africa, agrimony has been used as a medicinal herb since ancient times. Originally used for eye problems and diarrhoea or dysentery, it later became a favourite wound herb on the battlefield, and is used today for urinary disorders and poor digestion. A related Chinese variety, *Agrimonia pilosa*, is used in similar ways in the Far East.

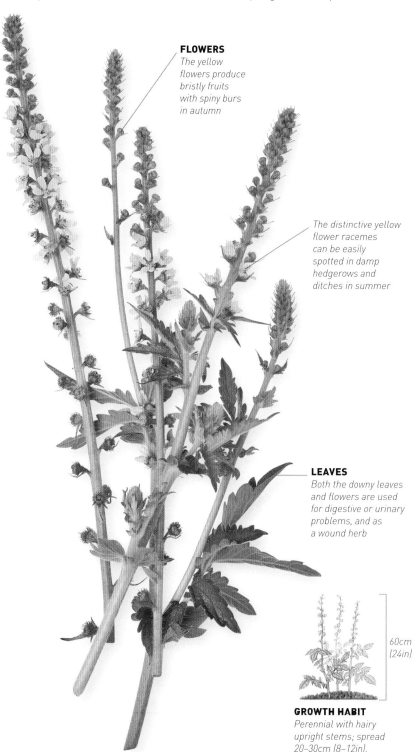

FLOWERS
The yellow flowers produce bristly fruits with spiny burs in autumn

The distinctive yellow flower racemes can be easily spotted in damp hedgerows and ditches in summer

LEAVES
Both the downy leaves and flowers are used for digestive or urinary problems, and as a wound herb

60cm
(24in)

GROWTH HABIT
Perennial with hairy upright stems; spread 20–30cm (8–12in).

PARTS USED Aerial parts
MAIN CONSTITUENTS Tannins, coumarins, volatile oil, flavonoids, minerals (incl. silica), vitamins B and K
ACTIONS Astringent, diuretic, tissue healer, haemostatic, cholagogue, some antiviral activity reported

HOW TO USE

INFUSION Take 1 cup of standard infusion (p.168) 3 times daily to improve sluggish digestion or to help strengthen the digestive system in cases of food intolerance. Agrimony is an ideal herb for children with diarrhoea (consult a herbalist for children's dosage), and can also be taken by nursing mothers to dose babies.
LOTION Use a standard infusion to bathe cuts, grazes, skin sores, weeping eczema, and varicose ulcers. It can be applied several times daily.
GARGLE Use 1 cup of standard infusion as a gargle for hoarseness, sore throats, and laryngitis.
TINCTURE Take 1–4ml (20–80 drops) 3 times daily for cystitis, urinary infections, or incontinence. For severe or persistent urinary symptoms, seek urgent medical advice to avoid potential kidney damage.

HOW TO SOURCE

GROW Prefers damp, fertile soil, and will tolerate partial shade or full sun. Sow the seeds in a cold frame in autumn or spring and transplant them when they are large enough to handle.
FORAGE Commonly found on wasteland or in damp hedgerows. It is easily noticeable because of its tall bright yellow flower spikes. Gather the whole aerial parts in summer.
HARVEST Gather in summer while in flower.

CAUTION This astringent herb is best avoided if constipated.

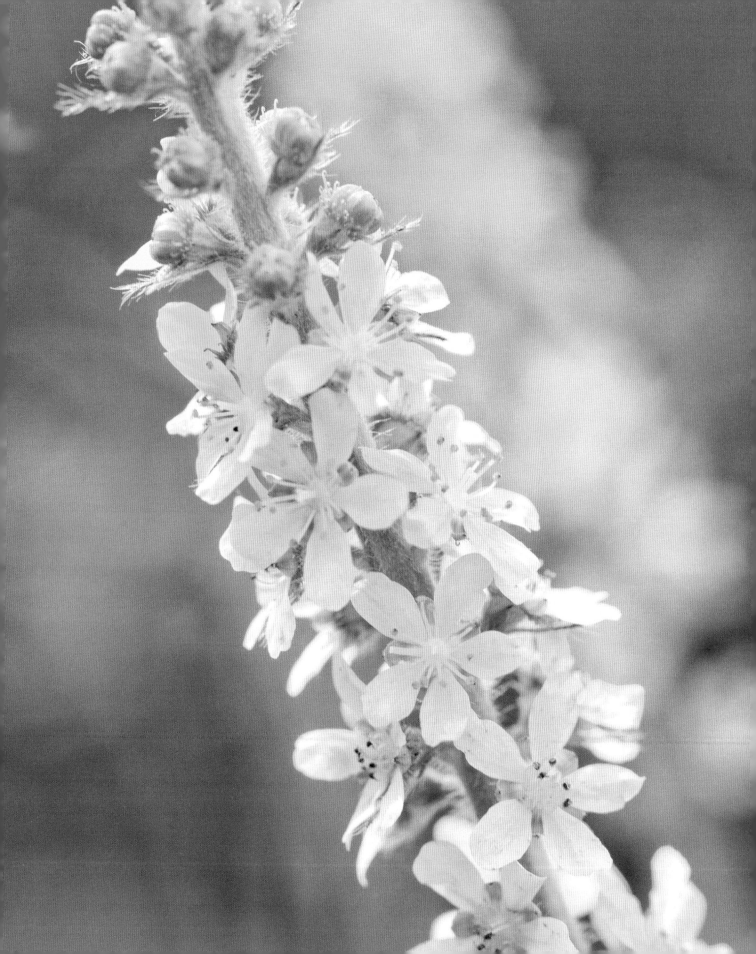

Alchemilla xanthochlora **Lady's mantle**

As its name suggests, lady's mantle has a long tradition of gynaecological uses and has been a remedy for menstrual irregularities, heavy menstrual bleeding, and to ease childbirth. The plant originated in northern Europe and mountainous regions further south. In recent years it has become a popular garden plant highly valued by flower arrangers for its flower stems.

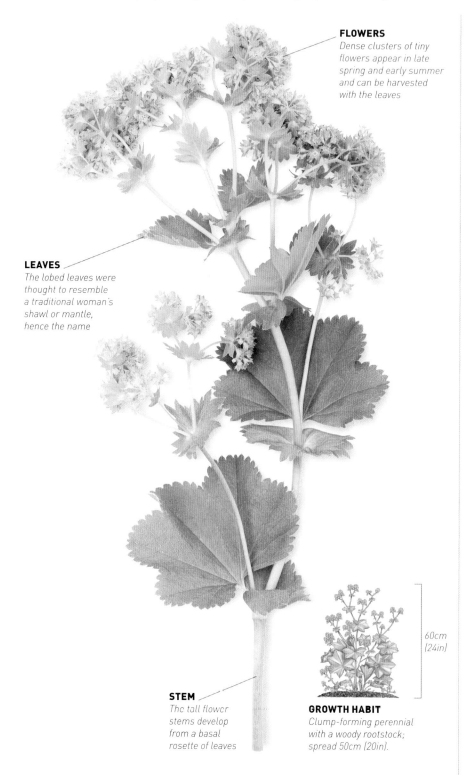

FLOWERS
Dense clusters of tiny flowers appear in late spring and early summer and can be harvested with the leaves

LEAVES
The lobed leaves were thought to resemble a traditional woman's shawl or mantle, hence the name

STEM
The tall flower stems develop from a basal rosette of leaves

GROWTH HABIT
Clump-forming perennial with a woody rootstock; spread 50cm (20in).

60cm (24in)

PARTS USED Aerial parts
MAIN CONSTITUENTS Tannins, salicylic acid, saponins, phytosterols, volatile oil, bitter principle
ACTIONS Astringent, menstrual regulator, digestive tonic, anti-inflammatory, wound herb

HOW TO USE

INFUSION Take 1 cup of a standard infusion (p.168) up to 5 times a day for acute diarrhoea or gastroenteritis, or to ease heavy menstrual bleeding or period pain.
TINCTURE Take 1–2ml (20–40 drops) 3 times daily to help regulate the menstrual cycle or, if combined with the same quantity of St John's wort, to ease period pains.
LOTION Use the standard infusion externally as a wash to bathe weeping eczema or skin sores.
GARGLE 1 cup of standard infusion can be used as a gargle for sore throats, laryngitis, or as a mouthwash for mouth ulcers.
CREAM/OINTMENT/PESSARIES Apply night and morning for vaginal discharges or itching. Insert 1 pessary at night. If symptoms do not improve in 2–3 days, seek advice from a genitourinary medicine clinic.

HOW TO SOURCE

GROW A hardy, clump-forming perennial, lady's mantle prefers moist, well-drained soil in full sun or dappled shade. The round, finely toothed leaves can have up to 11 distinct lobes. It can be grown from seed sown directly in spring or by division in spring or summer. Lady's mantle will self-seed enthusiastically.
FORAGE Found throughout northern Europe and the mountainous regions of central and southern Europe. It can also be found self-seeding outside gardens in other areas throughout the summer.
HARVEST Gather the whole aerial parts throughout the summer.

Allium sativum **Garlic**

Garlic is believed to have originated in south-west Siberia, but spread to much of Europe and Asia in ancient times. It has been used as a medicinal herb for at least 5,000 years, and is now known to reduce the risk of further heart attacks, as well as lower blood cholesterol levels. Also a strong antibiotic, garlic is used to treat colds, catarrh, and respiratory infections.

PARTS USED Bulb

MAIN CONSTITUENTS Volatile oil (incl. allicin, alliin, and ajoene), enzymes, vitamins A, B, C, and E, minerals (incl. selenium and germanium), flavonoids

ACTIONS Antibiotic, expectorant, diaphoretic, hypotensive, antithrombotic, hypolipidaemic, hypoglycaemic, antihistaminic, anthelmintic

HOW TO USE

JUICE Take up to 5ml (1 tsp) of juice in honey or water twice a day to combat infections, arteriosclerosis, or to reduce the risk of thrombosis.

FRESH CLOVES Rub the cut side of a fresh clove on acne pustules at night. Eat 2–3 cloves in cooked food each day to improve the cardiovascular system, lower cholesterol, or help prevent colds and flu.

CAPSULES Take 1 capsule before meals (check dosage on the packet) to help prevent seasonal infections.

TINCTURE Take 2–4ml (40–80 drops) in water 3 times daily for cardiovascular problems, respiratory disorders, or fungal infections.

POWDER For anyone who has suffered a heart attack, take up to 1 level teaspoon each day stirred into water or fruit juice to help prevent further attacks.

HOW TO SOURCE

GROW Prefers a warm site in deep, fertile, well-drained soil in full sun. Plant bulbs or individual cloves 5–10cm (2–4in) deep in the soil in autumn or winter.

FORAGE May be found growing wild in warm areas, but generally only likely to occur in cultivation.

HARVEST Gather the bulbs in late summer and early autumn and air-dry before storing in frost-free conditions.

CAUTION Garlic oil is a skin irritant and should only be taken in capsules. Garlic can cause gastric irritation in some people.

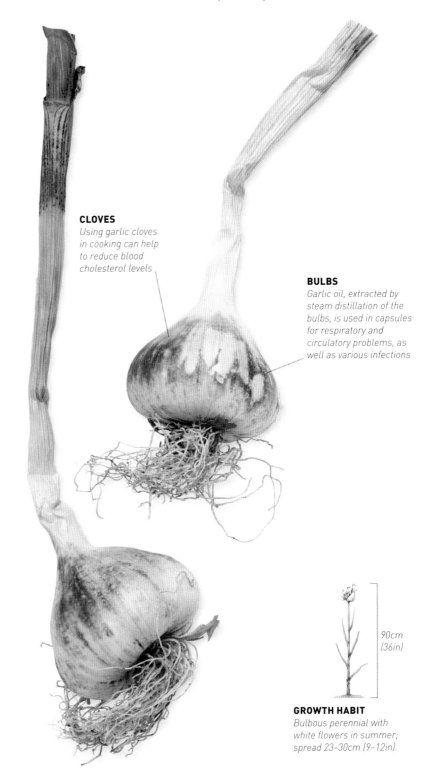

CLOVES
Using garlic cloves in cooking can help to reduce blood cholesterol levels

BULBS
Garlic oil, extracted by steam distillation of the bulbs, is used in capsules for respiratory and circulatory problems, as well as various infections

90cm
(36in)

GROWTH HABIT
Bulbous perennial with white flowers in summer; spread 23–30cm (9–12in).

Aloe vera **Aloe vera**

Native to tropical Africa, where it has been used as an antidote to poison arrow wounds, aloe vera reached Europe in ancient times and was well known to the Greeks and Romans as a wound herb. The sap is cooling and healing and for centuries has been used to treat burns, inflammation, and skin ulcers, while the whole leaf is purgative. Internal use is restricted in some countries.

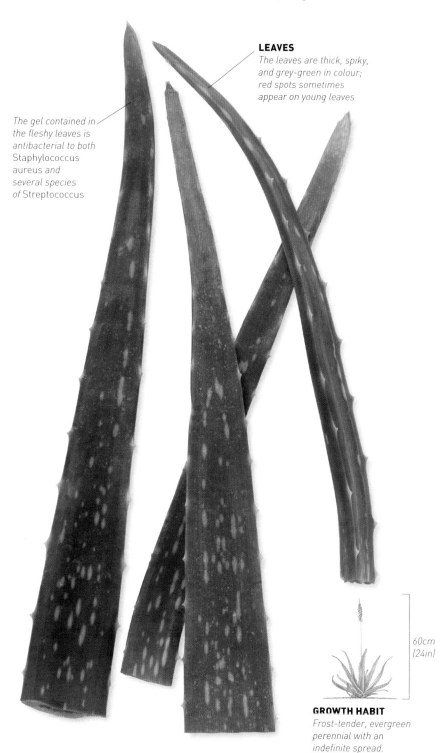

LEAVES
The leaves are thick, spiky, and grey-green in colour; red spots sometimes appear on young leaves

The gel contained in the fleshy leaves is antibacterial to both Staphylococcus aureus *and several species of* Streptococcus

60cm
(24in)

GROWTH HABIT
Frost-tender, evergreen perennial with an indefinite spread.

PARTS USED Leaves, gel
MAIN CONSTITUENTS Anthraquinone glycosides (incl. aloin and aloe-emodin), resins, polysaccharides, sterols, saponins, chromones
ACTIONS Purgative, cholagogue, wound healer, tonic, demulcent, antibacterial, antifungal, styptic, sedative, anthelmintic

HOW TO USE

FRESH GEL Split open a leaf and use the gel directly, or scrape it out with a blunt knife. Apply directly to burns, sunburn, dry skin, wounds, fungal infections, nappy rash, shingles, ringworm, insect bites, allergic rashes, eczema, or any itchy skin condition.
TINCTURE Made from the whole pulped leaf. Take 5ml (1 tsp) 3 times daily for constipation or take 0.5–3ml (10–60 drops) 3 times daily for poor appetite or to stimulate bile flow in sluggish digestion.
CAPSULES Commercially made from powdered leaf. Use in 100–500mg doses for constipation.
HAIR RINSE Combine 10ml (2 tsp) of gel with 120ml (4fl oz) of standard chamomile infusion (p.168) and use as a conditioner.

HOW TO SOURCE

GROW Prefers well-drained sandy soil in full sun with a moderate summer water supply and dry winters. Usually propagated by breaking off and replanting the small offsets that appear on mature plants, but can be grown from seeds sown in spring or early summer at 21°C (70°F). Grown as a houseplant in temperate areas; benefits from being kept outside in warm summers.
FORAGE Likely to be found growing wild in tropical regions only. Easily confused with many related, generally larger, species that grow outside in warmer regions.
HARVEST Collect the gel and leaves from plants as required throughout the year.

CAUTION Do not take aloe vera internally during pregnancy.

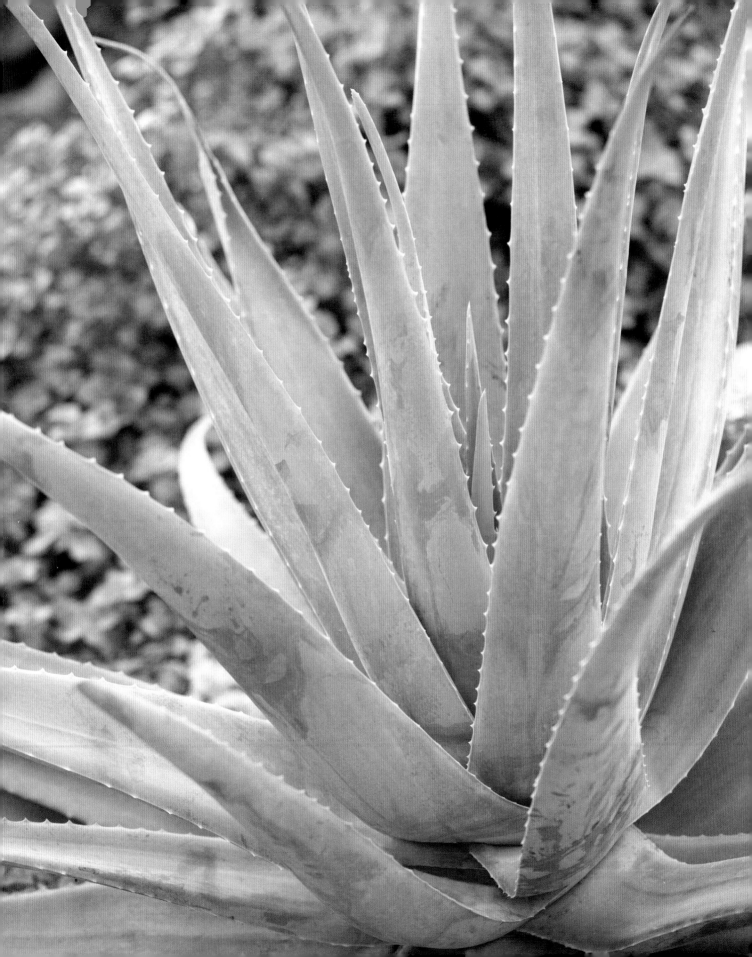

Aloysia triphylla **Lemon verbena**

Originally found growing in rocky areas of Chile and Argentina, lemon verbena is now cultivated worldwide both as a highly aromatic garden ornamental and for use in perfumery. It is also used in pot pourri or in cooking to give a strong lemony taste to desserts, marinades, and fruit drinks. It is traditionally regarded as both soothing and uplifting, so is used in restorative teas.

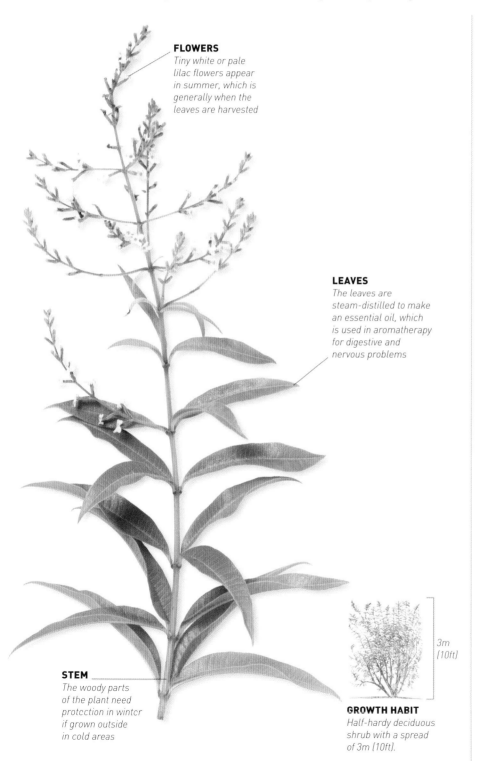

FLOWERS
Tiny white or pale lilac flowers appear in summer, which is generally when the leaves are harvested

LEAVES
The leaves are steam-distilled to make an essential oil, which is used in aromatherapy for digestive and nervous problems

STEM
The woody parts of the plant need protection in winter if grown outside in cold areas

3m (10ft)

GROWTH HABIT
Half-hardy deciduous shrub with a spread of 3m (10ft).

PARTS USED Leaves, essential oil
MAIN CONSTITUENTS Volatile oil (incl. citral, nerol, and geraniol)
ACTIONS Sedative, carminative, antispasmodic, febrifuge, stimulates liver and gall bladder function, some antifungal activity (to *Candida albicans*) reported

HOW TO USE

INFUSION Use ½ tsp dried leaves per cup (p.168) after meals for flatulence or at night for insomnia. Combine with dandelion leaves and drink 3 times daily to improve liver function. Can be used to ease feverish conditions in children; consult a herbalist for advice on dosage.
BATHS Add 1 cup of a standard infusion to bathwater to ease stress and tension.
MASSAGE OIL True lemon verbena oil is difficult to obtain, as it is often adulterated with other lemon-scented oils. Use 5 drops in 15ml (1 tbsp) of almond oil as a massage for cramps, indigestion, anxiety, insomnia, or other stress-related conditions.

HOW TO SOURCE

GROW Prefers full sun and moist but well-drained soil. Usually propagated by heeled softwood cuttings in summer; it also self-seeds if it sets fruit after a hot summer. It is not frost-hardy, so in colder areas is best grown in containers and over-wintered under glass. Alternatively, cut back to the wood, keep dry, and protect with fleece or straw lagging in winter (it should survive temperatures as low as -15°C/5°F).
FORAGE Unlikely to be found growing wild outside South America, although self-seeding in warmer areas is possible.
HARVEST Collect the leaves in summer.

CAUTION Prolonged use or large internal doses can cause gastric irritation. The oil can irritate sensitive skin and is photosensitizing, so avoid bright sunlight if using it externally.

Althaea officinalis **Marshmallow**

Originally found in coastal areas of Europe, marshmallow is now widely naturalized. The plant's botanical name comes from the Greek verb, *altho* (to heal), and it has been valued for its soothing and healing action, both internally and externally, for at least 3,500 years. As well as being used medicinally, both the root and leaves can be eaten as vegetables.

PARTS USED Root, leaves, flowers
MAIN CONSTITUENTS Root: asparagine, mucilage, polysaccharides, pectin, tannins
Leaves: mucilage, flavonoids, coumarin, salicylic, and other phenolic acids
ACTIONS Root: demulcent, expectorant, diuretic, wound herb
Leaves: expectorant, diuretic, demulcent
Flowers: expectorant

HOW TO USE

MACERATION Soak 30g (1oz) of root in 600ml (1 pint) of cold water overnight and strain: the result can often be very thick and mucilaginous and may need further dilution. Take ½–1 cup 3 times daily for acid reflux, gastric ulceration, cystitis, and dry coughs.
POULTICE Make a paste from 1 tsp of powdered root mixed with a little water and use on boils, abscesses, ulcers, or poorly healing infected wounds.
OINTMENT Use to draw pus, splinters, or thorns.
INFUSION Take 1 cup of a standard leaf infusion (p.168) 3 times daily for bronchitis, bronchial asthma, catarrh, or pleurisy.
SYRUP Make a syrup by combining 600ml (1 pint) of a standard infusion of fresh flowers with 450g (1lb) of honey or syrup; bring to the boil and simmer gently for 10–15 minutes. Take 5ml (1 tsp) doses as required.

HOW TO SOURCE

GROW Prefers fertile, moist, well-drained soil in full sun; tolerates other conditions. Sow seed in trays of compost in midsummer and transplant to 7.5cm (3in) pots when large enough to handle. Plant out the following spring. Alternatively, divide plants in autumn. Can self-seed enthusiastically in ideal conditions.
FORAGE Likely to be found in ditches, riversides, tidal zones, and pond margins, especially in coastal areas. Gather the flowers in summer to make a cough syrup, or the leaves during the growing period. The root can be boiled as a vegetable.
HARVEST Dig the root in autumn. Cut the aerial parts as the plant starts to flower.

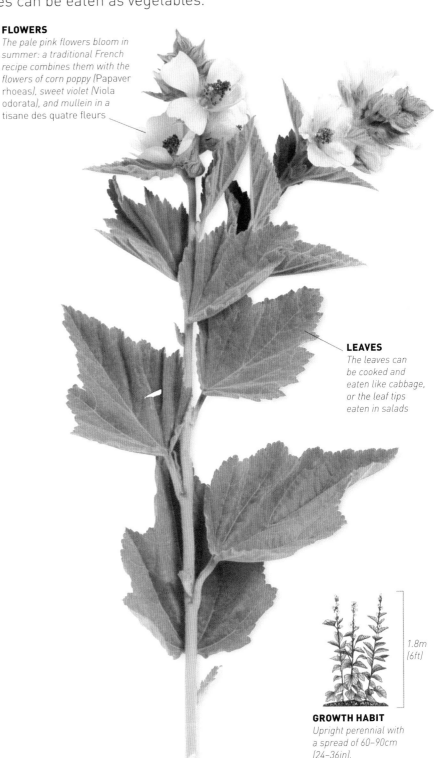

FLOWERS
The pale pink flowers bloom in summer: a traditional French recipe combines them with the flowers of corn poppy (Papaver rhoeas), sweet violet (Viola odorata), and mullein in a tisane des quatre fleurs

LEAVES
The leaves can be cooked and eaten like cabbage, or the leaf tips eaten in salads

1.8m (6ft)

GROWTH HABIT
Upright perennial with a spread of 60–90cm (24–36in).

Angelica archangelica **Angelica**

Native to northern Europe, angelica is a statuesque plant with striking flowerheads in summer. It reputedly takes its medieval Latin name (*herba angelica*) from a belief that it protects against evil spirits, and has been used for a wide range of ailments for centuries. The stems are also used in cooking, and the essential oil is used as a food flavouring.

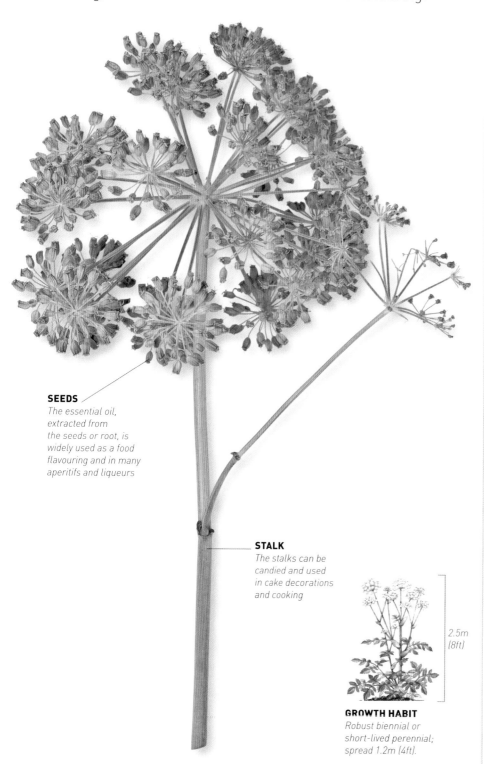

SEEDS
The essential oil, extracted from the seeds or root, is widely used as a food flavouring and in many aperitifs and liqueurs

STALK
The stalks can be candied and used in cake decorations and cooking

GROWTH HABIT
Robust biennial or short-lived perennial; spread 1.2m (4ft).

2.5m (8ft)

PARTS USED Leaves, root, essential oil
MAIN CONSTITUENTS Volatile oil (incl. phellandrene, pinene, borneol, linalol, and limonene), iridoids, resin, coumarins (incl. bergapten and angelicin), valerianic acid, tannins
ACTIONS Antispasmodic, diaphoretic, anti-inflammatory, expectorant, carminative, diuretic, antibacterial, digestive stimulant

HOW TO USE

INFUSION Take 1 cup of a standard infusion (p.168) of leaves after meals for indigestion.
DECOCTION Take ½–1 cup of a root decoction, made by simmering 15g (½oz) of root in 600ml (1 pint) of water for 5 minutes, for any cold condition where increased body heat is required, including arthritic and rheumatic problems in the elderly, poor circulation, or weak digestion.
TINCTURE Take 3ml (60 drops) 3 times daily of the leaf tincture for bronchitis or flatulent digestion. Take 1–2ml (20–40 drops) of the root tincture 3 times daily for bronchial catarrh, chesty coughs, digestive disorders including chronic indigestion and loss of appetite, or as a liver stimulant.
MASSAGE OIL Use 5 drops in 15ml (1 tbsp) of almond oil as a chest rub for bronchitis and coughs or to massage arthritic joints.

HOW TO SOURCE

GROW Prefers deep, fertile, moist soil in sun or partial shade. Surface-sow seeds when ripe or in spring. Thin out seedlings as required when they are large enough to handle. Self-seeds in the right conditions.
FORAGE Found in damp grassy places in northern and eastern Europe and into Asia.
HARVEST Gather leaves and stems in early summer, year-old roots in autumn, and seeds as they ripen.

CAUTION Avoid during pregnancy. Do not take therapeutic doses if diabetic, unless under professional guidance. Avoid exposure to sun if using externally (phototoxic).

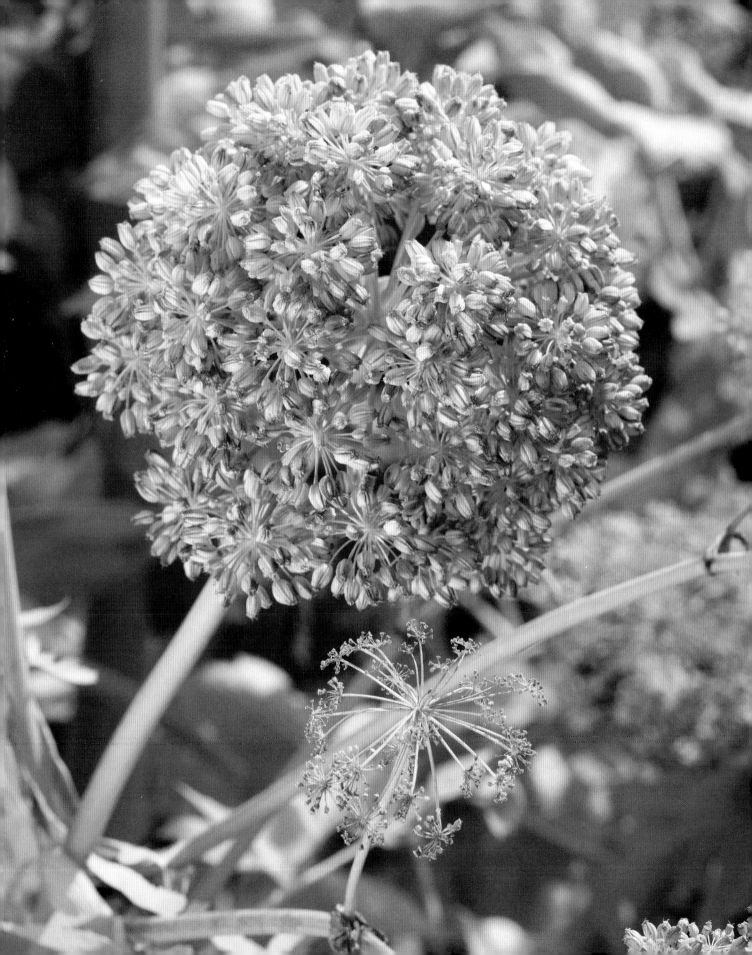

Apium graveolens **Wild celery**

Native to Europe, the Mediterranean region, and western Asia, celery has long been cultivated as a vegetable and cooked or used raw in dishes such as Waldorf salad (celery, walnuts, and apple). Medicinally, the seeds and essential oil of celery are used mainly for urinary and arthritic disorders, and also to help clear uric acid from joints affected by gout.

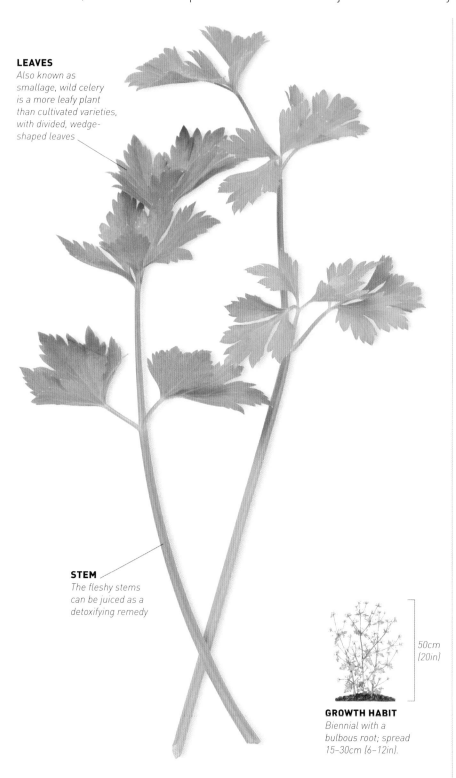

LEAVES
Also known as smallage, wild celery is a more leafy plant than cultivated varieties, with divided, wedge-shaped leaves

STEM
The fleshy stems can be juiced as a detoxifying remedy

GROWTH HABIT
Biennial with a bulbous root; spread 15–30cm (6–12in).

50cm (20in)

PARTS USED Seeds, stalks, essential oil
MAIN CONSTITUENTS Volatile oil (incl. limonene, apiol, selinene, and phthalides), coumarins, furanocoumarins, flavonoids, minerals (incl. iron, phosphorus, and potassium)
ACTIONS Antirheumatic, sedative, urinary antiseptic, diuretic, carminative, hypotensive, antispasmodic, galactagogue, anti-inflammatory, encourages elimination of uric acid, antifungal activity reported

HOW TO USE

DECOCTION Use 15g (½oz) of seeds to 600ml (1 pint) of water, simmer for 10 minutes and take in ½–1 cup doses 3 times daily for rheumatic disorders, gout, rheumatoid arthritis, and urinary tract inflammations.
MASSAGE OIL Use 1ml (20 drops) oil in 60ml (2fl oz) of almond oil and massage into the abdomen for indigestion, flatulence, and liver congestion. Use also for sciatica, rheumatism, and arthritis.
FOOTBATH Add 1ml (20 drops) oil to a bowl of warm water to soak feet or toe joints with very painful gout.
JUICE Liquidize the stalks and leaves and drink in wine-glass doses as a remedy for debility and nervous exhaustion.

HOW TO SOURCE

GROW Prefers moist, well-drained soil in full sun. Plant the seeds in seed trays in spring, cover with a thin layer of compost, and place in a heated propagator or on a warm window sill. Pot on to 7.5cm (3in) pots, and when 10cm (4in) tall plant in final growing positions 30cm (12in) apart.
FORAGE Grows wild in coastal areas.
HARVEST Pick the cultivated variety as a vegetable in the first year; collect the seeds when ripe in the second summer.

CAUTION Do not use seeds if pregnant. Do not use cultivated seeds medicinally, as they are often treated with fungicides. Do not take the essential oil internally unless under professional supervision.

Aralia racemosa **American spikenard**

Used by many Native Americans for a range of ailments including rheumatism, coughs, indigestion, asthma, and blood poisoning, American spikenard is found in many parts of the United States, from the Midwest to the eastern seaboard. The herb is known to encourage sweating and is detoxifying, but has otherwise been poorly researched.

PARTS USED Root
MAIN CONSTITUENTS Volatile oil, tannins, glycosides, diterpenes
ACTIONS Expectorant, diaphoretic, warming stimulant, detoxifying

HOW TO USE

DECOCTION Take ½ cup of a decoction made from 15g (½oz) dried root in 600ml (1pint) of water 3 times daily for rheumatic disorders.
SYRUP Combine 300ml (10fl oz) of strained decoction with 225g (8oz) of sugar or honey, bring to the boil, and simmer gently for 5–10 minutes to make a syrup. Take in 5ml (1 tsp) doses every 2–3 hours for coughs including bronchitis and whooping coughs.
LIQUID EXTRACT Take 1.5–3ml (30–60 drops) 3 times daily in a little water for rheumatic disorders, lumbago, and similar aches and pains.
POULTICE Mix 15g (½oz) of powdered root into a paste with a little water, spread on gauze, and use as a poultice for skin conditions including eczema.

HOW TO SOURCE

GROW Prefers partial shade, but tolerates sun. Sow the seeds where you want to grow them in autumn or in winter in a cold frame or unheated greenhouse; transplant into final positions the following spring.
FORAGE Largely found in woodland areas in the Midwest and eastern US; unlikely to occur growing wild in other areas. As well as their medicinal applications, the roots can be used in teas or to flavour beer.
HARVEST Dig up the roots in summer or autumn.

CAUTION Avoid during pregnancy.

FLOWERS
When fully in bloom in summer, the flowers are tiny, white-green, and carried in umbels

STEM
The stem is herbaceous, erect, and green to purple

LEAVES
The large, heart-shaped leaves, which can grow up to 20cm (8in) in length, are purple at the nodes

1.5m (5ft)

GROWTH HABIT
Herbaceous perennial with tiny flowers in summer and a spread of 60cm–2m (2–6ft).

Arctium lappa **Burdock**

Native to Europe and Asia, burdock is largely regarded as a cleansing remedy that helps to rid the body of toxins, including heavy metals, and is generally used for skin problems, arthritic conditions, and infections. The root and leaves are traditionally used in Europe, while the seeds are preferred in Chinese medicine and are often included in remedies for common colds.

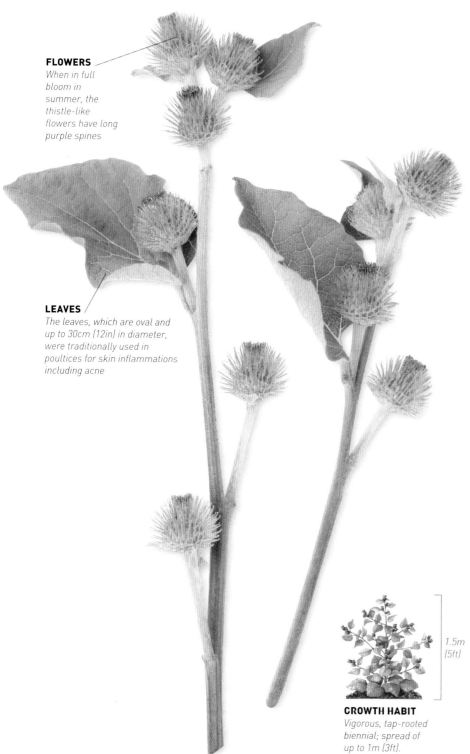

FLOWERS
When in full bloom in summer, the thistle-like flowers have long purple spines

LEAVES
The leaves, which are oval and up to 30cm (12in) in diameter, were traditionally used in poultices for skin inflammations including acne

GROWTH HABIT
Vigorous, tap-rooted biennial; spread of up to 1m (3ft).

1.5m (5ft)

PARTS USED Root, leaves, seeds
MAIN CONSTITUENTS Leaf/root: bitter glycosides (incl. arctiopictrin), flavonoids (incl. arctin), tannins, volatile oil, antibiotic polyacetylenes, resin, mucilage, inulin, alkaloids, sesquiterpenes
Seeds: essential fatty acids, vitamins A, B2
ACTIONS Root: cleansing, mild laxative, diuretic, diaphoretic, anti-rheumatic, antiseptic, antibiotic
Leaves: mild laxative, diuretic
Seeds: febrifuge, anti-inflammatory, anti-bacterial, hypoglycaemic

HOW TO USE

ROOT DECOCTION Take ½–1 cup of a standard decoction (p.168) of the root 3 times daily for skin disorders, including persistent boils, sores, and dry eczema. Use a cup of the mix as a wash for acne and fungal skin infections including athlete's foot or ringworm.
INFUSION Take 1 wineglass of a standard leaf infusion (p.168) before meals as a mild digestive stimulant to combat indigestion.
SEED DECOCTION Take 1 cup of a standard decoction of the seeds up to 3 times daily for feverish colds and infections with sore throat and cough; it is often combined with honeysuckle flowers or forsythia berries.
TINCTURE Take 5–10ml (1–2 tsp) root tincture 3 times daily to detoxify the system in arthritic conditions, for urinary stones and gravel, or to stimulate digestion. Usually used in combination with other herbs.
POULTICE Use a root poultice for skin sores and leg ulcers.

HOW TO SOURCE

GROW Prefers moist, neutral to alkaline soil in full sun to partial shade. Sow the seeds where you want to grow them in spring. Self-seeds prolifically and can be invasive. Harvest the plant before the fruits are ripe to reduce the spread.
FORAGE Easily spotted in hedgerows and waste areas in Europe and western Asia.
HARVEST The root is generally collected in late summer and the leaves when the plant is just starting to flower; the seeds should be gathered when ripe in autumn.

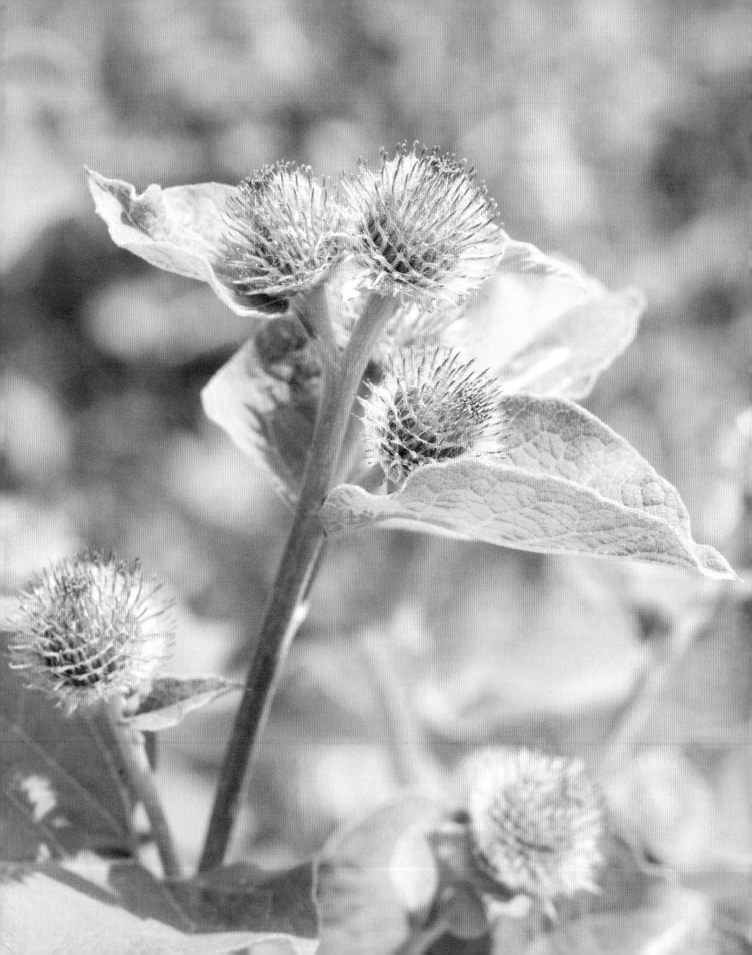

Arctostaphylos uva-ursi **Bearberry**

Native to moorland in Europe, Asia, and North America, this plant's fruits are a favourite food for bears – hence its common name, bearberry or uva-ursi (in Latin literally, "grape-bear"). It is highly regarded by herbalists as a urinary antiseptic largely due to the presence of chemicals called hydroquinones, which help to disinfect the urinary tract.

LEAVES
The small leaves need to be gathered and dried individually for use in remedies for cystitis and other urinary problems

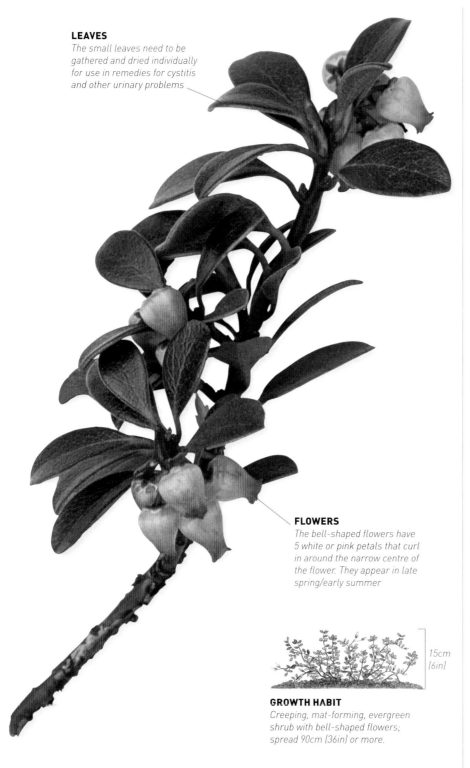

FLOWERS
The bell-shaped flowers have 5 white or pink petals that curl in around the narrow centre of the flower. They appear in late spring/early summer

GROWTH HABIT
Creeping, mat-forming, evergreen shrub with bell-shaped flowers; spread 90cm (36in) or more.

15cm (6in)

PARTS USED Leaves, berries
MAIN CONSTITUENTS Hydroquinones (incl. arbutin), ursolic acid, tannic acid, gallic acid, phenolic glycosides, flavonoids, volatile oil, resin, tannins
ACTIONS Astringent, antibacterial, urinary antiseptic, possibly diuretic, haemostatic, oxytocic

HOW TO USE

INFUSION Take 1 cup of a standard infusion (p.168) of leaves 3 times daily for temporary cystitis, urethritis, or burning pain when urinating. It is often combined with couch grass or cleavers. For any severe or persistent urinary symptoms, you should seek urgent medical advice to avoid any potential damage to the kidneys.
TINCTURE Take 2–4ml (40–80 drops) 3 times daily for urinary problems or leucorrhoea (a white or yellow vaginal discharge).
TABLETS Available commercially, often in combination with dandelion, as a remedy for fluid retention. Follow the directions on the pack.

HOW TO SOURCE

GROW A moorland plant, it prefers moist, fertile, acid soil in partial or dappled shade, and makes good ground cover in the right conditions. Requires lime-free (ericaceous) soil. Sow seeds in a cold frame in autumn and pot on as soon as the seedlings are large enough to handle.
FORAGE Found in moorland areas. The leaves can be harvested in summer. The berries are edible and can be gathered in autumn and made into jellies and jams.
HARVEST The leaves are mainly collected in spring or summer, and the berries are collected in autumn.

CAUTION Do not take in pregnancy, while breast-feeding, or if suffering from kidney disease. It should not be taken for more than 10 consecutive days without professional advice. Large doses may cause nausea and vomiting.

Artemisia absinthium **Wormwood**

An extremely bitter herb, wormwood is largely used today as a digestive stimulant. Native to Europe, it was once a popular remedy for treating parasitic worms, as its name implies, and is still occasionally used in this way today. Its botanical name highlights a link to the French drink, absinthe, a favourite with the 19th-century avant garde that was highly addictive.

PARTS USED Leaves, flowering tops
MAIN CONSTITUENTS Volatile oil (incl. sesquiterpene lactones, thujone, and azulenes), bitter principle, flavonoids, tannins, lignan, silica, antibiotic polyacetylenes, inulin, hydroxycoumarins
ACTIONS Bitter digestive tonic, anthelmintic, uterine stimulant, cholagogue, choleretic, carminative, anti-inflammatory, immune stimulant

HOW TO USE

NB: Use only under medical supervision.
TINCTURE Take 1 drop on the tongue to stimulate the digestion and combat any late-afternoon chocolate cravings.
MACERATION Add ½ level tsp of dried herb to 1 cup of cold water, steep overnight, strain, and drink in the morning for poor appetite, hepatitis, sluggish digestion, and stagnant liver syndromes.
COMPRESS Soak in a strained maceration and apply to bruises and insect bites.
WASH Use 1 cup of strained maceration as a wash for scabies or other parasitic skin infections.
FLUID EXTRACT Take 2ml (40 drops) well diluted with water on an empty stomach for parasitic worms; repeat fortnightly.

HOW TO SOURCE

GROW Prefers well-drained, fertile soil in full sun, but tolerates poor, dry soil. Sow seeds in a cold frame in autumn or spring and transplant to their final positions when large enough to handle. Alternatively, divide clumps in spring or take heeled semi-ripe cuttings in midsummer.
FORAGE Found in hedgerows and waste areas in Europe, central Asia, and parts of the US; gather the leaves in summer.
HARVEST Cut aerial parts while flowering.

CAUTION Avoid if pregnant or if blood pressure is high. Do not take for more than four to five weeks at a time. Take only under professional supervision and do not exceed stated dosages.

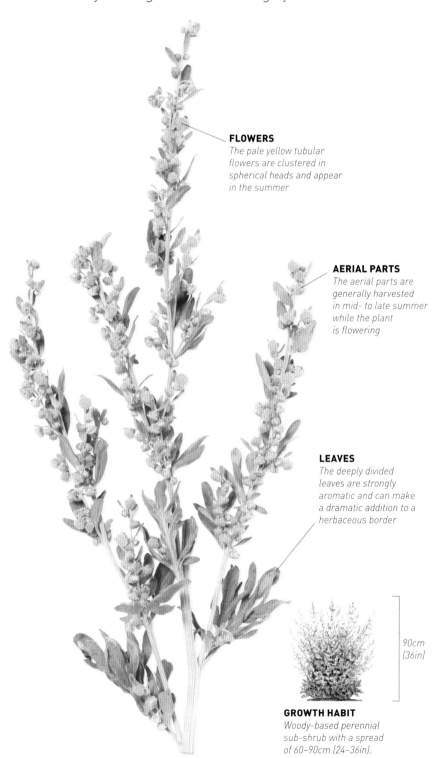

FLOWERS
The pale yellow tubular flowers are clustered in spherical heads and appear in the summer

AERIAL PARTS
The aerial parts are generally harvested in mid- to late summer while the plant is flowering

LEAVES
The deeply divided leaves are strongly aromatic and can make a dramatic addition to a herbaceous border

90cm
(36in)

GROWTH HABIT
Woody-based perennial sub-shrub with a spread of 60–90cm (24–36in).

Astragalus membranaceus **Astragalus**

One of China's most important medicinal herbs, astragalus – the English name is milk vetch – is generally used as a tonic for younger people (whereas ginseng is the preferred stimulant for older people). It is particularly effective at strengthening the immune system and boosting energy levels, and is also used to clear abscesses and ulcers.

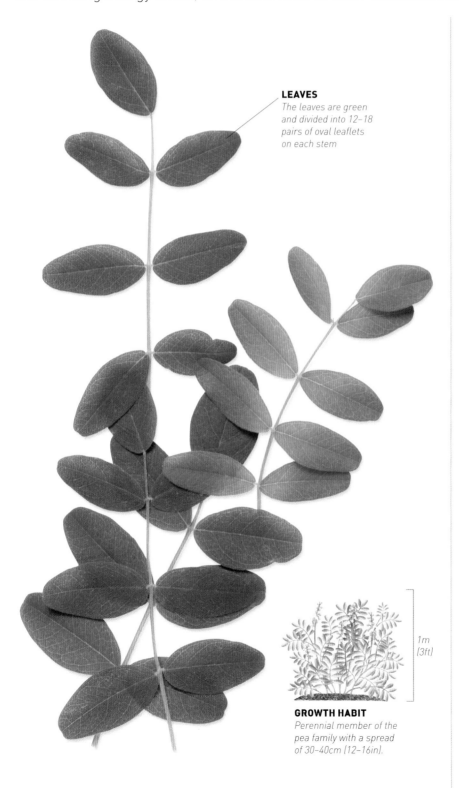

LEAVES
The leaves are green and divided into 12–18 pairs of oval leaflets on each stem

GROWTH HABIT
Perennial member of the pea family with a spread of 30–40cm (12–16in).

1m (3ft)

PARTS USED Root parts
MAIN CONSTITUENTS Flavonoids (mainly isoflavones), saponins (incl. astragalosides), polysaccharides (astragalans), asparagine, sterols
ACTIONS Antispasmodic, adaptogenic, diuretic, cholagogue, antibacterial, hypoglycaemic, nervous stimulant, hypotensive, immune stimulant

HOW TO USE

DECOCTION Generally used in combination with other herbs rather than by itself: typically 9–15g (⅓–½oz) is added to Chinese *tang* ("soup"), a therapeutic decoction generally taken once or twice a day. It is used with ginseng (*Panax ginseng*) for general debility and fatigue, or with Chinese angelica (*Angelica sinensis*) for low energy, blood loss, or some types of pain.
TINCTURE Take 2–4ml (40–80 drops) up to 3 times daily as a general tonic, to boost the immune system if suffering from fatigue with recurrent infections, or for conditions involving excess sweating.
CAPSULES Widely available in commercial products that are generally marketed as energy tonics. Follow the dosage directions on the pack.

HOW TO SOURCE

GROW Prefers full sun. Scarify seeds before planting 1cm (½in) deep and about 10cm (4in) apart in late winter/early spring in a prepared seed bed that contains sharp sand and is alkaline (above pH7). Thin to 30cm (12in) apart and only water when the soil dries out, as astragalus does not like wet ground.
FORAGE Only likely to be found growing wild in north-west China, Mongolia, or Manchuria.
HARVEST Dig the roots of four-year-old plants in autumn.

CAUTION Avoid in conditions involving excess heat and in acute stages of infections; may interfere with immune-suppressant or blood-thinning drugs.

Avena sativa **Oats**

Native to northern Europe, oats are cultivated worldwide as a cereal crop. Both oatmeal and oatbran are readily available and used in savoury dishes, oatcakes, porridge, or added to breakfast cereals. The whole plant is restorative for the nervous system, and can help to reduce blood cholesterol levels. Traditionally the green, newly harvested whole plant was used medicinally.

PARTS USED Seeds, bran, oatstraw (whole plant)

MAIN CONSTITUENTS Saponins, flavonoids, many minerals (incl. calcium), alkaloids, sterols, vitamins B1, B2, D, and E, carotene, silicic acid, protein (gluten), starch, fat

ACTIONS Antidepressant, restorative nerve tonic, diaphoretic, nutritive, reduces cholesterol levels

HOW TO USE

TINCTURE This should ideally be made from the fresh green whole plant. Take 1–5ml (20 drops–1 tsp) 3 times daily for nervous exhaustion, tension, anxiety, debility following illness, or depression. It combines well with vervain, wood betony, or valerian.

INFUSION Take 1 cup of a standard infusion (p.168) of oatstraw as required as a restorative for the nervous system.

FACIAL SCRUB For dull, greasy skin or a tendency for acne, mix ½ cup of fine oatmeal with water to make a paste. Apply to the face and leave for 10 minutes before rinsing.

BATH Strain 600ml (1 pint) of a standard decoction of the oatstraw or whole grains into the bath to ease itching and eczema.

HOW TO SOURCE

GROW Prefers neutral or slightly acidic soil and cool, damp conditions, but will tolerate dry spells. Winter oats are sown in autumn for a late summer harvest, or in spring as an early autumn crop.

FORAGE Do not trespass in a farmer's crop, but self-seeding plants are often found in hedgerows or field margins. Forage for dried stalks if they are not used for fodder. Wild oats are preferred by many herbalists as a more effective treatment.

HARVEST Harvest in late summer or early autumn as the grains turn to pale cream.

CAUTION For those sensitive to gluten, decoctions or tinctures should be allowed to settle and then the clear liquid only decanted for use.

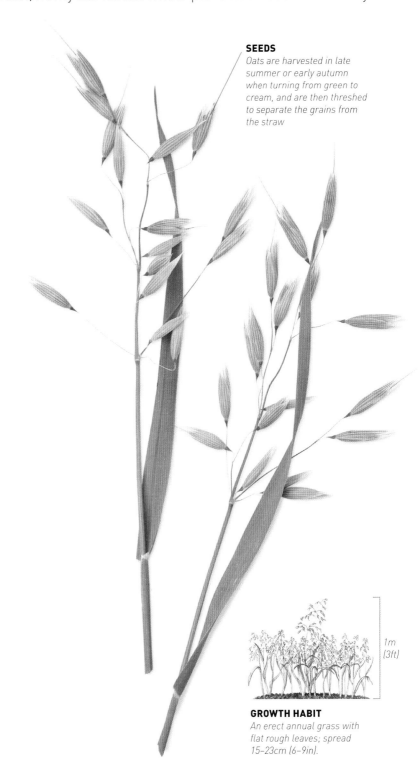

SEEDS
Oats are harvested in late summer or early autumn when turning from green to cream, and are then threshed to separate the grains from the straw

1m (3ft)

GROWTH HABIT
An erect annual grass with flat rough leaves; spread 15–23cm (6–9in).

Borago officinalis **Borage**

A native of Mediterranean regions and western Asia, borage has long been noted for its uplifting effects, and was called "the plant that cheers" (*euphrosynum*) by the Romans. This effect is in part due to its stimulant action on the adrenal glands to produce the "fight or flight" hormone, adrenaline. The seed oil is also produced commercially.

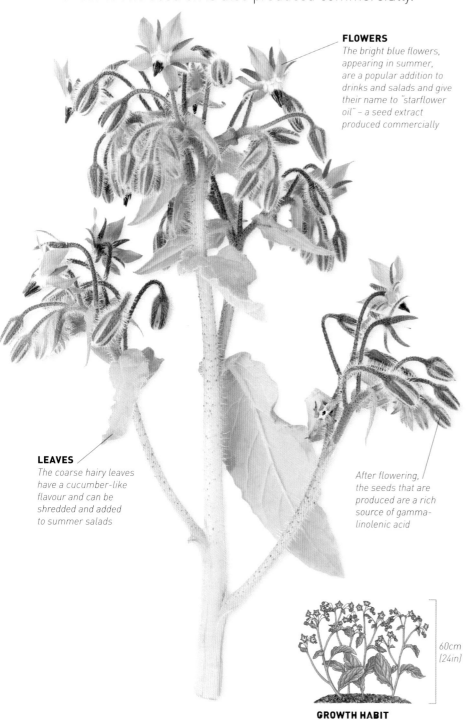

FLOWERS
The bright blue flowers, appearing in summer, are a popular addition to drinks and salads and give their name to "starflower oil" – a seed extract produced commercially

LEAVES
The coarse hairy leaves have a cucumber-like flavour and can be shredded and added to summer salads

After flowering, the seeds that are produced are a rich source of gamma-linolenic acid

GROWTH HABIT
Vigorous annual with upright, hollow stems; spread 15–30cm (6–12in).

60cm (24in)

PARTS USED Leaves, flowers, seeds
MAIN CONSTITUENTS Aerial parts/leaves: saponins, mucilage, tannins, vitamin C, calcium, potassium.
Seeds: cis-linoleic and gamma-linolenic acids
ACTIONS Adrenal stimulant, galactagogue, diuretic, diaphoretic, expectorant, antidepressant, anti-inflammatory

HOW TO USE

TINCTURE Use 2–5ml (40 drops–1 tsp) 3 times daily for 2–3 weeks only, to help combat the effects of stress, or following steroidal treatment.
LOTION Add an equal amount of water to the fresh juice and use to bathe itching skin or nervous rashes.
INFUSION Take 1 cup of a standard infusion (p.168) 3 times daily, combined with peppermint and elderflower for feverish colds.
CAPSULES The seed oil is widely available in capsules, which can be taken to help treat eczema, rheumatoid arthritis, menstrual irregularities, or irritable bowel syndrome.
SYRUP Make a standard infusion using either flowers or whole aerial parts and sweeten with honey or sugar (450g/1lb to every 600ml/1 pint of infusion) for coughs.

HOW TO SOURCE

GROW Prefers any type of well-drained soil, in dappled shade or sun. Plant the seeds in late summer, then thin to about 30cm (12in) apart when the seedlings are established. It self-seeds enthusiastically.
FORAGE Originally found growing in rocky places in Mediterranean regions, it now self-seeds in other areas.
HARVEST Gather aerial parts in summer.

CAUTION Avoid during pregnancy. Restricted in Australia and New Zealand, as it is related to comfrey, which is banned in these countries. Not recommended for prolonged treatment (2–3 weeks maximum).

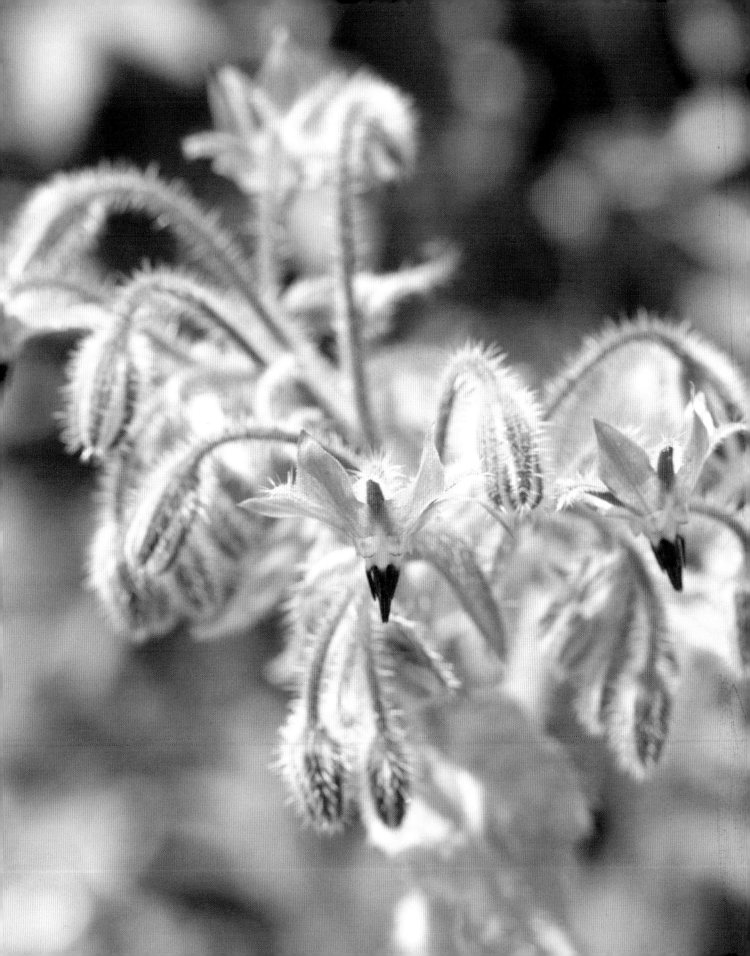

Calendula officinalis **Calendula or marigold**

Traditionally said to lift the spirits and encourage cheerfulness, calendula or marigold is one of the most popular and versatile medicinal herbs in current use. It is widely available in commercial calendula ointments and creams, and is also used internally for digestive and gynaecological problems or as a cleansing remedy in skin and rheumatic disorders.

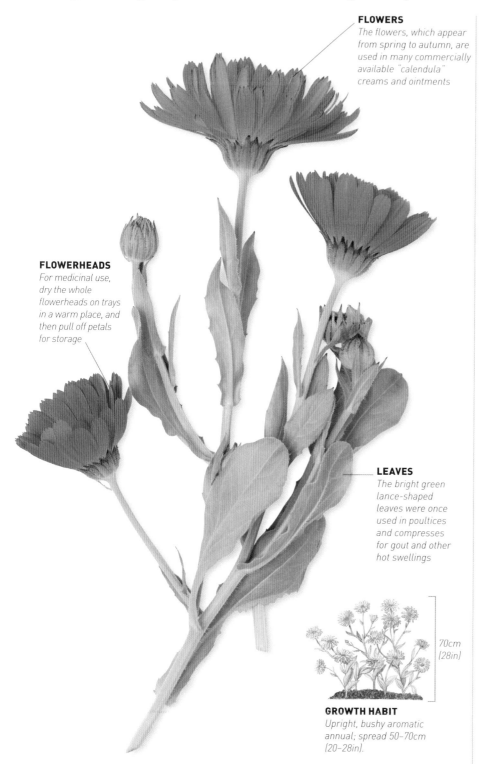

FLOWERS
The flowers, which appear from spring to autumn, are used in many commercially available "calendula" creams and ointments

FLOWERHEADS
For medicinal use, dry the whole flowerheads on trays in a warm place, and then pull off petals for storage

LEAVES
The bright green lance-shaped leaves were once used in poultices and compresses for gout and other hot swellings

70cm
(28in)

GROWTH HABIT
Upright, bushy aromatic annual; spread 50–70cm (20–28in).

PARTS USED Flowerheads, essential oil
MAIN CONSTITUENTS Flavonoids, mucilage, triterpenes, volatile oil, bitter glycosides, resin, sterols, carotenes
ACTIONS Astringent, antibacterial, antifungal, anti-inflammatory, wound herb, mildly oestrogenic, antispasmodic, menstrual regulator

HOW TO USE

Do not confuse with preparations made from French marigold (*Tagetes patula*).
INFUSION Take 1 cup of a standard infusion (p.168) 3 times daily for inflammatory digestive disorders. It also makes a suitable douche for vaginal thrush, or a mouthwash for gum disease and mouth ulcers.
CREAM/OINTMENT Use for minor cuts and grazes, and any inflamed or dry skin: eczema, chapped hands, chilblains, sore nipples in breast-feeding, acne, minor burns and scalds, sunburn, etc. It is also helpful for fungal infections such as ringworm, thrush, and athlete's foot.
MACERATED OIL Use as a cream or ointment on piles or broken capillaries; add up to 20% lavender oil for sunburn.
TINCTURE Take 2–5ml (40 drops–1 tsp) 3 times a day for menstrual problems, (irregular, heavy, or painful periods).

HOW TO SOURCE

GROW Prefers well-drained soil in a sunny site, but will tolerate partial shade. Sow seeds in autumn or spring, and thin or transplant seedlings when large enough to handle. Can also be grown in containers. It flowers throughout the summer and self-seeds enthusiastically, so gather flowers regularly to avoid excessive seeding.
FORAGE Most likely to be found naturalized in Mediterranean areas in rocky places or cultivated sites and on wasteland; elsewhere, self-seeded plants outside gardens are possible, but less common.
HARVEST Collect flowers in summer.

CAUTION Avoid internal use of calendula during pregnancy.

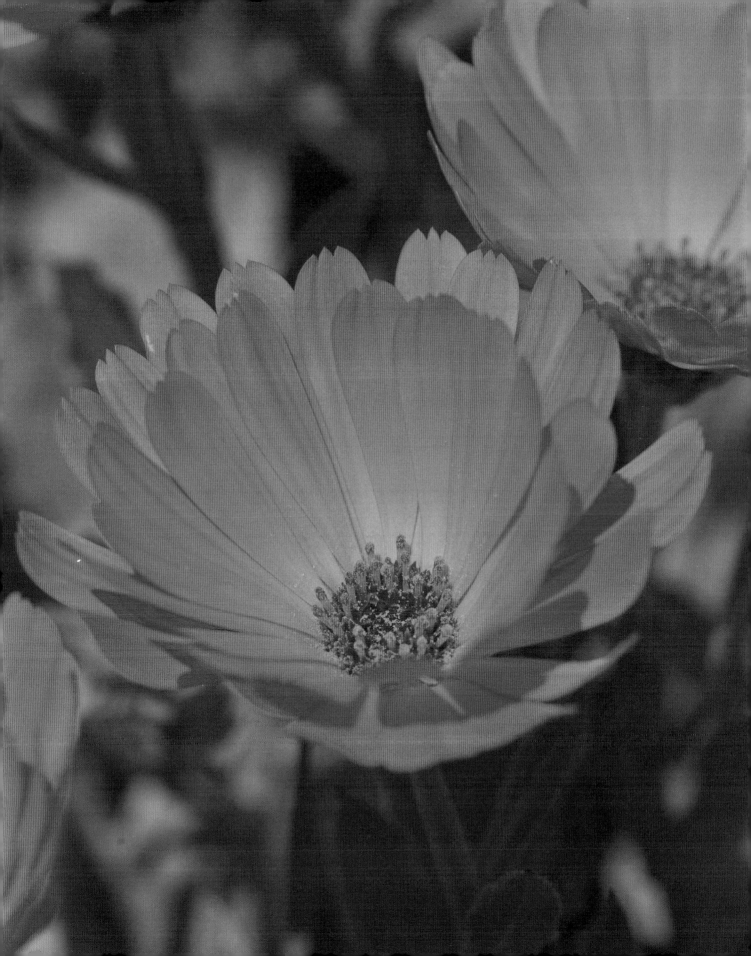

Capsicum annuum **Cayenne or chilli pepper**

Originally found in tropical America, cayenne was first described in 1493 by the physician accompanying the Portuguese explorer, Christopher Columbus. The plant was introduced into India and Africa by the Portuguese and reached Europe by the mid-16th century. It soon became an established culinary seasoning and medicinal herb. Today it is widely used as a warming remedy.

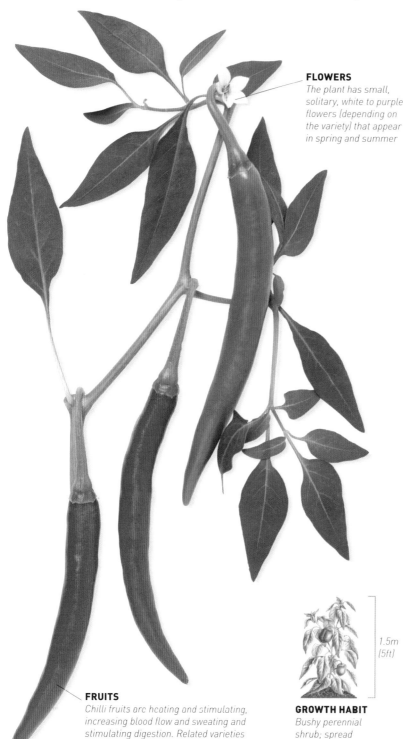

FLOWERS
The plant has small, solitary, white to purple flowers (depending on the variety) that appear in spring and summer

FRUITS
Chilli fruits are heating and stimulating, increasing blood flow and sweating and stimulating digestion. Related varieties of Capsicum may be in different shapes

GROWTH HABIT
Bushy perennial shrub; spread 50cm–2m (20in–6ft).

1.5m
(5ft)

PARTS USED Fruit
MAIN CONSTITUENTS Capsaicin, carotenoids, fatty acids, flavonoids, vitamins A, B1, and C, volatile oil, sugars
ACTIONS Circulatory stimulant, diaphoretic, gastric stimulant, carminative, antiseptic, antibacterial
Topically: counter-irritant, rubefacient

HOW TO USE

MACERATED OIL Heat 30g (1oz) of the powder, or 3–4 chopped fresh chillies, in 600ml (1 pint) of sunflower oil in a bowl over a saucepan of simmering water (bain-marie) for 2 hours. Use as a massage for rheumatism, lumbago, arthritis, and so on, or to relieve pain from shingles.
TINCTURE Take 1ml (20 drops) in a cup of warm water as a circulatory stimulant for cold hands and feet.
GARGLE Use ¼–½ml (5–10 drops) of tincture or a pinch (⅛ tsp) of cayenne powder to half a tumbler of warm water for sore throats or laryngitis.

HOW TO SOURCE

GROW Sow 2–3 seeds in each 7.5cm (3in) pot using good-quality compost. Plant out when the soil temperature reaches 15°C (59°F) or, in temperate regions, pot on into large containers and keep in a greenhouse.
FORAGE Unlikely to be found growing wild outside its native region, but self-seeded plants that grow outside gardens are possible; grown throughout the tropics in America, Africa, and India.
HARVEST Gather the fruits when ripe in summer and dry immediately in the shade.

CAUTION Do not exceed the stated dose: excess can lead to gastric irritation. Avoid touching the eyes or any cuts after handling chillies, as it can sting. Compresses left on the skin for long periods can cause blistering.

Carum carvi **Caraway**

Native to Mediterranean regions, caraway is now naturalized in parts of Asia and North America. Cultivated commercially, the oil is used in pharmaceuticals and toiletries such as toothpastes and mouthwashes, and as a food flavouring. Like its relatives anise and fennel, caraway is used for digestive and respiratory disorders, and is popular for treating colic in infants.

PARTS USED Seeds, essential oil
MAIN CONSTITUENTS Volatile oil (mainly carvone and limonene), flavonoids, polysaccharides
ACTIONS Antispasmodic, carminative, antimicrobial, expectorant, galactogogue, emmenagogue, diuretic, tonic

HOW TO USE

INFUSION Use a weak infusion (p.168) of the seeds 3 times daily for wind and colic in children. Reduce the dosage according to age. For children aged 1–2, use 10ml (2 tsp) of a standard infusion diluted with 100ml (3½fl oz) of warm water per dose; for children aged 3–4, use 20ml (4 tsp) of a standard infusion similarly diluted. Take a standard infusion 3 times daily for menstrual cramps or colic in adults, or drink 1 cup a day to improve milk flow when breastfeeding.
TINCTURE Take 3–5ml (60 drops–1 tsp) of a tincture of the seeds 3 times daily for poor appetite or flatulence.
ESSENTIAL OIL Add 5 drops of essential oil to 5ml (1 tsp) of almond oil and use as a chest rub for bronchitis and productive coughs (a cough that produces phlegm, rather than a dry cough).

HOW TO SOURCE

GROW Prefers deep, fertile, well-drained soil and full sun. Sow seeds where you want them to grow in spring, and thin out seedlings to 7.5–10cm (3–4in) if required. The plant is biennial, flowering in its second year. Caraway requires a long, hot growing season to set seed, so it may not produce as many seeds in cooler areas.
FORAGE Found in grassy areas or wastelands. In warmer zones it will set seed in late summer; in cooler areas seeds are likely only if the summer has been hot.
HARVEST Collect ripe seeds in late summer.

CAUTION The essential oil can cause skin irritation.

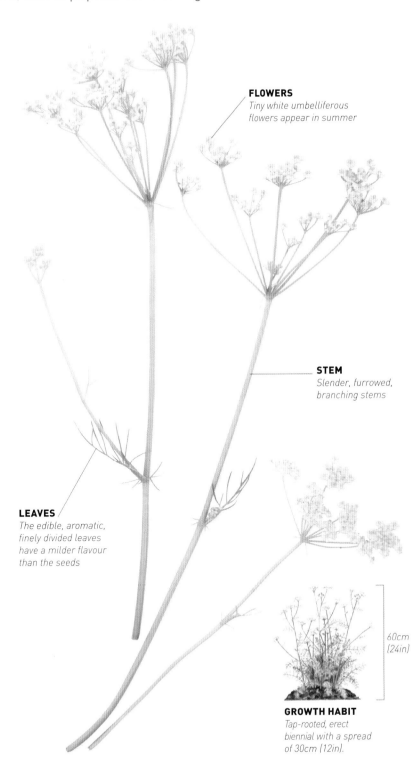

FLOWERS
Tiny white umbelliferous flowers appear in summer

STEM
Slender, furrowed, branching stems

LEAVES
The edible, aromatic, finely divided leaves have a milder flavour than the seeds

60cm (24in)

GROWTH HABIT
Tap-rooted, erect biennial with a spread of 30cm (12in).

Centella asiatica **Gotu kola**

Native to India, south-east Asia, and parts of northern Australia, gotu kola – a Sri Lankan name, which translates as "conical leaf" – is used as a fodder crop, green vegetable, or salad herb, and medicinal plant. In Ayurveda it is generally known as *brahmi* and used as a tonic remedy to improve longevity, memory, and intelligence. It is a restricted herb in some countries.

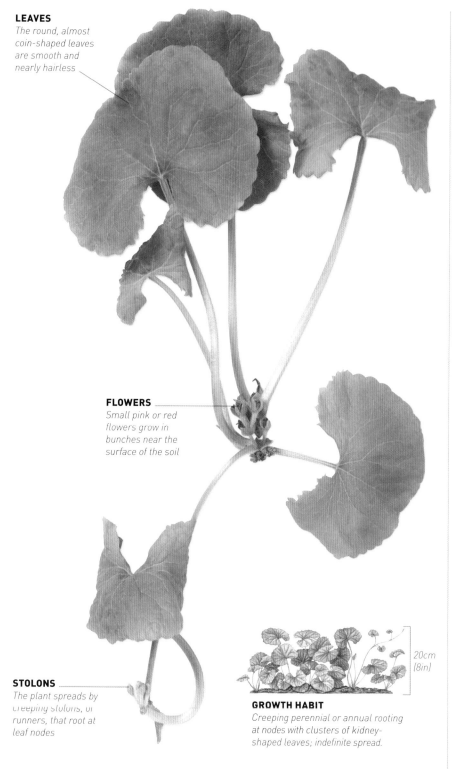

LEAVES
The round, almost coin-shaped leaves are smooth and nearly hairless

FLOWERS
Small pink or red flowers grow in bunches near the surface of the soil

STOLONS
The plant spreads by creeping stolons, or runners, that root at leaf nodes

GROWTH HABIT
Creeping perennial or annual rooting at nodes with clusters of kidney-shaped leaves; indefinite spread.

20cm (8in)

PARTS USED Whole plant
MAIN CONSTITUENTS Alkaloids (incl. hydrocotyline), terpenoid saponins, flavonoids, bitter principle, volatile oil
ACTIONS Tonic, antirheumatic, cleansing, adaptogen, relaxant, diuretic, laxative

HOW TO USE

INFUSION Use ½ tsp of the dried herb per cup of boiling water and take 1 cup daily for skin problems, rheumatism, or as a restorative for tiredness and depression.
TINCTURE Take 5ml (1 tsp) in water daily for poor memory, inability to concentrate, or general exhaustion.
LOTION/OINTMENT Use on poorly healing wounds or skin ulcers.
FRESH LEAVES Traditionally given to Indian children to combat dysentery, or included in salads as a restorative tonic.
FLUID EXTRACT Take 20 drops in water up to 3 times daily for rheumatic disorders and poor venous circulation.
POWDER Used in Ayurvedic medicine to make a paste (mixed with a little water) and applied to eczema and skin sores.

HOW TO SOURCE

GROW Generally gathered in the wild, but can be grown in warmer areas from seeds sown directly in the spring. It prefers marshy ditches and riverbanks, so is best grown in partial shade in moist soil. It has an indefinite spread, so can make useful ground cover with the right growing conditions, but can become invasive.
FORAGE The whole plant can be gathered at any time where it is naturalized (parts of southern Africa, South America, the southern United States, and its native Asia).
HARVEST The whole plant matures in three months and is gathered – including the roots – throughout the year.

CAUTION Can occasionally cause photosensitivity. Do not take for more than six weeks without a break.

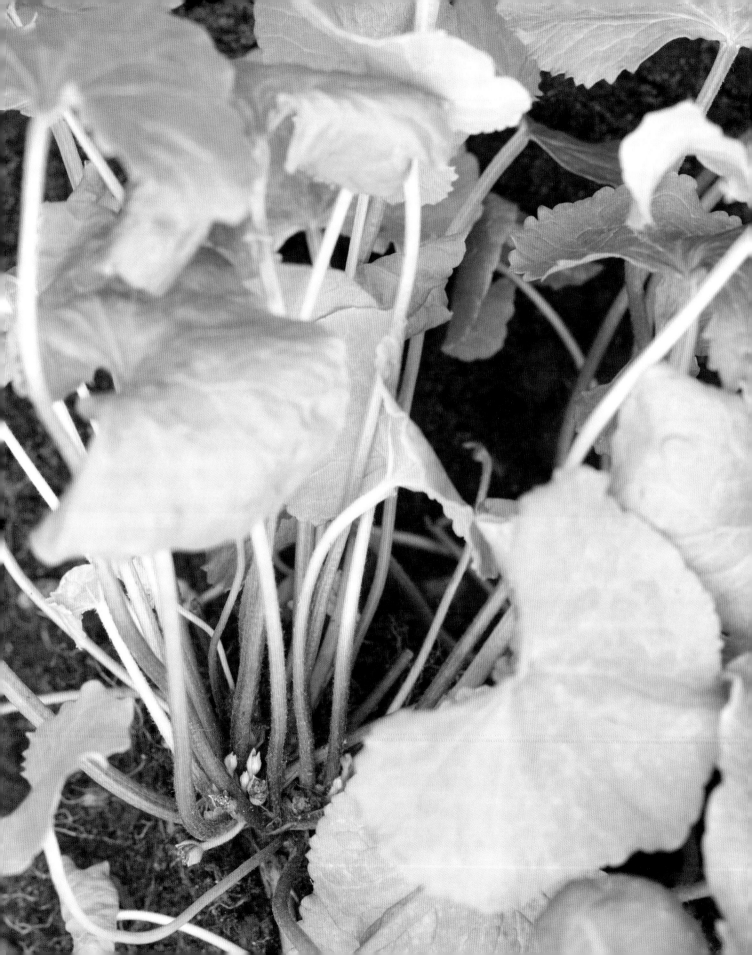

Cichorium intybus **Chicory**

Native to Mediterranean regions, chicory is now naturalized in many parts of Europe, North America, and Australia. It is cultivated as a vegetable – usually by producing chicons in complete darkness – and is also grown as a coffee substitute. The plant is extremely bitter, so it makes an excellent digestive stimulant and tonic, and is also a gentle laxative.

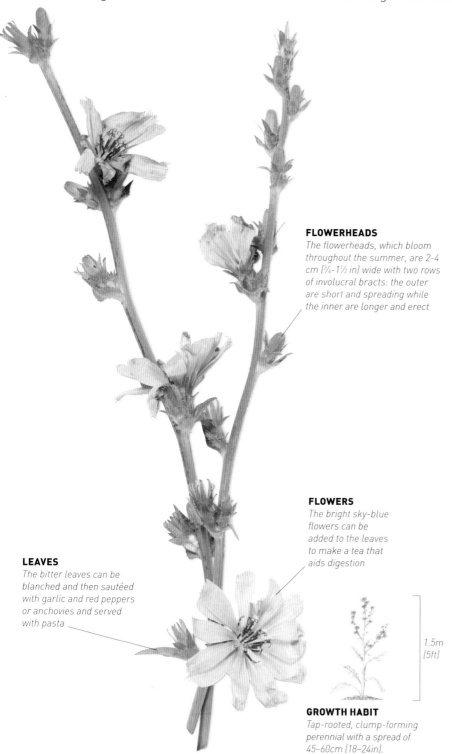

FLOWERHEADS
The flowerheads, which bloom throughout the summer, are 2-4 cm (¾-1½ in) wide with two rows of involucral bracts: the outer are short and spreading while the inner are longer and erect

FLOWERS
The bright sky-blue flowers can be added to the leaves to make a tea that aids digestion

LEAVES
The bitter leaves can be blanched and then sautéed with garlic and red peppers or anchovies and served with pasta

1.5m
(5ft)

GROWTH HABIT
Tap-rooted, clump-forming perennial with a spread of 45–60cm (18–24in).

PARTS USED Root, leaves, flowers
MAIN CONSTITUENTS Inulin (in the root), sesquiterpene lactones (lactucin and lactucopicrin), oligosaccharides, glycosides, vitamins, minerals
ACTIONS Laxative, diuretic, mild sedative, liver, and digestive tonic

HOW TO USE

DECOCTION Take ½–1 cup of a standard decoction (p.168) of chicory root 3 times daily as a stimulating tonic for the liver and digestive system. Use ½–1 cup of a quarter- to half-strength or less decoction 1–2 times a day for constipation. Chicory also contains oligosaccharides, which are probiotic and help to maintain healthy gastrointestinal flora.
INFUSION Combine the leaves and flowers in a standard infusion (p.168) and take 1 cup 3 times daily to improve digestion.
TINCTURE Take 1–2ml (20–40 drops) of the root tincture 3 times daily as an appetite stimulant.
FLUID EXTRACT Extracts have been successfully used for parasitic worm infections in sheep and cattle, although there is little research as to the effect on human parasites.

HOW TO SOURCE

GROW Prefers fertile, moist but well-drained, neutral to alkaline soil in full sun. Sow seeds in a cold frame in autumn or spring and when the seedlings are established transplant them to final positions in rows at least 60cm (24in) apart. Dead-head the flowers regularly, as the plant can be a prolific self-seeder.
FORAGE Sometimes found in hedgerows and field borders, especially in southern Europe. The leaves can be collected during summer. They have a bitter taste and can be boiled to improve their flavour.
HARVEST Lift the roots in early spring in the second year.

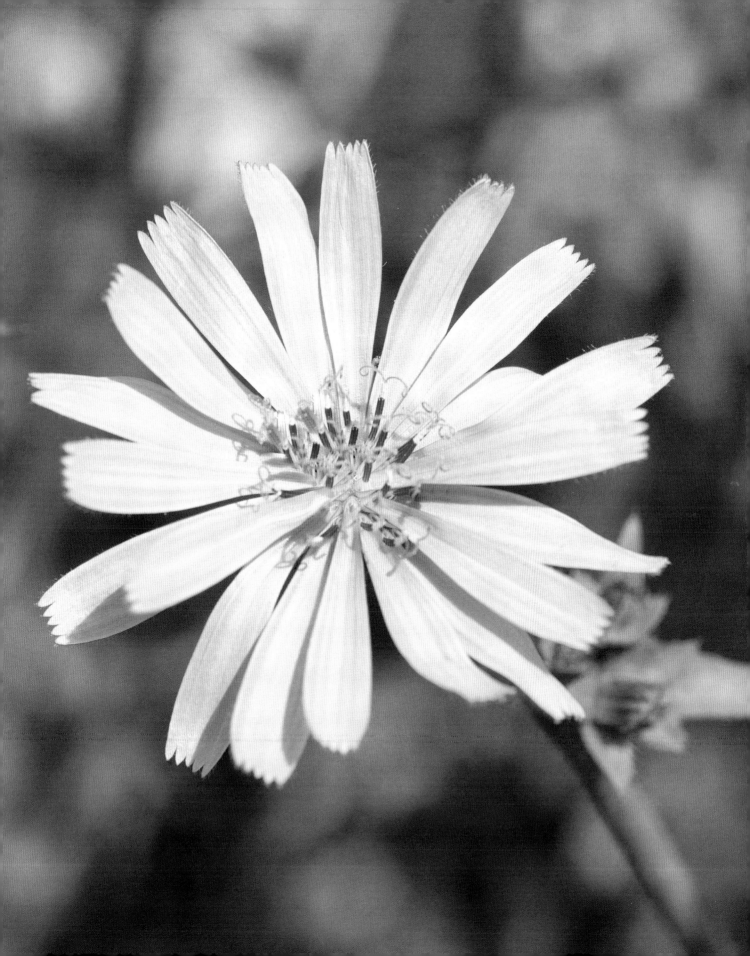

Crataegus laevigata **Hawthorn**

Thorny shrubs and trees from various species of hawthorn are found throughout northern temperate zones. *Crataegus laevigata* is the European species, but *Crataegus pinnatifida* is native to northern China, and is also used as a medicinal herb. The berries are traditionally made into a savoury jelly to eat with cheese, game, and cold meats.

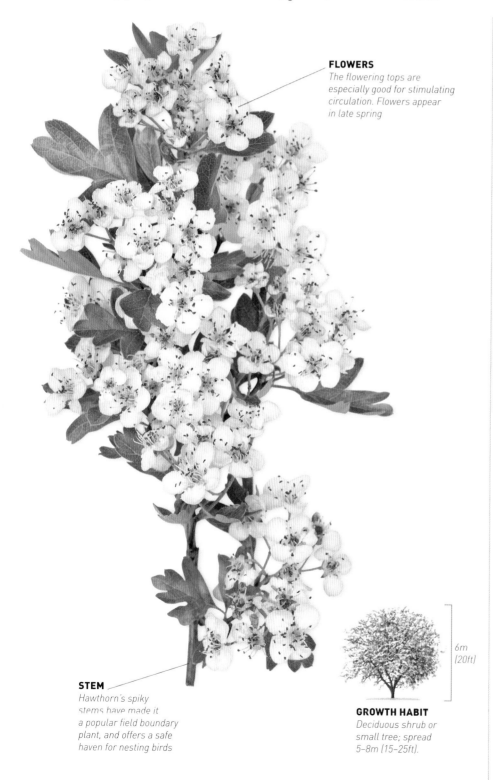

FLOWERS
The flowering tops are especially good for stimulating circulation. Flowers appear in late spring

STEM
Hawthorn's spiky stems have made it a popular field boundary plant, and offers a safe haven for nesting birds

GROWTH HABIT
Deciduous shrub or small tree; spread 5–8m (15–25ft).

6m (20ft)

PARTS USED Flowering tops, berries
MAIN CONSTITUENTS Bioflavonoid glycosides (incl. rutin and quercetin), triterpenoids, procyanidins, polyphenols, saponins, tannins, coumarins, minerals
ACTIONS Peripheral vasodilator, cardiac tonic, astringent, relaxant, antioxidant

HOW TO USE

INFUSION Take 1 cup of a standard infusion (p.168) of the flowering tops 3 times daily to improve peripheral circulation or to support treatments for high blood pressure.
DECOCTION Make a standard decoction of the berries and drink ½ cup up to 6 times daily for acute diarrhoea and digestive upsets. The same mixture can be used as a general tonic for the heart: take 2 cups daily.
TINCTURE Take 1–2ml (20–40 drops) of a standard tincture of either the berries or the flowering tops for high blood pressure; best combined with other herbs as appropriate.
JUICE Pulp the berries in a food processor, squeeze out the juice, and take in 10ml (2 tsp) doses twice daily for sluggish digestion and diarrhoea.

HOW TO SOURCE

GROW It can be grown from seed if planted in the autumn and allowed to over-winter in a cold frame, but is more often propagated from cuttings in spring. Plant heeled cuttings in a small pot and, once rooted, pot on into 20cm (8in) pots until sufficiently established to plant out. Will self-seed.
FORAGE A common hedgerow shrub found on field borders and roadsides. It is best to gather from shrubs within fields rather than those adjacent to roads. The flowering tops can be gathered in late spring/early summer for use in teas, and the berries in late autumn to make into jelly.
HARVEST Gather flowering tops in spring, and the red berries in autumn when ripe.

CAUTION Seek professional advice before self-medicating with hawthorn for heart disorders, or if using prescribed medication.

Curcuma longa **Turmeric**

Familiar to many people as a key ingredient in curry powder, turmeric, which originates in southern Asia, has a long history of use in both Ayurveda and traditional Chinese medicine. It is largely used for digestive and liver disorders, although modern research also suggests that it has potent antioxidant properties and can reduce cholesterol levels.

PARTS USED Rhizome
MAIN CONSTITUENTS Volatile oil, curcumin (yellow pigment), resin, vitamins, minerals, bitter principle
ACTIONS Carminative, cholagogue, antioxidant, choleretic, detoxifier, antibacterial, anti-inflammatory, antitumour activity, hypolipidaemic

HOW TO USE

DECOCTION Take ½ cup of a standard decoction (p.168) up to 3 times daily for digestive problems including nausea, gastritis, excessive stomach acid, indigestion, and liver or gall bladder disorders. Can also be combined with remedies for arthritis such as angelica or devil's claw and taken 3 times daily.
TINCTURE Take 2–4ml (40–80 drops) in a little water 3 times daily to help reduce blood cholesterol levels, or take 5ml (1 tsp) up to 3 times daily for period pain.
POWDER Take 1–2g (½–1 level tsp) stirred into a cup of water, fruit juice, or milk for arthritic problems or eczema.
OINTMENT Apply 2–3 times daily for athlete's foot, psoriasis, or ringworm.

HOW TO SOURCE

GROW Prefers moist, fertile soil with high humidity and partial shade. Will only grow in warm regions (minimum temperature 15–18°C/59–64°F), but can be cultivated under glass elsewhere. Sow seeds at 21°C (70°F) in autumn. Alternatively, propagate by root division while the plant is dormant in winter or by root cuttings in autumn.
FORAGE Unlikely to be found growing wild outside dry forest areas in India and some other parts of southern Asia.
HARVEST The rhizome is dug in autumn and is boiled and steamed before drying.

CAUTION May occasionally cause skin rashes or increase photosensitivity. Avoid therapeutic doses in pregnancy, but culinary quantities are perfectly safe. Seek professional advice if you suffer from gallstones.

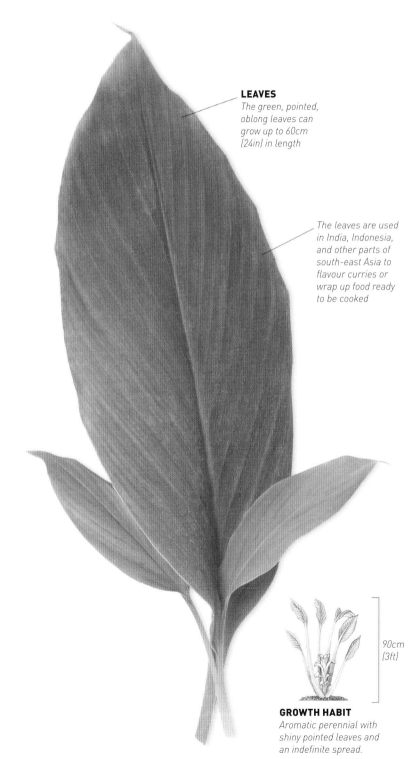

LEAVES
The green, pointed, oblong leaves can grow up to 60cm (24in) in length

The leaves are used in India, Indonesia, and other parts of south-east Asia to flavour curries or wrap up food ready to be cooked

90cm
(3ft)

GROWTH HABIT
Aromatic perennial with shiny pointed leaves and an indefinite spread.

Cymbopogon citratus **Lemon grass**

Originally native to grasslands in south-east Asia, lemon grass is now cultivated in many tropical regions, including Guatamala, the West Indies, and the Philippines, both as a culinary herb and for its essential oil. The herb is a popular digestive remedy in parts of Asia, and is used as a flavouring in perfumery and the food industry.

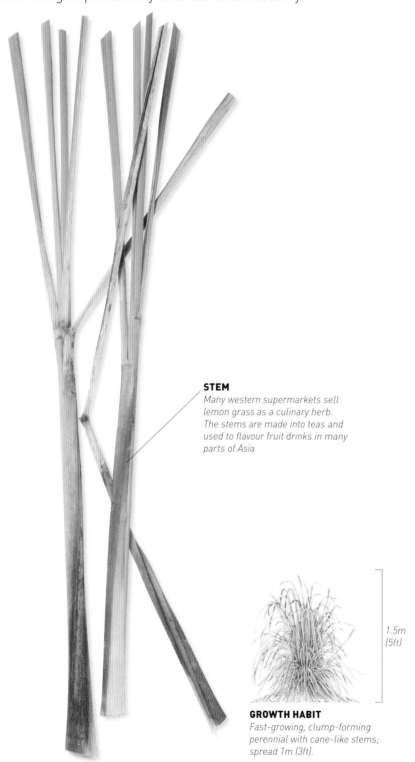

STEM
Many western supermarkets sell lemon grass as a culinary herb. The stems are made into teas and used to flavour fruit drinks in many parts of Asia

GROWTH HABIT
Fast-growing, clump-forming perennial with cane-like stems; spread 1m (3ft).

1.5m (5ft)

PARTS USED Leaves and stems, essential oil

MAIN CONSTITUENTS Volatile oil mostly citral (65–85%) as well as nerol, geraniol, citronellol, myrcene, and borneol

ACTIONS Antispasmodic, carminative, febrifuge, analgesic, antidepressant, antiseptic, astringent, antibacterial, antifungal, sedative, tonic

HOW TO USE

LOTION Dilute 30 drops of essential oil in 1 tbsp vodka, then add to 120ml (4fl oz) water and use in a spray bottle as an insect repellant (fleas, ticks, and lice), or as a deodorant and antiperspirant.

MASSAGE RUB Dilute 20 drops of essential oil in 60ml (2fl oz) of almond oil and massage into aching muscles, or use on the abdomen for stomach cramps.

INFUSION Take 1 cup of a standard infusion (p.168) 3 times daily for wind, flatulence, indigestion, or stomach cramps.

POULTICE Simmer a handful of chopped fresh lemon grass for 1–2 minutes in olive oil and use on arthritic or painful joints.

HOW TO SOURCE

GROW Grow in containers in cooler areas and over-winter in a conservatory or heated greenhouse, as not frost hardy (minimum temperature 7°C/45°F). In frost-free areas plant in fertile, moist, well-drained soil in full sun, keeping 60cm (24in) between plants. Sow seeds (at 18°C/64°F) in early spring in seed trays and transplant to 7cm (3.5in) pots when large enough. Alternatively, propagate by root division in late spring.

FORAGE Unlikely to be found growing wild other than in its native area of grassland in south-east Asia.

HARVEST Gather stems through the year.

CAUTION Do not take the essential oil internally without professional advice. Avoid therapeutic doses in pregnancy, but culinary quantities are safe.

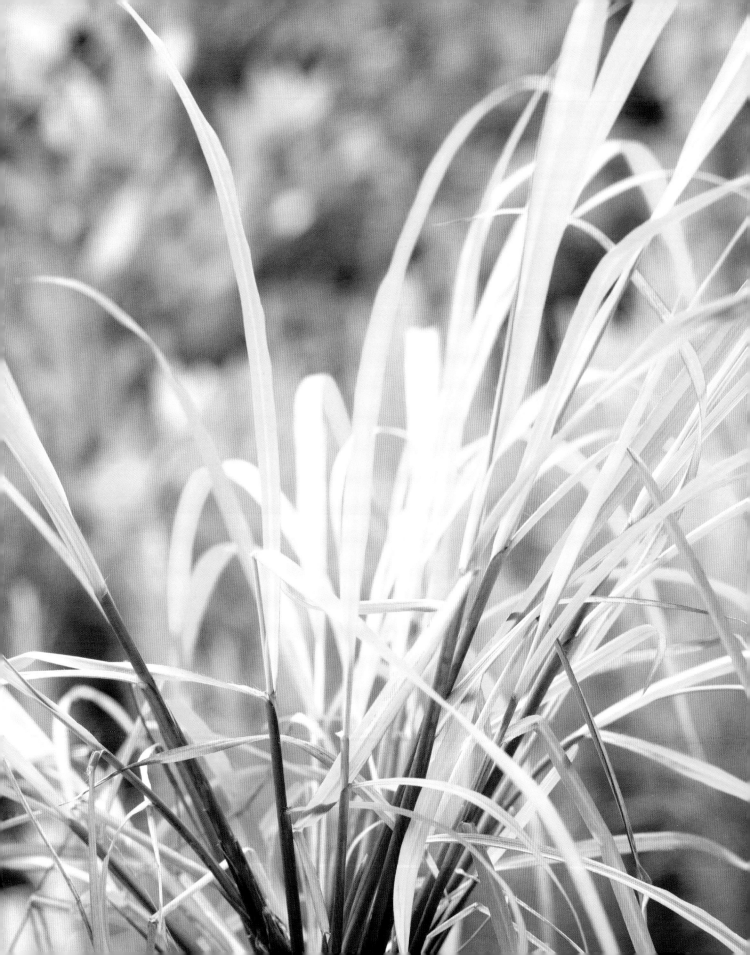

Cynara cardunculus Scolymus Group **Globe artichoke**

Originating in the Mediterranean region, the globe artichoke was probably developed from *Cynara cardunculus* in ancient times. The ball-like flowerheads, which are picked before they open, are valued as a vegetable, while the hearts can be used in salads. Medicinally, the plant is used as a liver remedy that helps to protect against toxins and infection and improve function.

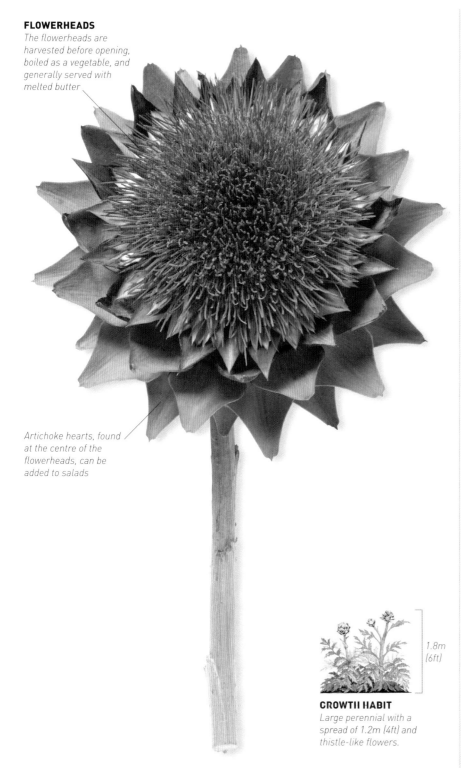

FLOWERHEADS
The flowerheads are harvested before opening, boiled as a vegetable, and generally served with melted butter

Artichoke hearts, found at the centre of the flowerheads, can be added to salads

GROWTH HABIT
Large perennial with a spread of 1.2m (4ft) and thistle-like flowers.

1.8m (6ft)

PARTS USED Flowerheads, leaves, root
MAIN CONSTITUENTS Sesquiterpene lactone (cynaropicrin), cynarin, inulin
ACTIONS Cholagogue, choleretic, liver restorative, hypoglycaemic, diuretic, hypolipidaemic

HOW TO USE

JUICE Mix an equal amount of juice from the leaves and flowerheads with water and drink 1 cup daily as a liver tonic.
INFUSION Take 1 cup of a standard infusion (p.168) of the leaves 3 times daily for liver and gall bladder disorders, including liver damage or jaundice, or for indigestion, nausea, or abdominal bloating. Also helps to reduce blood cholesterol levels and can be useful in the control of late-onset diabetes where treatment is focused on diet rather than medication.
DIET Eating artichoke hearts regularly can be helpful in the management of late-onset diabetes.
CAPSULES Take 3 x 250mg capsules containing powdered leaf before meals morning and evening to improve liver function.

HOW TO SOURCE

GROW Prefers an open but sheltered site in full sun in well-drained soil; add well-rotted manure to the soil before planting. Sow seeds in a cold frame in spring and transplant to their final growing positions when large enough to handle. Alternatively, propagate from suckers in spring or take root cuttings in winter.
FORAGE Unknown in the wild.
HARVEST Cut the leaves before flowering. Gather the flowerheads before the bracts open from the second year onwards to eat as a vegetable.

Dioscorea villosa **Wild yam**

Perhaps best known as the herb that gave rise to the first oral contraceptive pill, wild yam is native to the south and east USA and central America, although it is now naturalized in many semi-tropical areas worldwide. The chemical from the yam, diosgenin, was identified in the 1930s, and by 1960 was being used to manufacture the hormone progesterone.

PARTS USED Root and tuber
MAIN CONSTITUENTS Alkaloids, steroidal saponins (mainly dioscin, which breaks down to diosgenin), tannins, phytosterols, starch
ACTIONS Relaxant for smooth muscle, antispasmodic, cholagogue, anti-inflammatory, diaphoretic, antirheumatic, diuretic

HOW TO USE

DECOCTION Take ½–1 cup 3 times daily of a decoction made by simmering 10g (¼oz) in 600ml (1 pint) of water for 20 minutes for colicky pains associated with IBS or diverticulosis. Drink ½ cup every 3–4 hours for period pains, or sip cups constantly during labour to relieve pain.
TINCTURE Take 2–3ml (40–60 drops) 3 times daily for menopausal problems.
FLUID EXTRACT Take 1–2ml (20–40 drops) in a little water 3 times daily for arthritis: usually combined with other herbs such as black cohosh, cramp bark, meadowsweet, or white willow for rheumatoid arthritis. Also useful to stimulate liver function.

HOW TO SOURCE

GROW Prefers light to medium (sandy to loamy) soil that is moist but well drained, and requires partial shade. Usually grown from root cuttings, or from pea-sized tubers found growing in the leaf axils in late summer that can be collected and planted immediately. The plants are dioecious (have separate sexes), so both male and female plants are needed to set seeds, which can be sown in a cold frame in early spring and transplanted when large enough to handle.
FORAGE Generally found in damp woods, swamps, thickets, and hedgerows in central and southern USA and parts of central America.
HARVEST Dig tubers and roots in autumn, and wash and dry them.

CAUTION Saponin content may cause nausea in sensitive individuals.

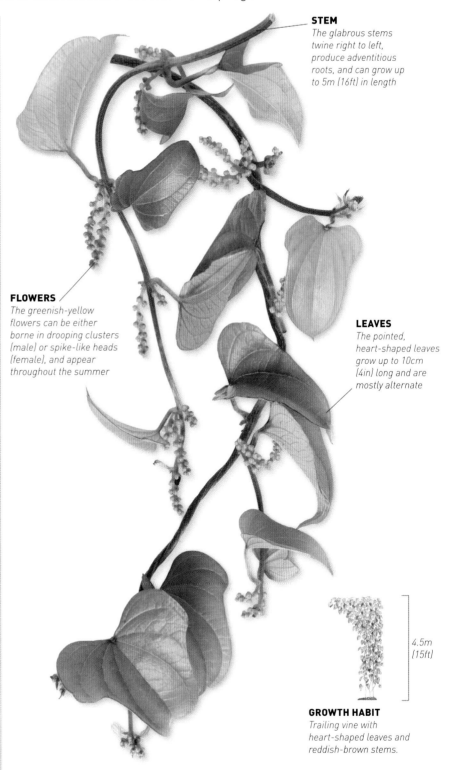

STEM
The glabrous stems twine right to left, produce adventitious roots, and can grow up to 5m (16ft) in length

FLOWERS
The greenish-yellow flowers can be either borne in drooping clusters (male) or spike-like heads (female), and appear throughout the summer

LEAVES
The pointed, heart-shaped leaves grow up to 10cm (4in) long and are mostly alternate

4.5m (15ft)

GROWTH HABIT
Trailing vine with heart-shaped leaves and reddish-brown stems.

Echinacea purpurea **Echinacea**

Native to the eastern states of the USA, echinacea was once known as "Missouri snakeroot" and was traditionally used by Native Americans for fevers and poorly healing wounds. It was introduced into Europe in the 19th century and has been extensively researched since, largely as an antibiotic remedy for treating a broad range of infections.

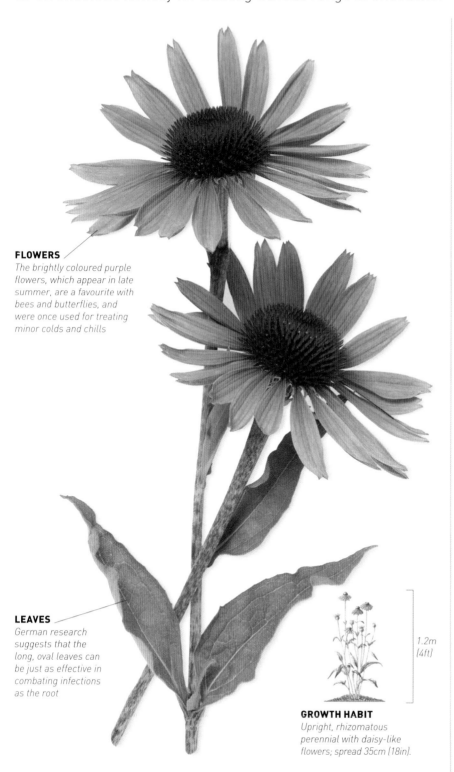

FLOWERS
The brightly coloured purple flowers, which appear in late summer, are a favourite with bees and butterflies, and were once used for treating minor colds and chills

LEAVES
German research suggests that the long, oval leaves can be just as effective in combating infections as the root

GROWTH HABIT
Upright, rhizomatous perennial with daisy-like flowers; spread 35cm (18in).

1.2m (4ft)

PARTS USED Root, leaves
MAIN CONSTITUENTS Volatile oil (incl. humulene), glycosides, alkamides, inulin, polysaccharides, antibiotic polyacetylenes
ACTIONS Immune stimulant, anti-allergenic, lymphatic tonic, antimicrobial, anti-inflammatory

HOW TO USE

INFUSION Take 1 cup of a standard infusion (p.168) of fresh leaves 3 times daily for common colds, chills, or influenza.
DECOCTION Take 10ml (2 tsp) of a standard decoction of the root every 2–4 hours for acute stages of infections. Combines well with hemp agrimony.
GARGLE/MOUTHWASH Use 1 cup of the root decoction or 10ml (2 tsp) of tincture in a cup of warm water 2–3 times daily for sore throats, mouth ulcers, and tonsillitis.
TINCTURE Take 5ml (1tsp) of tincture 3 times daily for urinary infections; combine with an equal amount of cleavers tincture for enlarged lymphatic nodes or glandular fever. For colds and influenza, take 10ml (2 tsp) of tincture as symptoms occur and repeat up to 4 times daily for 48 hours.
CREAM/OINTMENT Use on infected cuts, boils, acne, and skin sores.

HOW TO SOURCE

GROW Prefers fertile, moist, well-drained soil in full sun. Sow seeds in containers in spring and pot on; when well established, plant in permanent positions. Alternatively, divide established plants in autumn or spring or take root cuttings in late autumn or early winter.
FORAGE Unlikely to be found growing wild outside the USA. Over-cropping has caused it to become rare, so avoid foraging for the plant in its native habitat.
HARVEST The leaves can be gathered throughout the growing season, and the roots of four-year-old plants are lifted in autumn after flowering is over.

CAUTION High doses can occasionally cause nausea and dizziness.

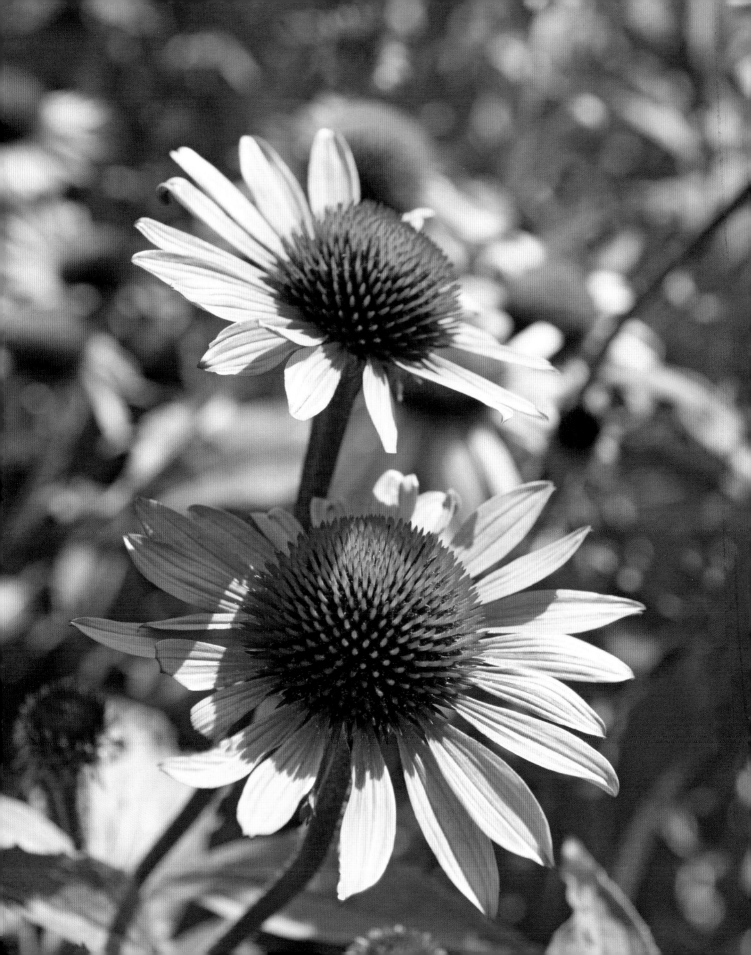

Equisetum arvense **Horsetail**

Native to Europe, Asia, and North America, horsetail is a survivor from prehistoric times. This early plant has been unchanged for millennia and once formed the vegetation that decomposed to produce coal seams. It encourages the healing of connective tissue, and has been used as a wound herb to stop bleeding since ancient times.

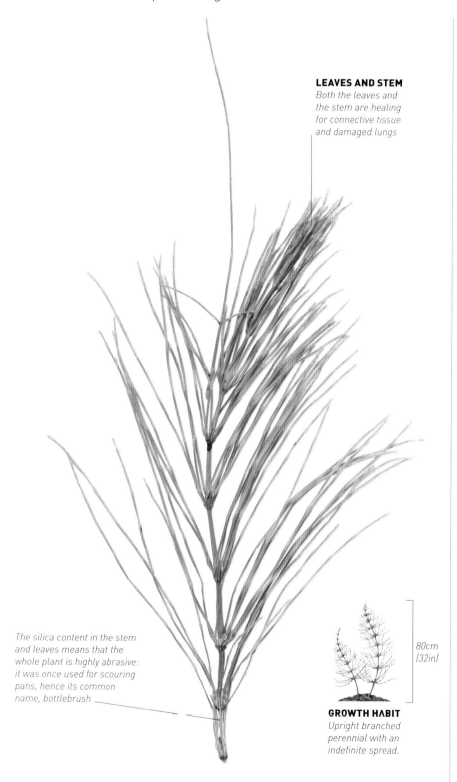

LEAVES AND STEM
Both the leaves and the stem are healing for connective tissue and damaged lungs

The silica content in the stem and leaves means that the whole plant is highly abrasive: it was once used for scouring pans, hence its common name, bottlebrush

80cm
(32in)

GROWTH HABIT
Upright branched perennial with an indefinite spread.

PARTS USED Aerial parts
MAIN CONSTITUENTS Silicic acid and silicates, alkaloids (incl. nicotine), tannins, saponins, flavonoids, bitter principles, other minerals (incl. potassium, manganese, magnesium), phytosterols
ACTIONS Astringent, haemostatic, diuretic, anti-inflammatory, tissue healer, increases coagulation

HOW TO USE

DECOCTION Take ½–1 cup of a decoction (p.168) made from 15g (½oz) of the herb to 600ml (1 pint) water 3 times daily for excessive menstruation, inflammation of the urinary tract, prostate problems, or chronic lung disorders.
JUICE Take 5–10ml (1–2 tsp) 3 times daily for damaged lungs or urinary disorders.
BATH Add 300ml (10fl oz) of the decoction to bath water for sprains, fractures, or irritable skin conditions including eczema.
POULTICE Use 1 tsp of powder made into a paste with a little water, or a handful of the fresh aerial parts sweated in a bowl over a saucepan of simmering water (bain marie); spread on gauze and use for leg ulcers, wounds, sores, or chilblains.
MOUTHWASH/GARGLE Use ½ cup of a decoction with an equal amount of water for mouth or gum infections or sore throats.

HOW TO SOURCE

GROW Prefers moist soil in full sun or partial shade. Usually propagated by root division in early spring. Under statutory control as an invasive weed in some countries.
FORAGE Found in meadows, field borders, hedgerows and waste ground. Don't confuse with marsh horsetail (*Equisetum palustre*), a larger plant that contains toxic alkaloids.
HARVEST Cut stems in the growing season.

CAUTION Seek professional guidance in all cases of blood in the urine, or for sudden changes in menstrual flow leading to heavy bleeding. Do not use for more than four weeks continuously without professional guidance.

Eucalyptus globulus **Eucalyptus**

Native to Australia and Tasmania, the eucalyptus, or "blue gum", tree is now cultivated worldwide both as a commercial crop and for its ability to absorb water and dry up marshes. It is an important remedy among the Australian Aboriginals, although in medicine the essential oil is more commonly used, largely as an antiseptic.

PARTS USED Leaves, essential oil
MAIN CONSTITUENTS Volatile oil (incl. cineole), tannins, aldehydes, bitter resin
ACTIONS Antiseptic, decongestant, antibiotic, antispasmodic, stimulant, febrifuge, hypoglycaemic, anthelmintic

HOW TO USE

DECOCTION Simmer 3–4 leaves per cup of water for 10 minutes in a covered pan and take ½–1 cup 3 times daily for the early stages of colds, chills, nasal catarrh, influenza, asthma, sinusitis, sore throats, and other respiratory disorders.
CHEST RUB Use ½ml (10 drops) of eucalyptus oil in 30ml (1fl oz) of almond oil as a chest rub for colds, bronchitis, asthma, and respiratory problems.
STEAM INHALATION Use ½ml (10 drops) of essential oil or 6 leaves in a bowl of boiling water as a steam inhalation for colds and chest infections.
COMPRESS Soak a pad in a mixture of 10 drops of essential oil and 60ml (2fl oz) of water and apply to inflammations, painful joints, or minor burns.

HOW TO SOURCE

GROW Prefers moisture-retentive soil that is neutral-to-slightly acid in a sunny site that is also sheltered from cold, dry winds. Sow the seeds at 21°C (70°F) in spring and grow on until large enough to transplant into final positions, although buying young trees from a nursery is a quicker process. As the plant absorbs so much water, it can deplete the soil over a significant area.
FORAGE Now found – often in commercial plantations – in many tropical, sub-tropical, and temperate areas worldwide, although it can also be found growing wild in marshy areas. Collect the leaves as required.
HARVEST Gather the leaves as required throughout the year.

CAUTION Do not take the essential oil internally; fatalities have been reported from comparatively low doses.

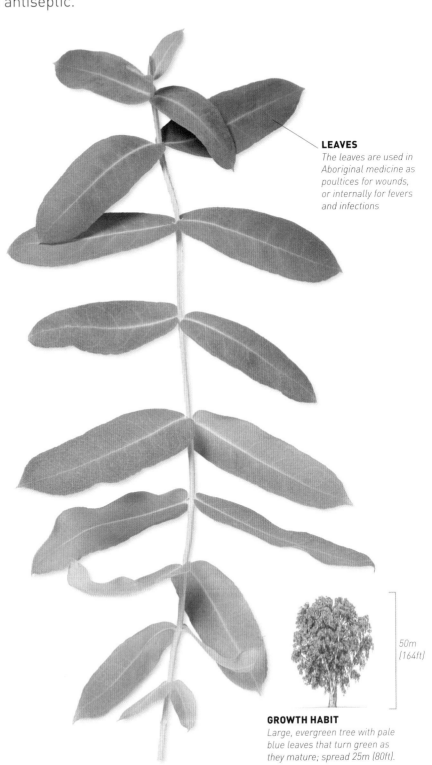

LEAVES
The leaves are used in Aboriginal medicine as poultices for wounds, or internally for fevers and infections

50m
(164ft)

GROWTH HABIT
Large, evergreen tree with pale blue leaves that turn green as they mature; spread 25m (80ft).

Eupatorium cannabinum **Hemp agrimony**

Native to Europe, hemp agrimony was traditionally used for feverish colds or as a poultice for skin sores. A bitter compound called eupatoriopicrin has now been identified in the plant and is believed to have an antitumour action. The plant also appears to be immunostimulant – increasing resistance in viral infections. However, it also contains toxic alkaloids, so must be used with caution.

LEAVES
The leaves can be pulped and the juice extracted to use as an insect repellent to rub into the coats of dogs and horses

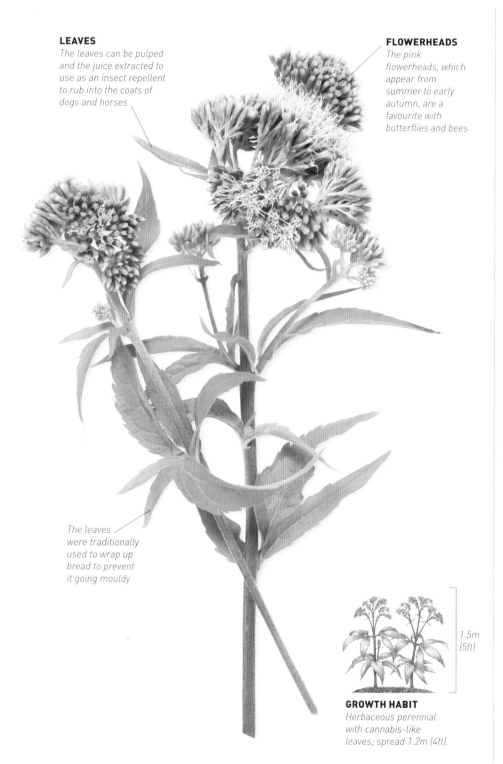

FLOWERHEADS
The pink flowerheads, which appear from summer to early autumn, are a favourite with butterflies and bees

The leaves were traditionally used to wrap up bread to prevent it going mouldy

GROWTH HABIT
Herbaceous perennial with cannabis-like leaves; spread 1.2m (4ft).

1.5m (5ft)

PARTS USED Aerial parts, root
MAIN CONSTITUENTS Volatile oil (incl. thymol, azulenes, alpha-terpinene), flavonoids, sesquiterpene lactones (incl. eupatoriopicrin), pyrrolizidine alkaloids
ACTIONS Febrifuge, diuretic, antiscorbutic, laxative, cholagogue, expectorant, immune stimulant, antirheumatic, diaphoretic, tonic

HOW TO USE

NB: Take for short periods and only under professional guidance.
INFUSION Traditionally used in the treatment of certain skin conditions, rheumatism, and arthritis, but use only under guidance from a qualified herbalist.
POULTICE Pulp a handful of fresh leaves in a blender, spread on gauze, and use on suppurating skin sores or ulcers.

HOW TO SOURCE

GROW Tolerates a range of soil conditions and grows in sun or partial shade, although prefers moist soil. Sow seeds in a cold frame in early spring and lightly cover with compost. Transplant to 7cm (3.5in) pots and plant out in early summer or when well established; allow 60cm (24in) between plants. Alternatively, sow seeds where you want them to grow in spring or autumn.
FORAGE Found in damp woods, ditches, waste ground, or marshy areas. Naturalized in parts of western Asia and North Africa.
HARVEST Cut flowering aerial parts in late summer/early autumn. Dig roots in autumn.

CAUTION Contains pyrrolizidine alkaloids, which are carcinogenic, so only use under professional guidance. High doses may cause nausea and vomiting. Avoid during pregnancy.

Eupatorium purpureum **Gravel root**

Originally found in damp thickets in the eastern USA, gravel root is grown as a statuesque garden ornamental in many parts of the world. Its other common name, Joe Pye weed, is reputedly named after a Native American medicine man who used it to cure typhus. The herb is used for clearing gravel and kidney stones and for other problems affecting the urinary tract.

PARTS USED Rhizome and root
MAIN CONSTITUENTS Eupatorin, volatile oil, flavonoids, resin
ACTIONS Soothing diuretic, antirheumatic, astringent

HOW TO USE

DECOCTION Take ½ cup of a decoction made of 1 tsp dried root to 1 cup water and simmered for 20 minutes for kidney stones, gravel, or painful urination. This mixture was traditionally used to ease the pain of childbirth. Gravel root is believed to enhance the removal of waste products by the kidneys, so the decoction is also useful in rheumatism and gout to improve the excretion of uric acid.

TINCTURE Use 2–4 ml (40–80 drops) 3 times daily for urinary disorders including cystitis and gravel, or discharges associated with infection. It combines well with white dead-nettle (*Lamium album*) for prostate problems and with parsley piert (*Aphanes arvensis*), pellitory-of-the-wall (*Parietaria judaica*), or hydrangea (*Hydrangea* spp.) for kidney stones.

HOW TO SOURCE

GROW Prefers moist, fertile soil in sun or partial shade. Sow seeds in spring in a cold frame and when the seedlings are large enough to handle transplant them to final positions. Allow at least 90cm (36in) between plants. It is best grown at the back of a border, but is popular in planting schemes as it flowers late in the season.

FORAGE Unlikely to be found growing wild beyond the eastern states of the USA, although it might occur as a garden escape. As the root is used, it is best not to collect from the wild. In Europe the related species *Eupatorium cannabinum* (hemp agrimony, p.54) is more likely to be found growing as a hedgerow plant.

HARVEST The roots of two-year-old, or older, plants are dug in autumn.

CAUTION Avoid during pregnancy.

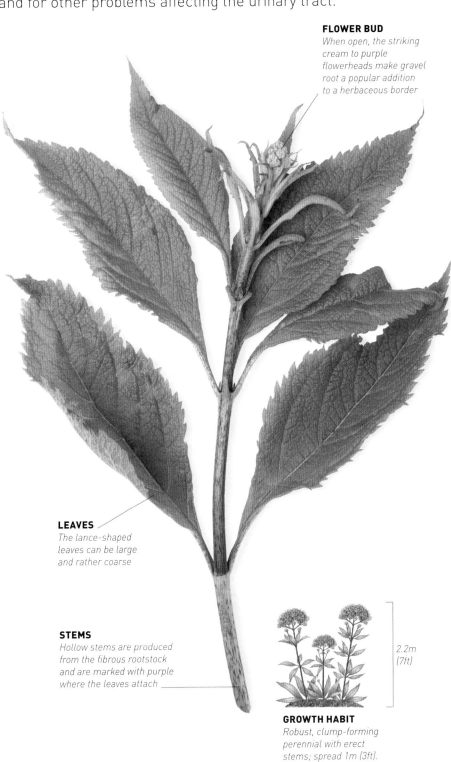

FLOWER BUD
When open, the striking cream to purple flowerheads make gravel root a popular addition to a herbaceous border

LEAVES
The lance-shaped leaves can be large and rather coarse

STEMS
Hollow stems are produced from the fibrous rootstock and are marked with purple where the leaves attach

2.2m (7ft)

GROWTH HABIT
Robust, clump-forming perennial with erect stems; spread 1m (3ft).

Filipendula ulmaria **Meadowsweet**

Growing in damp ditches throughout Europe and western Asia, meadowsweet takes its name from is original use of flavouring mead, or honey wine. Today it is highly regarded as an antacid herb, helping both to combat excess stomach acid leading to indigestion and gastritis and to reduce the body's acidity generally, so helping with arthritic conditions.

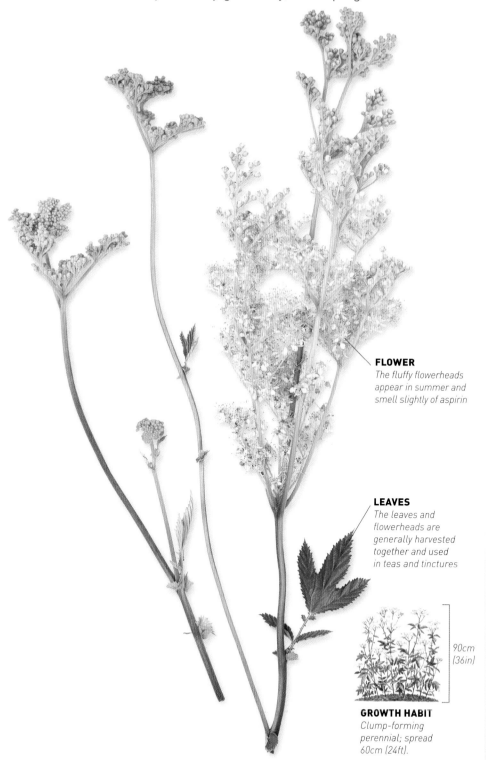

FLOWER
The fluffy flowerheads appear in summer and smell slightly of aspirin

LEAVES
The leaves and flowerheads are generally harvested together and used in teas and tinctures

90cm
(36in)

GROWTH HABIT
Clump-forming perennial; spread 60cm (24ft).

PARTS USED Aerial parts, flowers
MAIN CONSTITUENTS Salicylates, flavonoids (incl. rutin and hyperin), volatile oil (incl. salicylaldehyde), citric acid, mucilage, tannins
ACTIONS Antacid, anti-inflammatory, antirheumatic, soothing digestive remedy, diuretic, diaphoretic, anticoagulant

HOW TO USE

INFUSION Take 1 cup of a standard infusion (p.168) of leaves and flowers 3 times daily for feverish colds or mild rheumatic pains. Take ½ cup every 2 hours for acid reflux or indigestion. Can be given to children for stomach upsets; consult a herbalist for advice on dosage.
FLUID EXTRACT Take 2–5ml (40 drops– 1 tsp) 3 times daily for gastritis, gastric ulceration, or chronic rheumatism. Combine with angelica, bogbean (*Menyanthes trifoliata*), or willow for arthritis.
COMPRESS Soak a pad in dilute tincture and apply to painful arthritic joints or for rheumatism or neuralgia.

HOW TO SOURCE

GROW Prefers fertile, non-acid, moist-to-boggy soil in a sunny or lightly shaded position. Sow seeds in autumn in a cold frame and transplant the following spring when the seedlings are established. Allow 60cm (24in) between plants. Alternatively, propagate by division in autumn or spring, or by root cuttings in winter.
FORAGE Found in damp meadows and hedgerow ditches throughout Europe and western Asia. The aerial parts can be collected as flowering begins, or the flowers harvested separately when in full bloom.
HARVEST Collect in summer just before, or at, flowering.

CAUTION Avoid meadowsweet during pregnancy. Avoid in cases of salicylate (or aspirin) sensitivity.

Foeniculum vulgare **Fennel**

Cultivated as both a herb and a vegetable since Roman times, fennel originated in Mediterranean areas, but by the 8th century AD had spread to northern Europe. It is widely available as an after-dinner herbal drink in teabags to improve the digestion, and has been used as a culinary herb with fish for centuries.

PARTS USED Seeds, root, leaves, essential oil

MAIN CONSTITUENTS Volatile oil (incl. estragole, anethole), essential fatty acids, flavonoids (incl. rutin), vitamins, minerals

ACTIONS Carminative, circulatory stimulant, anti-inflammatory, encourages milk flow, mild expectorant, diuretic

HOW TO USE

INFUSION 1/2–1 tsp of seeds to 1 cup of boiling water as an after-dinner tea to combat wind and indigestion. A standard infusion (p.168) taken 3 times daily can increase milk flow when breast-feeding.

MOUTHWASH/GARGLE Use 1 cup of a standard infusion of seeds as a wash for gum disorders or a gargle for sore throats.

TINCTURE 1/4–1/2ml (5–10 drops) as a remedy for constipation to combat griping pains.

DECOCTION Take 1 cup of a standard decoction of the root 3 times daily for disorders linked to high uric acid levels.

CHEST RUB Add 1/4–1/2ml (5–10 drops) each of fennel, thyme, and eucalyptus essential oil to 20ml (4 tsp) of almond oil and massage into the chest for coughs and bronchitis.

HOW TO SOURCE

GROW Sow fennel seeds where you want them to grow in spring and thin to 30cm (12in), or transplant self-sown seedlings. Generally fairly hardy, but may suffer in severe winters. Can be treated as a biennial. The *dulce* variety is grown as a vegetable.

FORAGE Generally grows on waste ground and in coastal areas, but self-seeded plants growing outside gardens can be found in many places. Gather the leaves in summer for culinary use and the seeds in autumn for teas and medicinal use.

HARVEST Collect the leaves in summer and the seeds in autumn. Lift the root, if using, once the leaves have died down.

CAUTION Essential oils should not be taken internally except under professional advice.

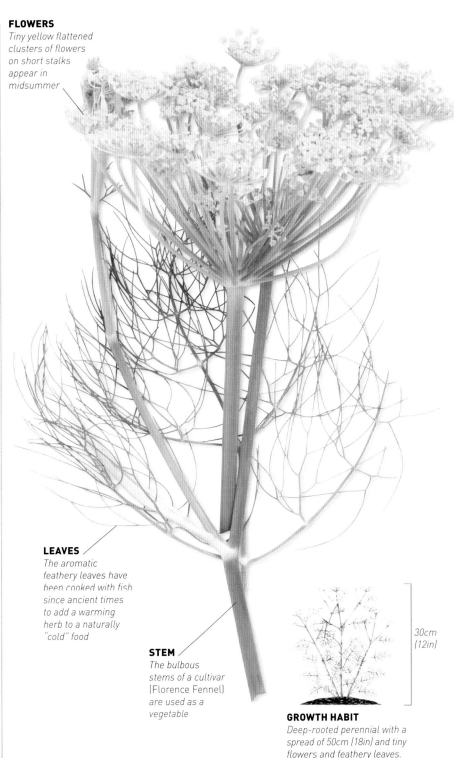

FLOWERS
Tiny yellow flattened clusters of flowers on short stalks appear in midsummer

LEAVES
The aromatic feathery leaves have been cooked with fish since ancient times to add a warming herb to a naturally "cold" food

STEM
The bulbous stems of a cultivar (Florence Fennel) are used as a vegetable

30cm (12in)

GROWTH HABIT
Deep-rooted perennial with a spread of 50cm (18in) and tiny flowers and feathery leaves.

Fragaria vesca **Wild strawberry**

Alpine strawberries, now grown worldwide, originated from this wild strawberry and have smaller, more aromatic fruits than "cultivated" strawberries (which were developed in the 18th century from an American hybrid). Wild strawberry is found in woodlands and grassy areas of Europe, western Asia, and North America. Its leaves and fruits are used medicinally – mainly in astringent teas.

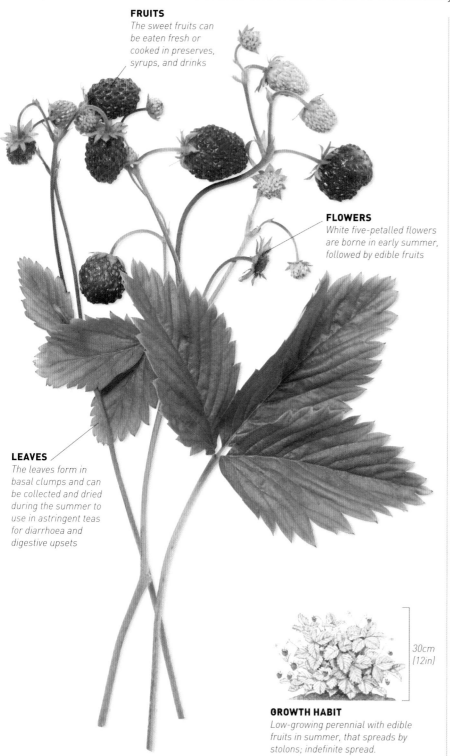

FRUITS
The sweet fruits can be eaten fresh or cooked in preserves, syrups, and drinks

FLOWERS
White five-petalled flowers are borne in early summer, followed by edible fruits

LEAVES
The leaves form in basal clumps and can be collected and dried during the summer to use in astringent teas for diarrhoea and digestive upsets

GROWTH HABIT
Low-growing perennial with edible fruits in summer, that spreads by stolons; indefinite spread.

30cm (12in)

PARTS USED Leaves, fruit
MAIN CONSTITUENTS
Leaf: Volatile oil, flavonoids tannins
Fruit: Fruit acids, salicylates, sugar, vitamins B, C, and E
ACTIONS Astringent, wound herb, diuretic, laxative, liver tonic, cleansing

HOW TO USE

INFUSION Take 1 cup of a standard infusion (p.168) of the leaves 3 times daily for diarrhoea.
MOUTHWASH/GARGLE Use 1 cup of the standard infusion of the leaves for sore throats and gum disease.
LOTION Use the standard infusion of the leaves as a lotion to bathe minor burns, cuts, and grazes.
FRESH BERRIES Traditionally regarded as cooling, strawberries have, in the past, been prescribed for gout, arthritis, rheumatism, and tuberculosis. They can also be soothing for gastritis and in convalescence.
JUICE Juice some fresh berries and take in 10ml (2 tsp) doses 3 times daily to combat infections and as a mild, cleansing laxative in constipation and arthritic disorders.
POULTICE The crushed fresh berries can be used as a poultice to soothe sunburn and skin inflammations.

HOW TO SOURCE

GROW Prefers moist but well-drained fertile soil, which is rich in organic matter, in sun or partial shade. Propagate by sowing seeds in trays in spring or autumn and lightly covering them with soil. Keep moist and transplant to 7.5cm (3in) pots when large enough to handle. Alternatively, grow from rooted stolons (horizontal shoots) separated from the mother plant in late summer. It can be grown as an edging plant in a herb garden.
FORAGE Can be found in hedgerows, woodlands, and grassy areas in many parts of the world. Gather the berries when ripe and the leaves throughout the summer.
HARVEST Collect the fruit as it ripens in the summer and gather the leaves throughout the growing period.

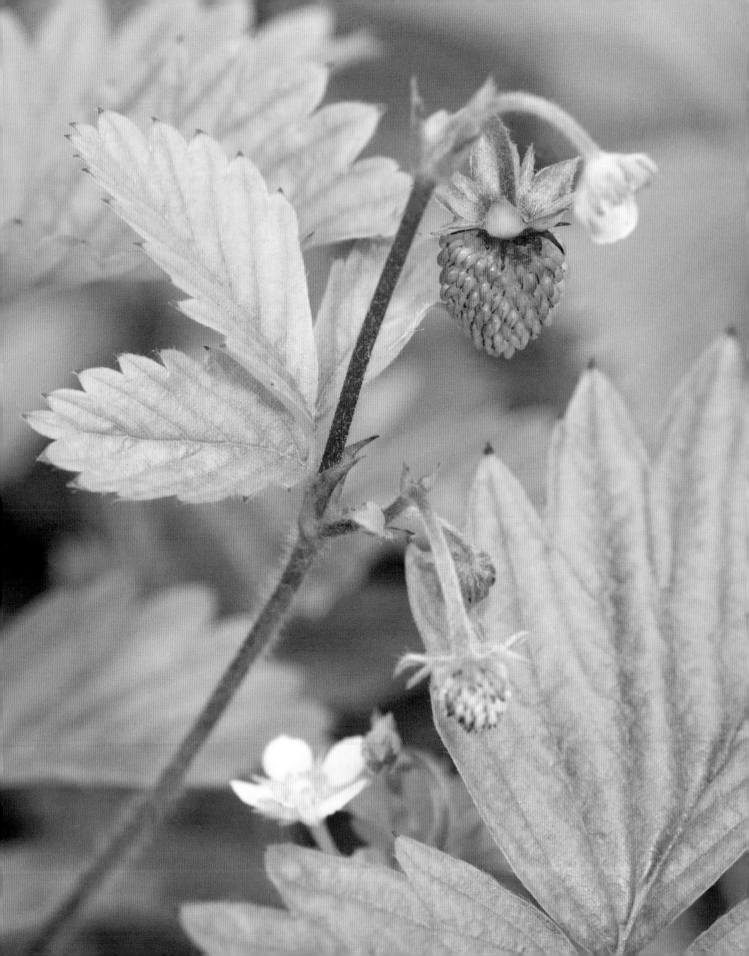

Galium aparine **Cleavers**

A familiar garden weed, cleavers is found throughout Europe and northern and western Asia. In China the whole plant is sometimes eaten as a vegetable. It has been used in cancer treatments since ancient times, although its efficacy has not been confirmed by modern research. It is, however, highly regarded as a cleanser for the lymphatic system.

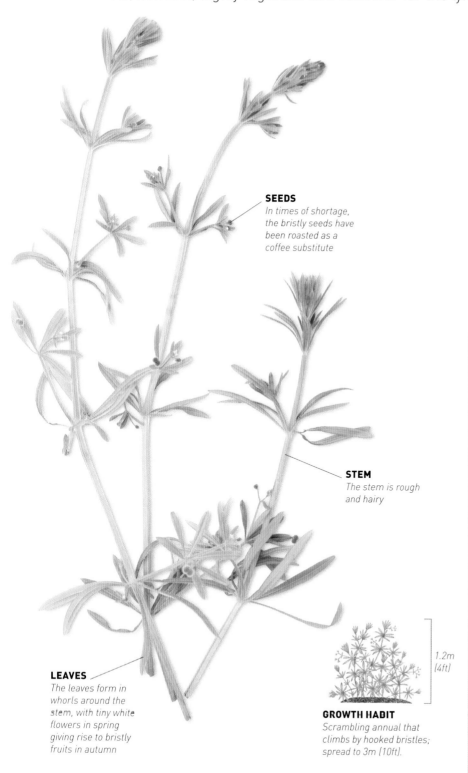

SEEDS
In times of shortage, the bristly seeds have been roasted as a coffee substitute

STEM
The stem is rough and hairy

LEAVES
The leaves form in whorls around the stem, with tiny white flowers in spring giving rise to bristly fruits in autumn

1.2m (4ft)

GROWTH HABIT
Scrambling annual that climbs by hooked bristles; spread to 3m (10ft).

PARTS USED Whole plant
MAIN CONSTITUENTS Flavonoids, anthraquinone derivatives (in the root), iridoids, coumarins, tannins, polyphenolic acids
ACTIONS Diuretic, lymphatic cleanser and detoxifier, astringent tonic, anti-inflammatory

HOW TO USE

JUICE Take 10ml (2 tsp) of freshly made juice up to 3 times daily as a lymphatic cleanser and diuretic for conditions such as glandular fever, tonsillitis, and prostate disorders.
CREAM Use frequently for psoriasis; it is most effective if treatment begins early when the skin patches are still small.
INFUSION Take 1 cup of a standard infusion (p.168) of the fresh herb 3 times daily for urinary problems, such as cystitis and stones in the urinary tract. Usually combined with other urinary remedies, such as yarrow, couchgrass (*Elymus repens*), marshmallow, or buchu (*Agathosma* spp.).
TINCTURE Take up to 5ml (1 tsp) 3 times daily as a lymphatic cleanser and detoxifier for any enlargement of the lymph nodes.
COMPRESS Apply a pad soaked in a standard infusion to grazes, skin ulcers, and inflammations.

HOW TO SOURCE

GROW Regarded by most gardeners as an irritating annual weed, cleavers climbs by means of hooked bristles through shrubs to reach heights of 1.2m (4ft), and spreads to 3m (10ft). It is not a plant many would choose to cultivate, as it usually grows anywhere and everywhere, but the bristly fruits that appear in autumn can be collected and immediately scattered where the plant is to grow the following year.
FORAGE From spring to autumn, cleavers can be found scrambling through banks, hedgerows, and garden borders. The whole plant can be gathered, and is best used fresh.
HARVEST The whole plant is best gathered in the spring just before flowering.

Ginkgo biloba **Ginkgo**

A survivor of the fossil age, the ginkgo or maidenhair tree is the sole member of its genus and dates back at least 200 million years. The trees are either male or female and only flower when in close proximity. The edible seeds are used in traditional Chinese medicine for some types of asthma, while the leaves have become popular in the West for circulatory disorders.

PARTS USED Leaves, seeds

MAIN CONSTITUENTS Leaves: flavone glycosides, bioflavones, beta-sitosterol, lactones, anthocyanin
Seeds: fatty acids, minerals, bioflavones

ACTIONS Leaves: vasodilator, circulatory stimulant
Seeds: astringent, antifungal, antibacterial

HOW TO USE

FLUID EXTRACT Take 1–3ml (20–60 drops) up to 3 times daily for diseases involving the peripheral circulation, or for cerebral arteriosclerosis in the elderly.

TINCTURE Take 3–5ml (60 drops–1 tsp) 3 times daily for cardiovascular system disorders. It is generally combined with periwinkle (*Vinca* spp.) and lime flowers for circulatory problems, or melilot for venous disorders.

DECOCTION Take 1 cup of a decoction of the seeds, made from 3–4 seeds to 600ml (1 pint) of water, 3 times daily for wheeziness, persistent coughs, or asthmatic conditions. This can be combined with an infusion of coltsfoot and mulberry leaves (*Morus* spp.).

TABLETS Widely available and generally recommended for poor circulation, varicose veins, or memory loss.

HOW TO SOURCE

GROW Most commercially available trees are grown from cuttings from male trees; so female trees can be hard to find. Prefers fertile, moist, but well-drained soil in full sun. Grow from ripe seeds collected from a female tree in autumn and plant in a cold frame, or take semi-ripe cuttings in summer. Avoid pruning.

FORAGE Rarely found in the wild, but widely cultivated as a specimen tree in parks and gardens.

HARVEST Collect leaves and fruits in autumn.

CAUTION Avoid if taking aspirin or warfarin. High doses of the seeds can lead to skin disorders and headaches. Restricted in some countries.

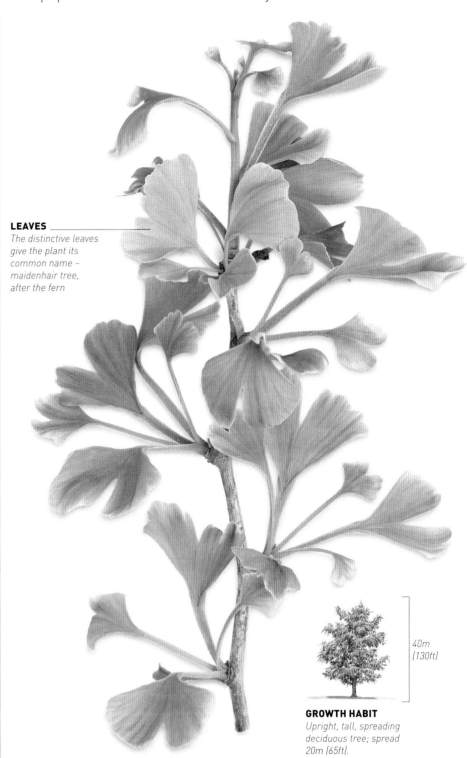

LEAVES
The distinctive leaves give the plant its common name – maidenhair tree, after the fern

40m
(130ft)

GROWTH HABIT
Upright, tall, spreading deciduous tree; spread 20m (65ft).

Glycyrrhiza glabra **Liquorice**

A native of the Mediterranean region and south-west Asia, liquorice has been valued for its sweet taste since ancient times. The Romans also used it as a remedy for asthma and coughs. Its cultivation spread to northern Europe in the 15th century. A related Asian species (*Glycyrrhiza uralensis*) is known as "the grandfather of herbs", and is widely used in Chinese medicine.

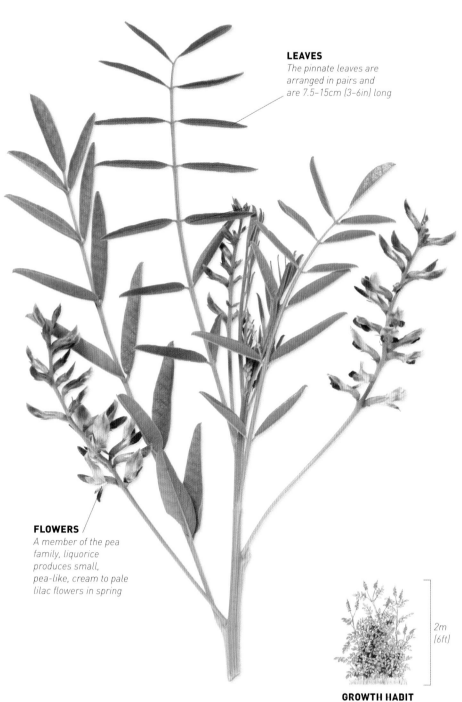

LEAVES
The pinnate leaves are arranged in pairs and are 7.5–15cm (3–6in) long

FLOWERS
A member of the pea family, liquorice produces small, pea-like, cream to pale lilac flowers in spring

GROWTH HABIT
Tap-rooted perennial with oblong pods; spread 1m (3ft).

2m (6ft)

PARTS USED Root
MAIN CONSTITUENTS Saponins, glycyrrhizin, oestrogenous substances, coumarins, flavonoids, sterols, asparagine
ACTIONS Anti-inflammatory, demulcent, tonic stimulant for adrenal cortex, mild laxative, expectorant, lowers cholesterol levels, soothing for gastric mucosa

HOW TO USE

TINCTURE Take 2–5ml (40 drops–1 tsp) 3 times daily for gastritis, peptic ulceration, mouth ulcers, or excessive stomach acid. Add a similar amount to cough syrups.
FLUID EXTRACT Take 1–2ml (20–40 drops) 3 times a day to strengthen the adrenal glands, especially after steroidal therapy, or as a digestive tonic.
DECOCTION Take 1 cup of a standard decoction (p.168) up to 3 times daily to reduce stomach acid and ease any inflammation or ulceration. Take 1 cup last thing at night for mild constipation.
SYRUP Combine the decoction with an equal amount of honey to make a cough syrup. Combines well with thyme, hyssop, or elecampane for chest problems including bronchitis, asthma, and chest infections.
WASH Add 5ml (1 tsp) of tincture to 50ml (1¾fl oz) of warm water to bathe skin inflammations and irritant skin rashes.

HOW TO SOURCE

GROW Prefers deep, neutral to alkaline, well-drained soil in full sun. Sow seeds in autumn or spring and transplant into 7.5cm (3in) pots when large enough. Grow on in containers until sturdy enough to plant out.
FORAGE Grows wild in southern Europe. Collecting wild roots is not recommended. Gather the seed pods to cultivate at home.
HARVEST Gather the roots of three- or four-year-old plants in autumn.

CAUTION Do not take therapeutic doses if pregnant. Avoid if you have high blood pressure or take digoxin-based drugs. Do not take for prolonged periods except under professional advice.

Hamamelis virginiana **Witch hazel**

Used by Native Americans for traumatic injuries and aching muscles, Virginian witch hazel was originally found in North America's moist woodland areas, from Nova Scotia to Florida. Today it is widely cultivated for its medicinal properties, and as an attractive garden ornamental with heavily scented autumn flowers. Distilled Virginian witch hazel is a familiar first aid remedy.

PARTS USED Leaves, twigs

MAIN CONSTITUENTS Tannins, flavonoids (incl. kaempferol and quercetin), saponins, bitters, volatile oil (incl. eugenol and safrole), choline, gallic acid

ACTIONS Astringent, stops internal and external bleeding, anti-inflammatory

HOW TO USE

DISTILLATE/HYDROSOL The leaves and twigs are distilled commercially to produce a mixture of water and essential oil (sometimes preserved with alcohol). It can be used to stop bleeding from cuts, grazes, or nosebleeds, to bathe varicose veins and irritant skin rashes, and in compresses for sprains or sore eyes.

INFUSION Take 1 cup of a standard infusion (p.168) of leaves up to 3 times daily for diarrhoea, bleeding piles, or capillary fragility.

MOUTHWASH/GARGLE Use 1 cup of a standard infusion of the leaves for sore throats, mouth ulcers, tonsillitis, pharyngitis, and spongy or bleeding gums.

TINCTURE Add 5ml (1 tsp) of the bark tincture to 50ml (1¾fl oz) of water and use as an alternative to distilled witch hazel.

CREAM/OINTMENT Use the bark for minor cuts, grazes, bruises, piles, or varicose veins.

HOW TO SOURCE

GROW Prefers fertile, well-drained, slightly acidic soil in sun or dappled shade, but will tolerate deep soil over chalk. Sow ripe seeds in a cold frame in autumn. The seeds can be slow to germinate, but grow on in larger pots until the young tree is large enough to plant out. Alternatively, take softwood cuttings in summer or hardwood cuttings in autumn.

FORAGE Virginian witch hazel may be found growing wild in woodlands on the eastern side of North America. Gathering bark from wild trees is not recommended, as it can damage the tree, although leaves and a few twigs can be harvested in summer and early autumn before flowering.

HARVEST The leaves are gathered in summer and the bark in autumn. The twigs can be cropped when the tree is dormant.

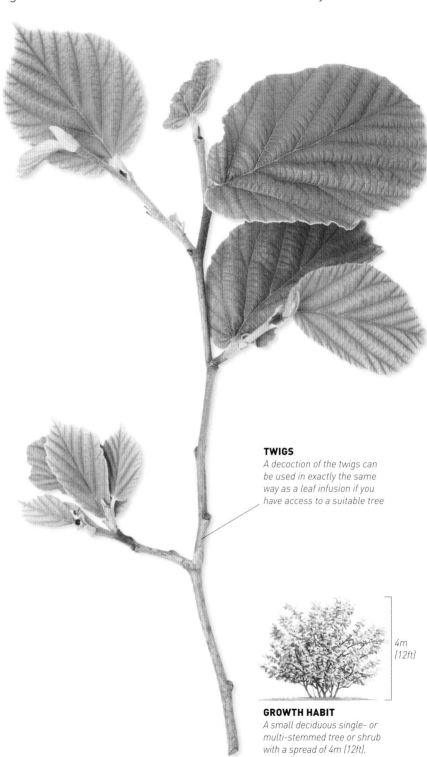

TWIGS
A decoction of the twigs can be used in exactly the same way as a leaf infusion if you have access to a suitable tree

4m
(12ft)

GROWTH HABIT
A small deciduous single- or multi-stemmed tree or shrub with a spread of 4m (12ft).

Houttuynia cordata **Dokudami**

This plant was once used as an antidote to poisons and its common name, dokudami, translates as "poison blocking" in Japanese. Its Chinese name, *yu xing cao*, means "fish-smelling plant", and houttuynia is a common addition to savoury dishes. One of the most popular medicinal herbs in Japan, dokudami is used widely as a cleanser and detoxifier.

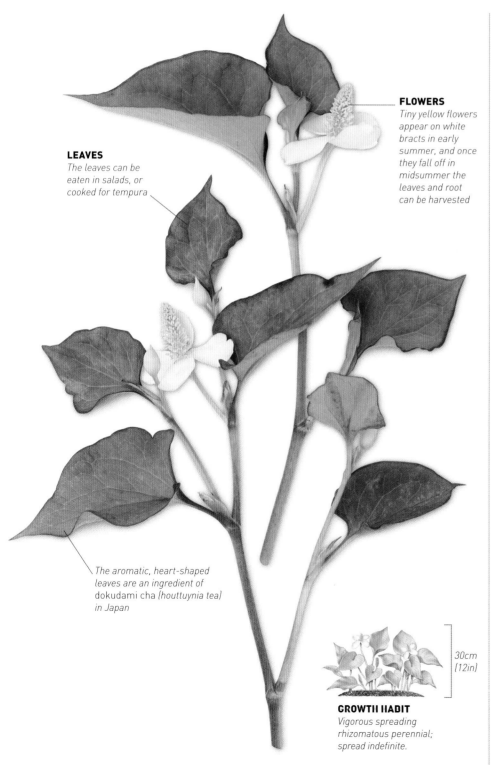

LEAVES
The leaves can be eaten in salads, or cooked for tempura

FLOWERS
Tiny yellow flowers appear on white bracts in early summer, and once they fall off in midsummer the leaves and root can be harvested

The aromatic, heart-shaped leaves are an ingredient of dokudami cha (houttuynia tea) in Japan

30cm (12in)

GROWTH HABIT
Vigorous spreading rhizomatous perennial; spread indefinite.

PARTS USED Leaves, root
MAIN CONSTITUENTS Flavonoids (incl. quercetin and hyperin), terpenes (incl. limonene and camphene), linalool, sitosterols, potassium salts, volatile oil (incl. decanol-acetaldehyde)
ACTIONS Astringent, diuretic, antibacterial, laxative, urinary antiseptic, anti-inflammatory, antitussive, wound herb

HOW TO USE

TINCTURE Take up to 10ml (2 tsp) 3 times daily for urinary infections or pain on urination. For severe or persistent urinary symptoms, seek urgent medical advice to avoid any potential kidney damage.
INFUSION Make a standard infusion (p.168), using the fresh herb when available, and take 1–2 cups on 1 day each month as a general detoxifier.
SYRUP Add 450g (1lb) of honey to 600ml (1 pint) of a standard infusion containing equal amounts of dokudami and Chinese balloon flower and take in 5ml (1 tsp) doses 4–5 times daily for coughs with thick, yellow-green sputum.
DECOCTION Make a standard decoction of the whole plant and take 1–2 cups daily for boils and abscesses, although abscesses will not improve unless drained.
LOTION/OINTMENT Use on cuts, grazes, acne, boils, athlete's foot, or insect bites.

HOW TO SOURCE

GROW Prefers damp, fertile soil in full sun or dappled shade, but will grow in dry conditions, and may require protection in cold areas in winter. Sow seeds in trays in the summer, pot on, and transplant to their final growing positions in spring when well established. Can be invasive.
FORAGE Native to marginal aquatic and marshy areas in China, Japan, Laos, and Vietnam. It is classified as an alien invasive species in North America and Australia.
HARVEST Cut after flowering in summer.

CAUTION A cooling herb, so avoid in cold syndromes.

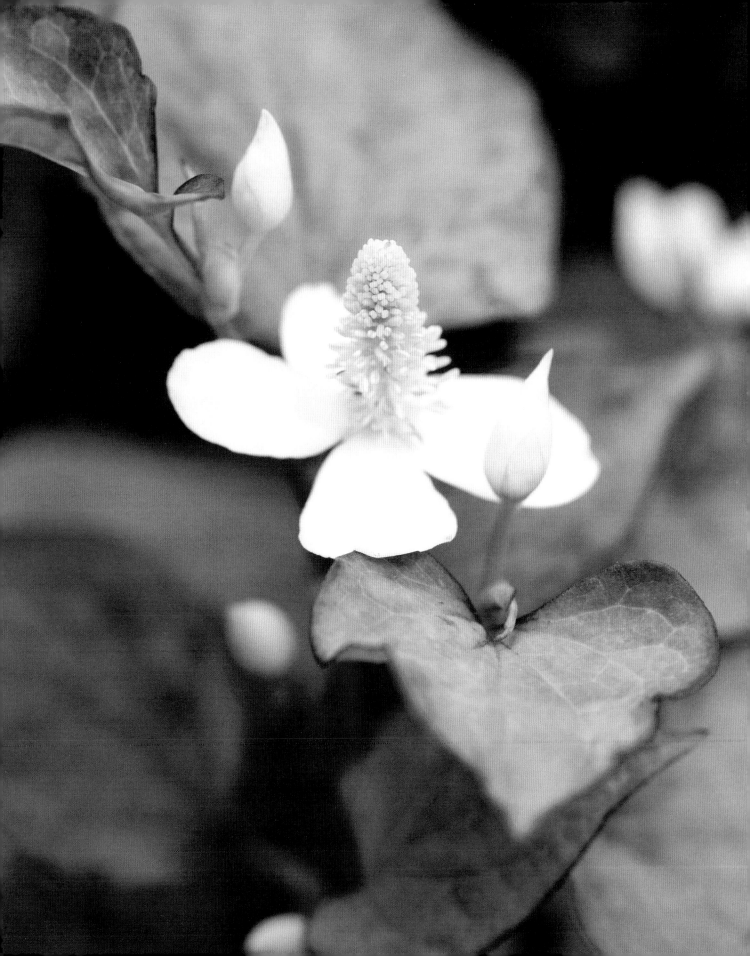

Humulus lupulus **Hops**

The strobiles, or female flowers, of the hop plant have been used since the 11th century for brewing beer, while the Romans used the leaves as a salad herb. The plant, which is native to Europe, is sedative and bitter, so it is used medicinally both for nervous disorders and digestive problems. It is also oestrogenic, leading to a loss of libido in men who regularly drink large amounts of beer.

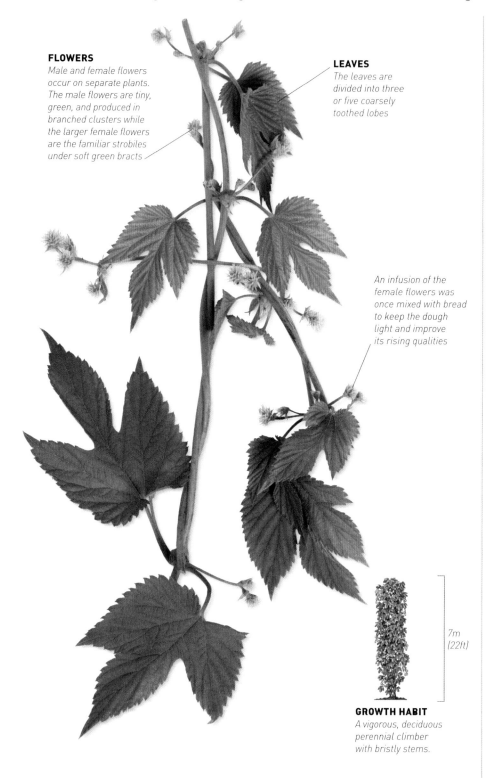

FLOWERS
Male and female flowers occur on separate plants. The male flowers are tiny, green, and produced in branched clusters while the larger female flowers are the familiar strobiles under soft green bracts

LEAVES
The leaves are divided into three or five coarsely toothed lobes

An infusion of the female flowers was once mixed with bread to keep the dough light and improve its rising qualities

7m (22ft)

GROWTH HABIT
A vigorous, deciduous perennial climber with bristly stems.

PARTS USED Strobiles (female flowers)
MAIN CONSTITUENTS Bitter principles (incl. humulon and valerianic acid), tannins, volatile oil (incl. humulene), oestrogenic substances, asparagine, flavonoids
ACTIONS Sedative, anaphrodisiac, restoring tonic for the nervous system, bitter digestive stimulant, diuretic, soporific, astringent

HOW TO USE

TINCTURE Take 1–2ml (20–40 drops) in water 3 times a day as a sedative for nervous tension and anxiety, to stimulate the digestion in poor appetite, and to ease gut spasms and colic.
INFUSION For insomnia, use 2–4 fresh strobiles per cup of boiling water, infuse for 5 minutes, and drink 30 minutes before bedtime. Freshly dried hops can also be used (older plant material is less effective).
WASH Use a standard infusion of fresh or freshly dried hops (above) as a wash for chronic ulcers, skin eruptions, or wounds.
COMPRESS Add 10ml (2 tsp) of tincture to 120ml (4fl oz) of water, soak a pad in the mixture, and use as a compress on varicose ulcers.

HOW TO SOURCE

GROW Prefers fertile, well-drained soil in sun or partial shade, and must be supported on canes or trellises. Sow the seeds in spring in trays in a propagator at 15°C (59°F) and transplant to their final growing positions when established. Alternatively, propagate by softwood cuttings in spring or early summer. Cut down old growth in winter.
FORAGE Likely to be found in hedgerows or waste ground, especially if plants have self-seeded outside commercial hop-growing areas. Collect the female flowers.
HARVEST Collect the strobiles in summer.

CAUTION Do not take if suffering from depression. The growing plant can cause contact dermatitis. Harvesting large amounts can disrupt a menstrual cycle.

Hydrastis canadensis **Goldenseal**

Used by Native Americans for a wide range of ailments, including whooping cough, liver disorders, and heart problems, goldenseal originated in mountain woodlands in North America, and today is used mainly for ulceration and inflammations affecting the mucous membranes. By the 20th century over-harvesting caused the plant to become endangered.

PARTS USED Rhizome
MAIN CONSTITUENTS Alkaloids (incl. hydrastine, canadine, and berberine), volatile oil, resin
ACTIONS Astringent, tonic, digestive, bile stimulant, anti-inflammatory, antibacterial, anticatarrhal, laxative, healing to gastric mucosa, uterine stimulant, stops internal bleeding

HOW TO USE

TINCTURE Take 0.5–2ml (10–40 drops) 3 times a day for catarrhal conditions, mucous colitis, gastroenteritis, or vaginal discharge, as a liver tonic for sluggish digestion, or to help control heavy menstrual and postpartum bleeding.
MOUTHWASH/GARGLE Use 2–3ml (40–60 drops) of tincture in 100ml (3½fl oz) of warm water for mouth ulcers, gum disease, sore throats, and catarrhal conditions.
CAPSULES Use 1 x 300mg capsule 3 times daily for catarrh, infections, or with powdered eyebright to relieve hay fever symptoms.

HOW TO SOURCE

GROW Prefers moist, well-drained slightly acid to neutral soil in shade. Plant seeds in a cold frame in small pots when ripe. Pot on and plant out when large enough, or propagate by root division in autumn.
FORAGE The plant is on the CITES list of endangered species and should not be harvested from the wild.
HARVEST Roots of mature plants are lifted in the autumn and dried.

CAUTION A uterine stimulant, so avoid during pregnancy and lactation.
Avoid if you have high blood pressure.
Prolonged use can reduce absorption of B vitamins.

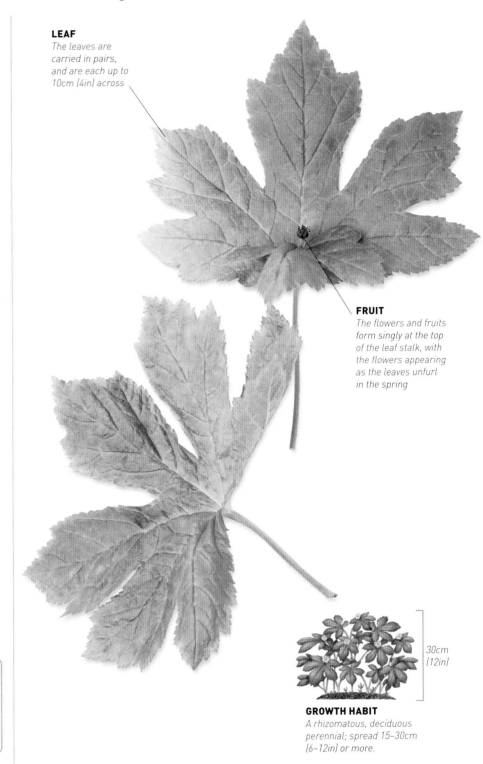

LEAF
The leaves are carried in pairs, and are each up to 10cm (4in) across

FRUIT
The flowers and fruits form singly at the top of the leaf stalk, with the flowers appearing as the leaves unfurl in the spring

30cm (12in)

GROWTH HABIT
A rhizomatous, deciduous perennial; spread 15–30cm (6–12in) or more.

Hypericum perforatum **St John's wort**

Native to temperate zones in Europe and Asia, St John's wort has been used as a wound herb since the Crusades, and was widely regarded as a cure-all in earlier centuries. It was also used for treating hysteria and mental illness. Today it is widely prescribed in parts of Europe for depression; the quality of commercial preparations, readily available to purchase, can vary.

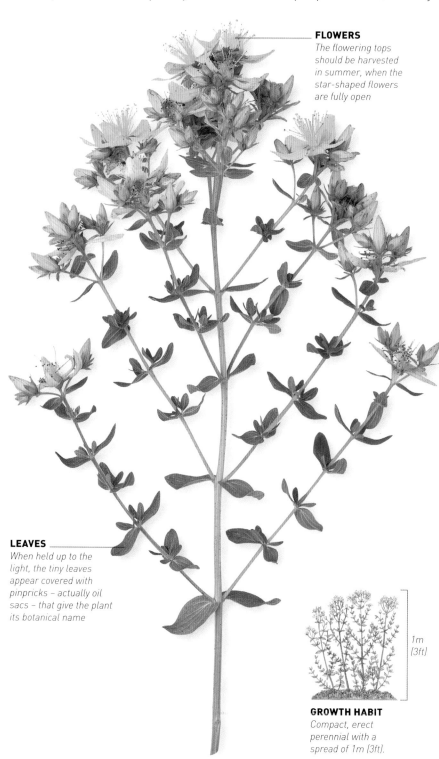

FLOWERS
The flowering tops should be harvested in summer, when the star-shaped flowers are fully open

LEAVES
When held up to the light, the tiny leaves appear covered with pinpricks – actually oil sacs – that give the plant its botanical name

GROWTH HABIT
Compact, erect perennial with a spread of 1m (3ft).

1m (3ft)

PARTS USED Aerial parts, flowering tops
MAIN CONSTITUENTS Hypericin, pseudohypericin, flavonoids (incl. rutin), volatile oil, tannins, resins
ACTIONS Astringent, analgesic, antiviral, anti-inflammatory, sedative, restoring tonic for the nervous system

HOW TO USE

INFUSION Take 1 cup of a standard infusion (p.168) of the aerial parts 3 times daily for anxiety, nervous tension, irritability, or emotional upsets associated with menopause or PMS.
TINCTURE Take 2–5ml (40 drops–1 tsp) 3 times daily for nervous tension leading to exhaustion and depression. 5–10 drops of tincture at night can be useful for childhood bed-wetting.
WASH Use 1 cup of a standard infusion to bathe wounds, skin sores, and bruises.
MACERATED OIL Apply a little oil 2–3 times daily to minor burns, sunburn, cuts, or grazes. Massage gently to relieve inflamed joints and tendonitis, and to ease nerve pains. Up to 10 drops of lavender or yarrow essential oil with 5ml (1 tsp) of the oil increases efficacy.

HOW TO SOURCE

GROW Prefers a sunny position and well-drained, alkaline soil. Sow seeds in seed trays in autumn or spring and pot up when large enough to handle. Harden off before planting in final positions.
FORAGE Found growing wild, often in hedgerows, in many parts of the world. A number of closely related species can be easily mistaken for *Hypericum perforatum*.
HARVEST Gather the whole plant just before flowering, or just the flowering tops in midsummer.

CAUTION Avoid during pregnancy. May cause gastrointestinal disturbances and allergic reactions. Interacts with many prescription medicines, including the contraceptive pill. Photosensitive: do not apply topically before sun exposure.

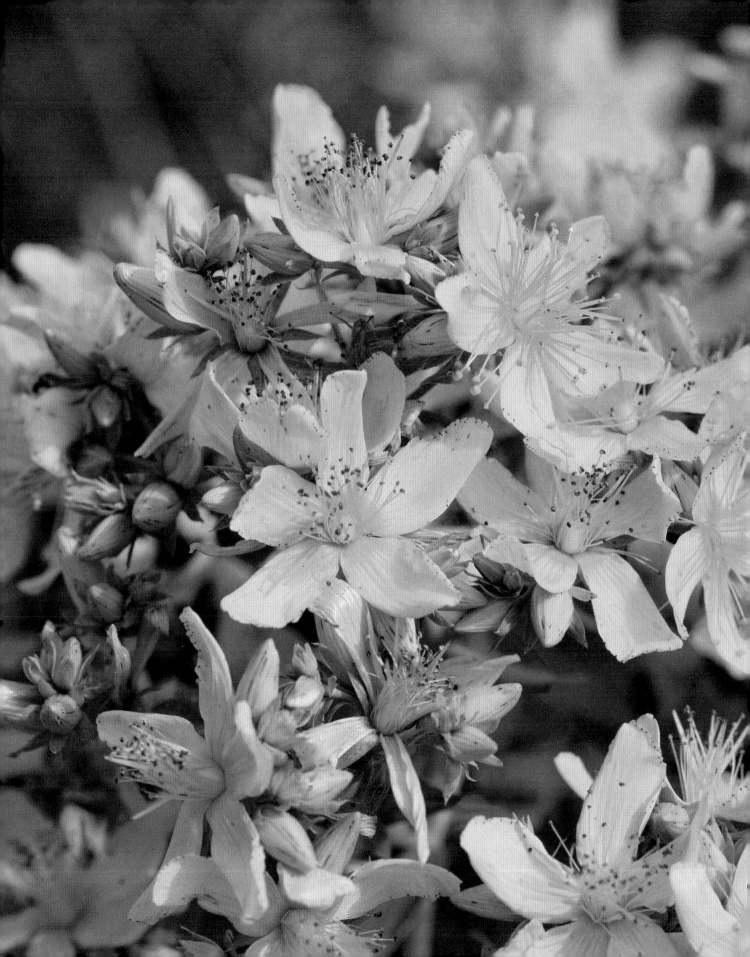

Jasminum officinale **Jasmine**

Native to Himalayan regions, India, Pakistan, and parts of China, jasmine is widely grown as a garden ornamental and is also extensively cultivated for its essential oil, which is used mainly as a sedative and antidepressant. Its close relation, *Jasminum grandiflorum*, is known as *jati* in India and is considered an important spiritual tonic to emphasize love and compassion.

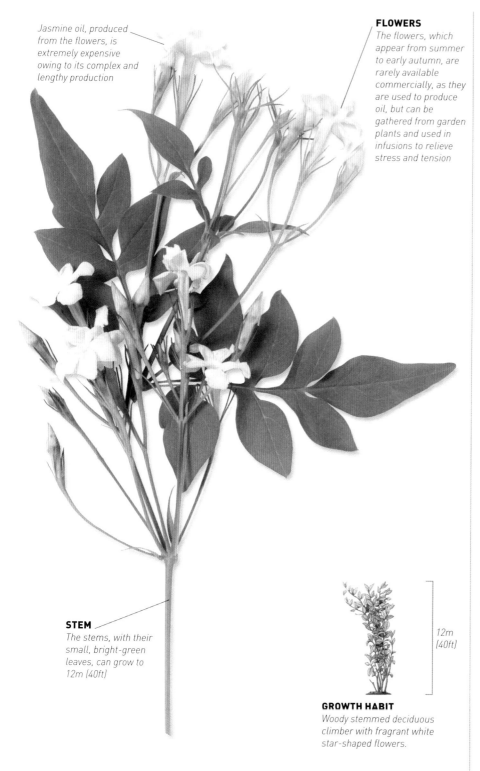

Jasmine oil, produced from the flowers, is extremely expensive owing to its complex and lengthy production

FLOWERS
The flowers, which appear from summer to early autumn, are rarely available commercially, as they are used to produce oil, but can be gathered from garden plants and used in infusions to relieve stress and tension

STEM
The stems, with their small, bright-green leaves, can grow to 12m (40ft)

GROWTH HABIT
Woody stemmed deciduous climber with fragrant white star-shaped flowers.

12m (40ft)

PARTS USED Flowers, essential oil
MAIN CONSTITUENTS Alkaloids (incl. jasminine), volatile oil (incl. benzyl alcohol, linalool, and linyl acetate), salicylic acid
ACTIONS Aphrodisiac, astringent, bitter, relaxing nervine, sedative, mild analgesic, galactagogue, antidepressant, antiseptic, antispasmodic, uterine tonic, encourages parturition

HOW TO USE

INFUSION Use 4–6 fresh flowers in 1 cup of boiling water, infuse for 5 minutes, and drink 2–3 times a day to relieve stress and tension, or for mild depression.
MASSAGE OIL Add 1–2 drops of essential oil to 5ml (1tsp) of almond oil for massage rubs to relieve anxiety, insomnia, or depression. Use 20 drops of essential oil in 30ml (1fl oz) of almond oil to massage the abdomen during the first stages of labour. The same mixture can be used for period pains.
DIFFUSER Use 2–3 drops of essential oil in a diffuser to scent a bedroom for problems with impotence or frigidity; a mutual massage between partners using 1–2 drops of jasmine oil in 5ml (1 tsp) of almond oil before lovemaking can help.

HOW TO SOURCE

GROW Prefers fertile, well-drained soil in a sun or partial shade. Prune after flowering if necessary. Usually grown from semi-ripe cuttings in summer, although established plants will frequently self-seed.
FORAGE Rarely found in the wild outside its native area, although cultivated commercially worldwide.
HARVEST The flowers are traditionally gathered in the evening when their scent is greatest while in full bloom.

Juniperus communis **Juniper**

Native to Europe, North America, and many parts of Asia, juniper has long been associated with ritual cleansing and has been burned in various temples throughout history. Today the herb is mainly used as remedy for urinary disorders, while its essential oil is included in various massage rubs for muscle and joint pains.

PARTS USED Fruits, essential oil, cade oil
MAIN CONSTITUENTS Volatile oil (incl. myrcene and cineole), flavonoids, sugars, glycosides, tannins, vitamin C
ACTIONS Urinary antiseptic, diuretic, carminative, digestive tonic, emmenagogue, antirheumatic

HOW TO USE

TINCTURE Take 1–2ml (20–40 drops) in a little water 3 times daily for urinary tract problems including cystitis, or to stimulate the digestion and ease flatulence.
INFUSION Infuse 15g (½oz) of crushed berries in 600ml (1 pint) of boiling water for 30 minutes and take ½–1 cup 3 times daily for gastric upsets, stomach chills, or period pains. The infusion can also be sipped during the first stages of labour.
MASSAGE OIL Use 10 drops of juniper essential oil in 5ml (2 tsp) of almond oil as a massage for arthritic pains.
HAIR RINSE Use 10 drops of cade oil in 1 tbsp almond oil, add to 600ml (1 pint) of hot water, mix well, and apply for psoriasis affecting the scalp. Leave for 15 minutes or longer, and rinse thoroughly.

HOW TO SOURCE

GROW Tolerates almost all conditions including both acid and alkaline soils, sun and partial shade or exposed positions, but dislikes water-logged soil. Usually grown from seed sown in a propagator in autumn or spring or by heeled cuttings in autumn. Grow on until the plants are well established and can be moved to their final positions.
FORAGE Found on moors, heaths, conifer woods, and scrubland in temperate regions throughout the northern hemisphere.
HARVEST Collect the "berries" – actually small cones –by shaking the branches over a groundsheet to dislodge them.

CAUTION Avoid during pregnancy. May irritate the kidneys after long-term use, so do not take for more than six weeks internally without a break or if there is already kidney damage.

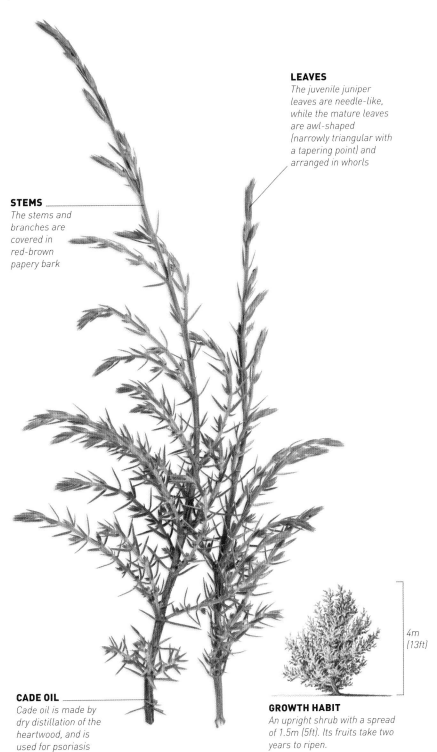

LEAVES
The juvenile juniper leaves are needle-like, while the mature leaves are awl-shaped (narrowly triangular with a tapering point) and arranged in whorls

STEMS
The stems and branches are covered in red-brown papery bark

CADE OIL
Cade oil is made by dry distillation of the heartwood, and is used for psoriasis

GROWTH HABIT
An upright shrub with a spread of 1.5m (5ft). Its fruits take two years to ripen.

4m (13ft)

Lavandula angustifolia **Lavender**

Lavender takes it name from the Latin *lavare* (to wash), and has been used to scent bath oils and soaps for centuries. It originates in Mediterranean regions and is still closely associated with the perfume industry in southern France. The flowers are valued for their soothing and sedating properties, and the essential oil is used for muscle aches and respiratory problems.

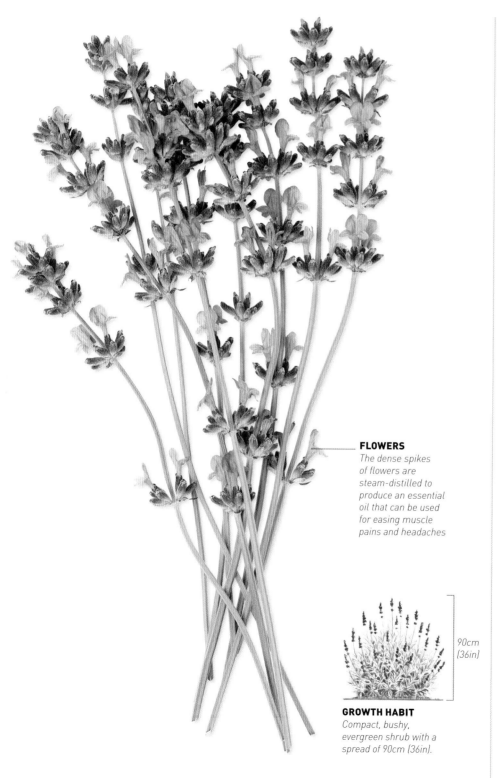

FLOWERS
The dense spikes of flowers are steam-distilled to produce an essential oil that can be used for easing muscle pains and headaches

90cm (36in)

GROWTH HABIT
Compact, bushy, evergreen shrub with a spread of 90cm (36in).

PARTS USED Flowers, essential oil
MAIN CONSTITUENTS Volatile oil (mostly linalyl acetate and cineole), tannins, coumarins, flavonoids, triterpenoids
ACTIONS Relaxant, antispasmodic, tonic for the nervous system, circulatory stimulant, antibacterial, analgesic, carminative, cholagogue, antidepressant

HOW TO USE

INFUSION Take 1 cup of a standard infusion (p.168) of the flowers up to 3 times daily for nervous exhaustion tension headaches. A cup before bedtime can also help with insomnia, or after meals with indigestion.
TINCTURE Take up to 5ml (1 tsp) twice a day for headaches, depression, or nervous tension. Can also help ease asthma, especially where attacks are triggered by nervousness or stress.
MASSAGE OIL Dilute 2ml (40 drops) of essential oil in 10ml (2 tsp) carrier oil. Use for muscular pains, or rub into the temples and the nape of the neck for tension headaches or at the first sign of a migraine.
HAIR RINSE Dilute 1ml (20 drops) of essential oil in a jug of water as a final hair rinse for head lice, and use a few drops of neat oil on a fine-toothed comb run through the hair to remove both lice and nits.
ESSENTIAL OIL Use neat on insect bites or stings, or add 10 drops to 50ml (1¾fl oz) of water to use as a lotion for sunburn. Add 3–4 drops to a tissue and place on the pillow to aid sleep.

HOW TO SOURCE

GROW Prefers well-drained, moderately fertile soil in full sun. Germination from seed can be erratic; alternatively, take semi-ripe cuttings in summer.
FORAGE Native to dry, rocky regions in the Mediterranean and south-west Asia; may grow wild in other areas.
HARVEST Flowers are usually harvested in the mornings on sunny days in summer.

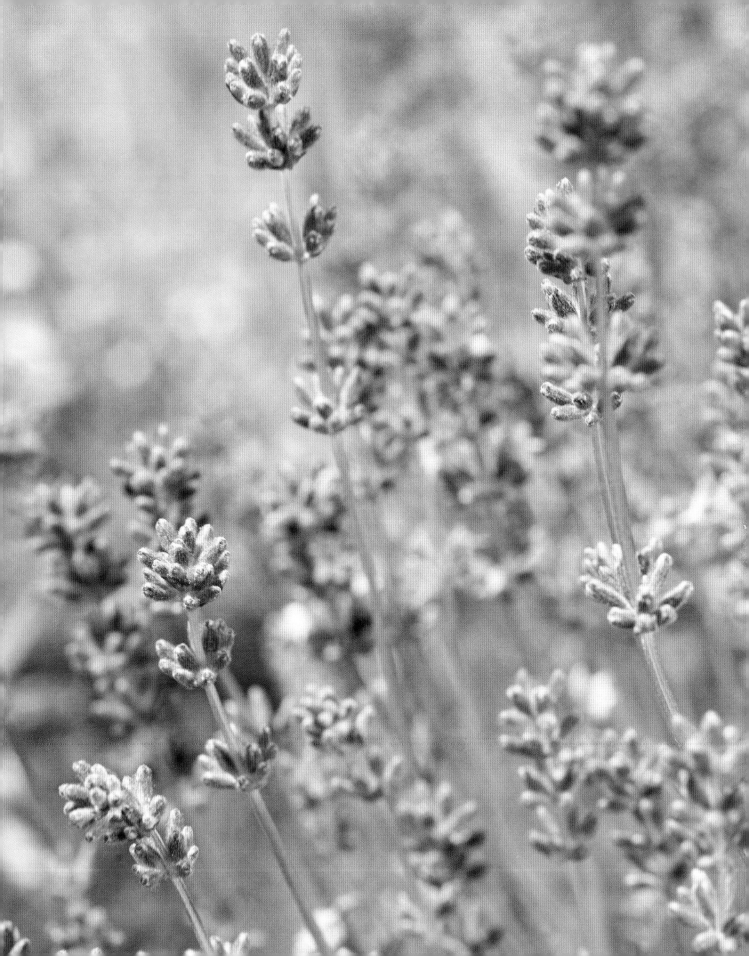

Leonurus cardiaca **Motherwort**

As its name suggests, motherwort has a long tradition as a woman's herb and was used both to calm the mother in childbirth and encourage contractions. Native to much of Europe, the plant has striking foliage and is sometimes grown as a garden ornamental. It is also used in treating heart conditions and it is commonly given for palpitations and to improve heart function.

PARTS USED Aerial parts
MAIN CONSTITUENTS Alkaloids (incl. stachydrine), iridoid (leonurine), flavonoids, diterpenes, volatile oil, tannins, vitamin A
ACTIONS Uterine stimulant, relaxant, cardiac tonic, carminative, antispasmodic, hypotensive, diaphoretic

HOW TO USE

INFUSION Take ½ cup of a standard infusion (p.168) 3 times daily for anxiety, menopausal problems, or heart weakness. Sip the tea flavoured with cloves (*Syzygium aromaticum*) during labour, and after childbirth to help restore the womb and reduce the risk of bleeding. Combine with lemon balm and lime flowers and use 2–4 tsp per cup to relieve symptoms of angina pectoris.
TINCTURE Take 5ml (1 tsp) 3 times daily for palpitations, menopausal problems such as hot flushes and emotional ability, rapid heartbeat, or PMS.
CAPSULES/POWDER Use as an alternative to the bitter infusion. Blend 1 level tsp of powdered herb with 1 tsp of honey, or take 2 x 500mg capsules, 2–3 times daily.

HOW TO SOURCE

GROW Prefers moist but well-drained soil in sun or partial shade. Sow seeds in a cold frame in spring and transplant to their final position when the seedlings are well-established; allow 45cm (18in) between plants. Alternatively, propagate by division in spring or autumn. It can self-seed enthusiastically and become invasive.
FORAGE May be found growing on waste ground, at woodland edges, or by roadsides across Europe. Avoid plants from busy roadsides to minimize pollutants.
HARVEST Gather in summer while the plant is flowering.

CAUTION A uterine stimulant, so avoid in pregnancy (except during labour) and heavy menstruation. Seek professional advice for all heart conditions.

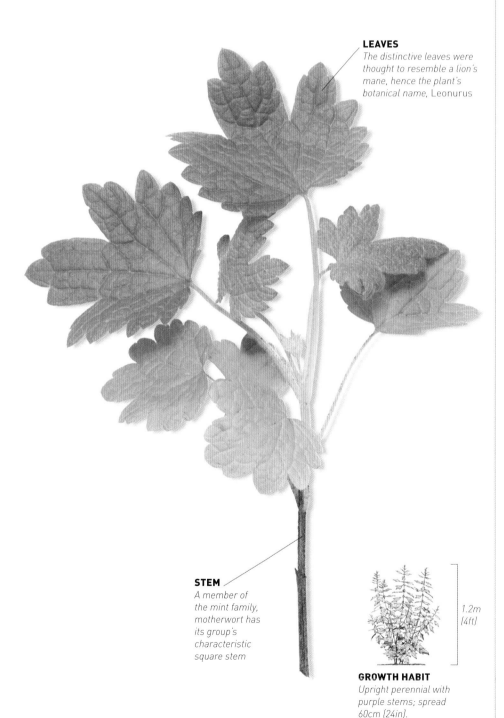

LEAVES
The distinctive leaves were thought to resemble a lion's mane, hence the plant's botanical name, Leonurus

STEM
A member of the mint family, motherwort has its group's characteristic square stem

1.2m (4ft)

GROWTH HABIT
Upright perennial with purple stems; spread 60cm (24in).

Levisticum officinale **Lovage**

Traditionally associated with love potions and aphrodisiacs, lovage was originally called *luveshe* (Old French) or "loveache". It originates in the eastern Mediterranean, although it is now widely naturalized. A culinary herb used in stock cubes, lovage is also used for treating various digestive, respiratory, and urinary problems, and is generally warming for the circulation.

PARTS USED Root, leaves, seeds
MAIN CONSTITUENTS Volatile oil (mostly phthalides), coumarins (incl. bergapten), beta-sitosterol, resins, and gums
ACTIONS Mild antibiotic, anticatarrhal, antispasmodic, diaphoretic, expectorant, sedative, carminative, mild diuretic, emmenagogue

HOW TO USE

DECOCTION Add 15g (½oz) of the root to 900ml (1½ pints) of water and simmer to reduce the volume by one third. Take ½–1 cup up to 3 times daily for indigestion, cystitis, rheumatism, gout, poor appetite, or painful menstruation. Combines well with an equal amount of agrimony infusion for indigestion.
TINCTURE Take 1–3ml (20–60 drops) of the root tincture in warm water 3 times daily for indigestion, poor appetite, urinary tract problems, or period pain. Take every 2 hours for colic.
GARGLE Use 1 cup of the root decoction as a mouthwash for mouth ulcers or as a gargle for tonsillitis.
SEEDS Chew 2–3 seeds to relieve flatulence and indigestion.
FRESH LEAVES AND STEMS Chop and add to casseroles to flavour the stock.

HOW TO SOURCE

GROW Prefers fertile, moist, well-drained soil in full sun and an open position; tolerates other conditions. Sow seeds when ripe in early autumn and transplant into position when large enough, or propagate by dividing established plants in spring.
FORAGE Sometimes found growing wild; harvest the leaves and seeds to use in cooking throughout the growing period. Lovage shoots appear early in the year, so can be useful when little else is available.
HARVEST Gather leaves through spring and early summer, seeds in late summer or autumn, and the root in late autumn.

CAUTION Avoid during pregnancy. The foliage can irritate skin.

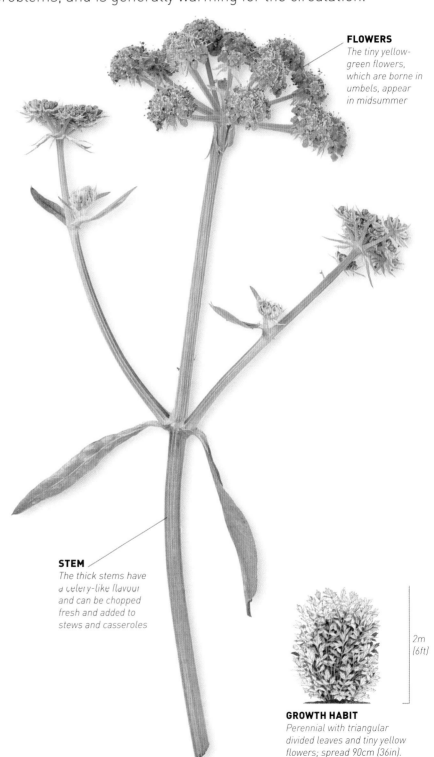

FLOWERS
The tiny yellow-green flowers, which are borne in umbels, appear in midsummer

STEM
The thick stems have a celery-like flavour and can be chopped fresh and added to stews and casseroles

2m
(6ft)

GROWTH HABIT
Perennial with triangular divided leaves and tiny yellow flowers; spread 90cm (36in).

Linum perenne **Perennial flax**

Perennial flax is very similar to a related species, common flax or linseed *(Linum usitatissimum)*, which is the more commonly cultivated form. Both are native to Europe, although linseed also grows from the Mediterranean to India. The seeds of perennial flax are used much like linseed, although – unlike common flax – the fresh aerial parts are also a traditional remedy.

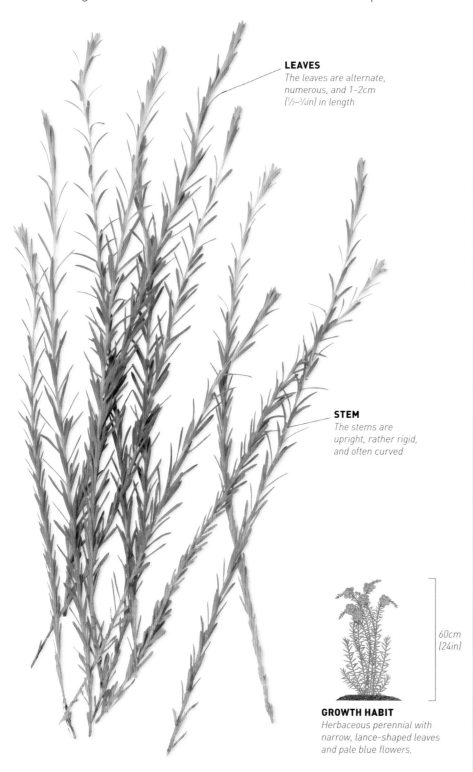

LEAVES
The leaves are alternate, numerous, and 1–2cm (½–¾in) in length

STEM
The stems are upright, rather rigid, and often curved

60cm (24in)

GROWTH HABIT
Herbaceous perennial with narrow, lance-shaped leaves and pale blue flowers.

PARTS USED Aerial parts, seeds, seed oil
MAIN CONSTITUENTS Mucilage, linoleic acid, cyanogenic glycosides, bitter principle, fixed oil incl. linolenic acid, vitamins A, B, D, and E, minerals, and amino acids
ACTIONS Antirheumatic, diuretic, anti-inflammatory, demulcent, soothing antitussive, antiseptic, laxative

HOW TO USE

INFUSION Add 60g (2oz) of fresh chopped aerial parts to 600ml (1 pint) of boiling water and take 1 cup 3 times daily for colds.
POULTICE The seeds can be used as linseeds: crush or pulp in a blender or food processor, spread on gauze, and apply to boils, abscesses, or skin ulcers.
CRUSHED SEEDS Crush 30g (1oz) in a pestle and mortar or food processor and mix with yoghurt as a dietary supplement providing essential fatty acids to support treatments for eczema, menstrual disorders, rheumatoid arthritis, or atherosclerosis.
SEEDS For constipation, mix 1–2 tsp of dried seeds with muesli, porridge, or yoghurt and eat at breakfast. Then drink 300ml (10fl oz) of water or fruit juice.

HOW TO SOURCE

GROW Prefers well-drained light or sandy soil in full sun. Sow seeds in trays in early spring in a cold frame and transplant out after the last frosts; alternatively, sow seeds directly in spring after all danger of frost is past, or in late summer, and cover with a light dusting of compost. Transplant out, leaving 25cm (10in) between plants.
FORAGE Commonly found at higher altitudes (eg, the Alps) and northern regions. Only collect seeds from sustainable populations. Collect the aerial parts while flowering in summer for use in infusions.
HARVEST Gather seeds in summer and aerial parts through the growing season.

CAUTION The seeds contain traces of prussic acid (which are potentially toxic in large quantities). Do not exceed stated dosages.

Lycium barbarum **Goji**

Native to China and Tibet, goji – variously known as wolfberry, matrimony vine, or Chinese boxthorn – is used as a hedging shrub. Both the root bark and berries have been used in China for more than 2,000 years as remedies for various problems associated with weakened liver or kidney energy, including impotence and eye disorders.

PARTS USED Fruit

MAIN CONSTITUENTS Fruit: vitamins, minerals, amino acids, essential fatty acids
Bark: alkaloids, saponins, tannins

ACTIONS Hypotensive, hypoglycaemic, hypolipidaemic, immune stimulant, liver tonic and restorative

HOW TO USE

FRESH BERRIES Add up to 30g (1oz) to breakfast cereal or yoghurt to increase vitamin and mineral intake, enhance energy and well-being, or stimulate the immune system.

DRIED BERRIES Add up to 30g (1oz) to soups and stews, or add to cakes and desserts as alternatives to blueberries.

TINCTURE Take 1–2ml (20–40 drops) up to 3 times daily as a general energy tonic.

PATENT CHINESE REMEDIES Various products such as *qi ju di huang wan* (pills that include lycium and chrysanthemum) are used as a tonic for blood and *yin* energy, but are best prescribed by professional practitioners.

HOW TO SOURCE

GROW Prefers average soil in a sunny position and is drought tolerant. Sow fresh seeds 1cm (½in) deep in compost. Keep in a warm place until germinated, and pot on when the leaves develop. Pinch out the tops when 10cm (4in) high to ensure bushy growth. Will produce fruit from the second year.

FORAGE Introduced into Europe in the 18th century, it can sometimes be found naturalized in hedgerows.

HARVEST Gather berries in autumn. They discolour if touched by hand, so shake them into a cloth.

CAUTION Avoid therapeutic doses in pregnancy – small doses in cooking are perfectly safe. Avoid during colds or flu, if suffering from diarrhoea and/or if digestion is poor. Ensure that your supplies are of good quality.

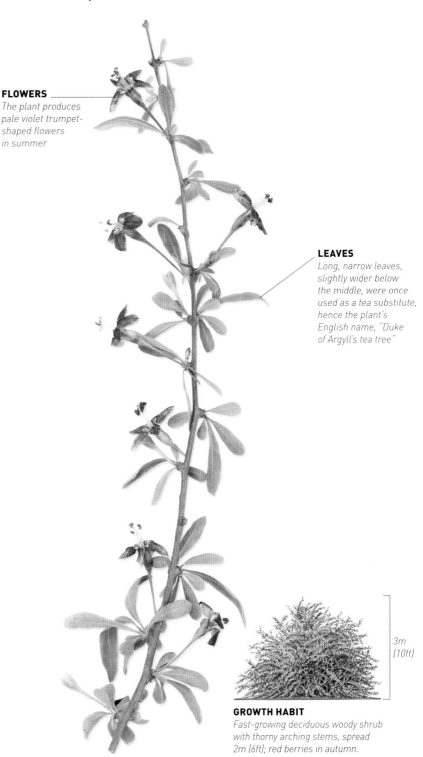

FLOWERS
The plant produces pale violet trumpet-shaped flowers in summer

LEAVES
Long, narrow leaves, slightly wider below the middle, were once used as a tea substitute, hence the plant's English name, "Duke of Argyll's tea tree"

3m
(10ft)

GROWTH HABIT
Fast-growing deciduous woody shrub with thorny arching stems, spread 2m (6ft); red berries in autumn.

Matricaria recutita **German chamomile**

Also known as scented mayweed, German chamomile's apple-scented fragrance is familiar to herbal tea drinkers, and is used both for digestive disorders and nervous problems and as an ingredient in anti-inflammatory creams and ointments. Its close relation, Roman chamomile (*Chamaemelum nobile*), is used in similar ways. It is native to Europe, western Asia, and India.

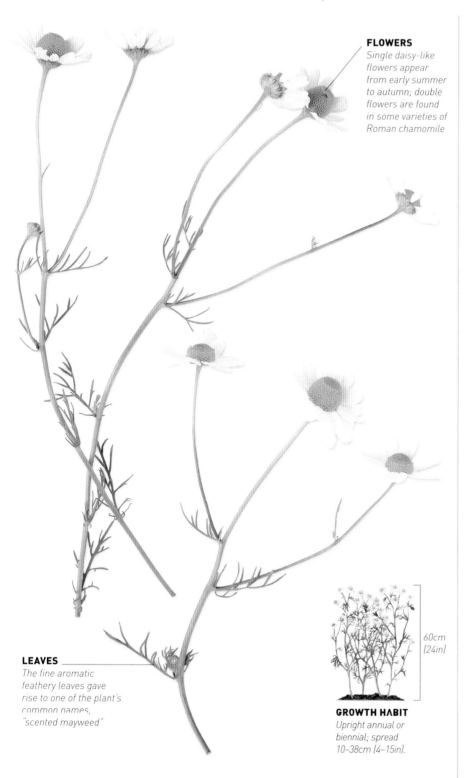

FLOWERS
Single daisy-like flowers appear from early summer to autumn; double flowers are found in some varieties of Roman chamomile

LEAVES
The fine aromatic feathery leaves gave rise to one of the plant's common names, "scented mayweed"

GROWTH HABIT
Upright annual or biennial; spread 10–38cm (4–15in).

60cm (24in)

PARTS USED Flowers, essential oil
MAIN CONSTITUENTS Volatile oil (incl. proazulenes), flavonoids (incl. rutin), valerianic acid, coumarins, tannins, salicylates, cyanogenic glycosides
ACTIONS Anti-inflammatory, antispasmodic, bitter, sedative, anti-emetic, carminative, anti-allergenic

HOW TO USE

INFUSION Take 1 cup of standard infusion (p.168) of the flowers for mild digestive problems or insomnia. German chamomile is a gentle herb that is suitable for children at reduced doses.
STEAM INHALATION Add 10ml (2 tsp) of flowers or 5 drops of essential oil to a basin of boiling water for hay fever or mild asthma.
TINCTURE Take 10ml (2 tsp) of the flower tincture 3 times daily for irritable bowel syndrome or nervous tension.
BATHS Add 4–5 drops of essential oil to the bath to heal wounds or soothe the skin. Add 1 cup of strained infusion to a baby's bath at night to encourage sleep.
CREAM/OINTMENT/LOTION Use on insect bites, wounds, or eczema.
MOUTHWASH/GARGLE Use 10ml (2 tsp) of tincture in a glass of warm water, or 1 cup of standard infusion for gum disease and mouth inflammations or as a gargle for sore throats.

HOW TO SOURCE

GROW Prefers well-drained, neutral to slightly acid soil, and a sunny site. Sow seeds where you want them to grow in autumn or spring. It self-seeds freely.
FORAGE Found growing in Europe, western Asia, and India. Easily confused with other daisies, so be familiar with its distinctive smell before gathering.
HARVEST Gather flowers in summer.

CAUTION Can cause contact dermatitis. Avoid if you are allergic to the Compositae family.

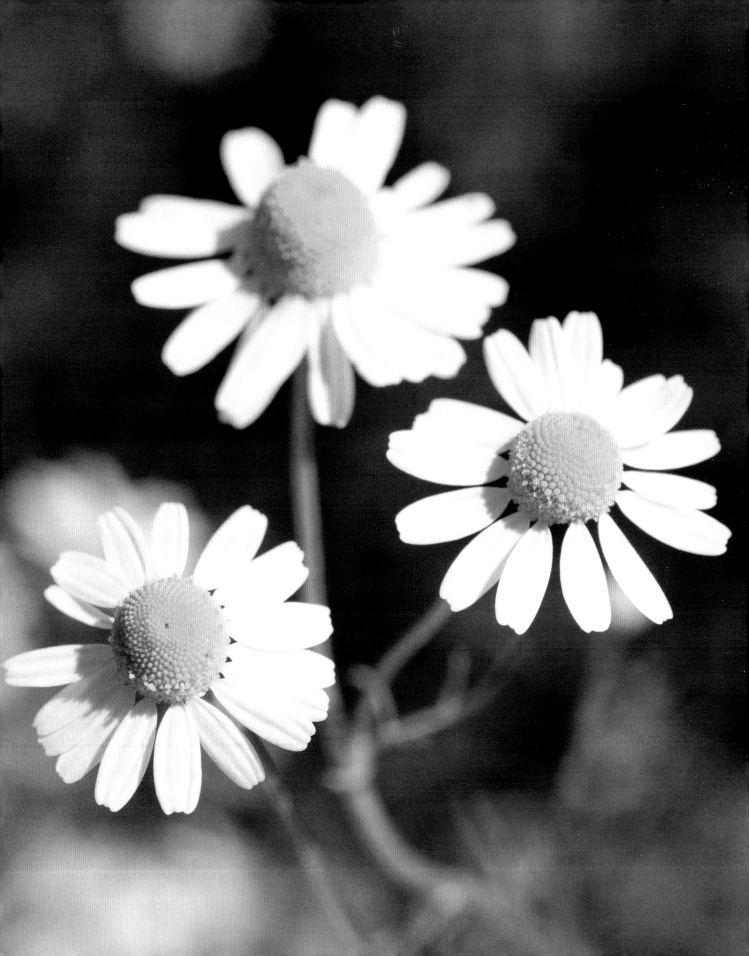

Melilotus officinalis **Melilot**

Also known as king's clover, melilot is native to Europe, north Africa, and temperate regions of Asia, and is widely cultivated as a fodder crop for silage. Today it is largely used for problems associated with venous circulation, including thrombosis and varicose veins, although in the past it was a popular remedy for indigestion, bronchitis, and insomnia in children.

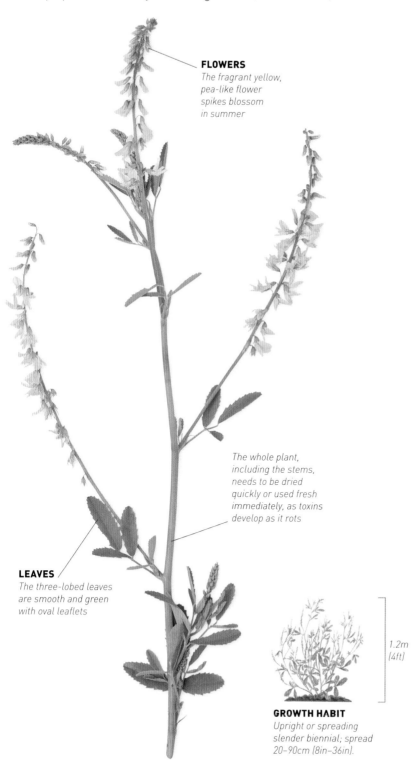

FLOWERS
The fragrant yellow, pea-like flower spikes blossom in summer

The whole plant, including the stems, needs to be dried quickly or used fresh immediately, as toxins develop as it rots

LEAVES
The three-lobed leaves are smooth and green with oval leaflets

GROWTH HABIT
Upright or spreading slender biennial; spread 20–90cm (8in–36in).

1.2m (4ft)

PARTS USED Aerial parts
MAIN CONSTITUENTS Flavonoids, coumarins, resin, tannins, volatile oil; dicoumarol (an anti-coagulant) is produced as the plant ages and rots
ACTIONS Antispasmodic, anti-inflammatory, diuretic, expectorant, sedative, styptic, mild analgesic

HOW TO USE

INFUSION Take ½–1 cup of a standard infusion (p.168) of the aerial parts up to 3 times daily for varicose veins, lymphatic swellings, piles, anxiety, menopausal disorders, insomnia, or to reduce the risk of thrombosis. Can be used for insomnia in children; consult a herbalist for advice on dosage.
CREAM Combine with an equal amount of calendula cream and apply 3–4 times daily for varicose eczema.
OINTMENT Use several times daily for piles (haemorrhoids).
COMPRESS Apply a pad soaked in 1 cup of infusion for facial or intercostal neuralgia.
EYEBATH Simmer 1 cup of well-strained standard infusion gently for 2–3 minutes to sterilize the mix; allow to cool thoroughly and used as an eyebath for conjunctivitis.

HOW TO SOURCE

GROW Prefers sun and well-drained neutral to alkaline soil; tolerates other conditions. Sow seeds in spring or summer where you want to grow them, then thin out to 60cm (24in) apart. Self-seeds in ideal conditions.
FORAGE Found in meadow borders, dry waste ground, and hedgerows. Collect the whole plant in late spring or early summer and use fresh, or dry immediately while still flowering. Collect the flowers separately to use in cold macerated oils.
HARVEST Gather while flowering in late spring or early summer.

CAUTION Do not take if on anti-coagulant medication (such as warfarin or heparin); can be emetic in large doses.

Melissa officinalis **Lemon balm**

A European native, also known as "bee balm", this herb takes its botanical name from the Greek word for "honey bee" as it was regarded as being as healing and curative as honey. Both relaxing and tonifying for the nervous system, lemon balm is largely used today for anxiety, depression, nervous tension, and related digestive disorders.

PARTS USED Aerial parts, essential oil
MAIN CONSTITUENTS Volatile oil (incl. citronellal, linalool, and citral), polyphenols, tannins, bitter principle, flavonoids, rosmarinic acid
ACTIONS Sedative, antidepressant, digestive stimulant, peripheral vasodilator, diaphoretic, relaxing restorative for nervous system, carminative, antiviral, antibacterial

HOW TO USE

INFUSION Take 1 standard infusion (p.168) of fresh or dried leaves 3 times daily for depression, nervous exhaustion, indigestion or nausea; use a dilute infusion for children suffering from chicken pox.
CREAM/OINTMENT Use on sores, cold sores, poorly healing wounds, or insect bites.
LOTION Add 1ml (20 drops) of essential oil to 100ml (3½fl oz) of water in a spray bottle and spray on skin to repel biting insects.
TINCTURE Take 10–20 drops in water 3–5 times daily for depression, tension headaches, and anxiety. Best made from fresh leaves.
MASSAGE OIL Add 5–6 drops of essential oil to 15ml (1 tbsp) of almond oil and use as a massage for depression, tension, asthma, and bronchitis, or dab on cold sores at the first sign of symptoms.

HOW TO SOURCE

GROW Prefers moist, well-drained soil, but thrives in poor soil and tolerates full sun or shade. Sow seeds in a cold frame in spring and transplant when well established, or divide roots in spring when growth starts to appear in autumn. Self-seeds, and can be invasive. Less vigorous variegated or golden cultivars are an alternative option.
FORAGE Grows in scrubby, partially shaded areas across Europe, or as cultivated plants that have self-seeded elsewhere.
HARVEST Gather the aerial parts just before the flowers open in summer, and the leaves throughout the growing period.

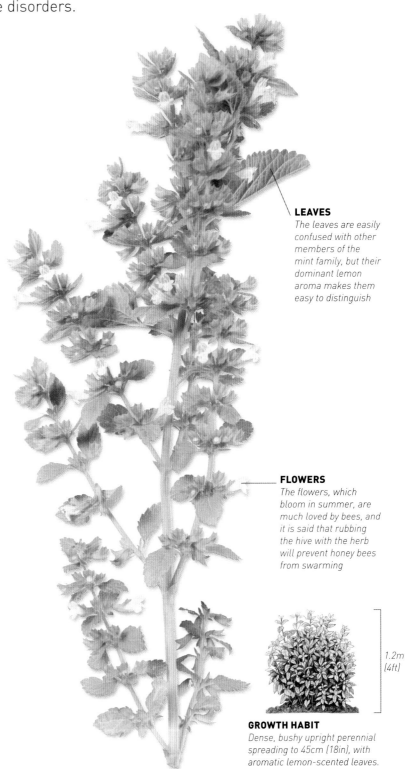

LEAVES
The leaves are easily confused with other members of the mint family, but their dominant lemon aroma makes them easy to distinguish

FLOWERS
The flowers, which bloom in summer, are much loved by bees, and it is said that rubbing the hive with the herb will prevent honey bees from swarming

1.2m
(4ft)

GROWTH HABIT
Dense, bushy upright perennial spreading to 45cm (18in), with aromatic lemon-scented leaves.

Mentha x *piperita* **Peppermint**

There are more than 25 different types of mint, many of which cross-pollinate readily to produce variable hybrids. Peppermint, which originates in Europe, was the result of one such cross, possibly in ancient times, and is now naturalized worldwide. It is widely cultivated for its oil, which is used in flavourings and to scent perfumes and toiletries.

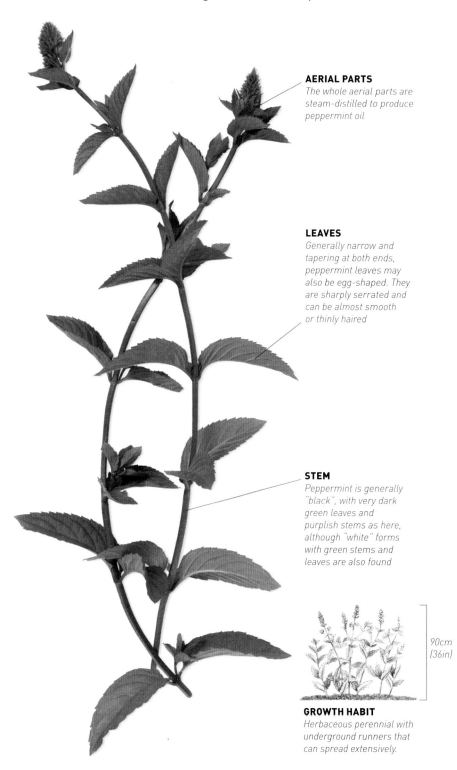

AERIAL PARTS
The whole aerial parts are steam-distilled to produce peppermint oil

LEAVES
Generally narrow and tapering at both ends, peppermint leaves may also be egg-shaped. They are sharply serrated and can be almost smooth or thinly haired

STEM
Peppermint is generally "black", with very dark green leaves and purplish stems as here, although "white" forms with green stems and leaves are also found

90cm
(36in)

GROWTH HABIT
Herbaceous perennial with underground runners that can spread extensively.

PARTS USED Aerial parts, essential oil
MAIN CONSTITUENTS Volatile oil (mainly menthol), tannins, flavonoids (incl. luteolin), tocopherols, choline, bitter principle, triterpenes
ACTIONS Antispasmodic, digestive tonic, anti-emetic, carminative, peripheral vasodilator, diaphoretic, cholagogue, analgesic, antiseptic

HOW TO USE

TEA Add 2–3 fresh leaves to 1 cup of boiling water and infuse for 5 minutes for everyday drinking; especially suitable after meals.
STEAM INHALATION Add a few fresh sprigs to a basin of boiling water and use as an inhalant to ease nasal congestion.
INFUSION Use 15g (½oz) to 600ml (1pint) of boiling water and take ½–1 cup 2–3 times daily for nausea, indigestion, flatulence, or colic, or with other herbs for colds or catarrh.
LOTION Add 30 drops of essential oil to 120ml (4fl oz) vegetable oil and massage into aching muscles and joints, or use for scabies or ringworm. Use in a spray bottle as a mosquito repellent or foot deodorant.

HOW TO SOURCE

GROW Prefers fertile, moist soil in full sun or partial shade. Can be invasive if growing conditions are ideal. Propagated by division in spring or autumn or by tip cuttings in spring or summer; easy to root if the sprigs are kept standing in water for a few days. As a hybrid, it is sterile and produces no seeds. In general, mints should not be grown from seed, as they cross-pollinate readily and may not come true.
FORAGE Generally found in moist areas. Native to Europe and the Mediterranean area; classified as invasive in parts of North America. Collect the leaves for tea throughout the growing season.
HARVEST Cut aerial parts before flowering.

CAUTION Do not use peppermint oil for children under the age of five.

Nepeta cataria **Catnip**

Also known as catmint, catnip – as the name implies – is much loved by cats, who will roll ecstatically in the young plants. Native to Europe and Mediterranean regions, but now naturalized in many parts of the world, the herb is used for digestive disorders or feverish chills. As a gentle remedy, it is also safe to use for many childhood disorders.

PARTS USED Aerial parts

MAIN CONSTITUENTS Volatile oil (incl. citronellol, geraniol, and nepetalactone), glycosides

ACTIONS Antispasmodic, antidiarrhoeal, emmenagogue, diaphoretic, carminative, nerve relaxant

HOW TO USE

INFUSION Take ¹/₂–1 cup of a standard infusion (p.168) 3 times a day for colds, flu, stomach upsets, and indigestion. Reduce the dose, depending on age, for children and use for childhood illnesses, colic, or emotional upsets.

TINCTURE Take up to 5ml (1 tsp) 3 times daily with the infusion for headaches associated with digestive disturbances. Use 5–10ml (1–2 tsp) neat externally as a friction rub for rheumatism and arthritis.

ENEMA Use up to 1 litre (1³/₄ pints) of a well-strained standard infusion to clear toxic wastes from the colon.

OINTMENT Apply 2–3 times daily for piles (haemorrhoids).

HOW TO SOURCE

GROW Prefers moist but well-drained soil in full sun. Sow the seeds in autumn in trays of compost in a cold fame and transplant to 7.5cm (3in) pots when large enough to handle. Plant out in early summer in their final growing positions. Alternatively, propagate by root division in autumn or spring or take cuttings in spring or early summer. Self-seeds in favourable conditions, especially in gardens where there are no cats. Said to repel aphids, cucumber beetles, and other pests in companion planting.

FORAGE Found in scrubby, waste ground and wayside places in many parts of Europe and Asia, and now naturalized in North America. Collect the aerial parts in summer.

HARVEST Cut the aerial parts just as the plant is starting to flower.

CAUTION Avoid during pregnancy.

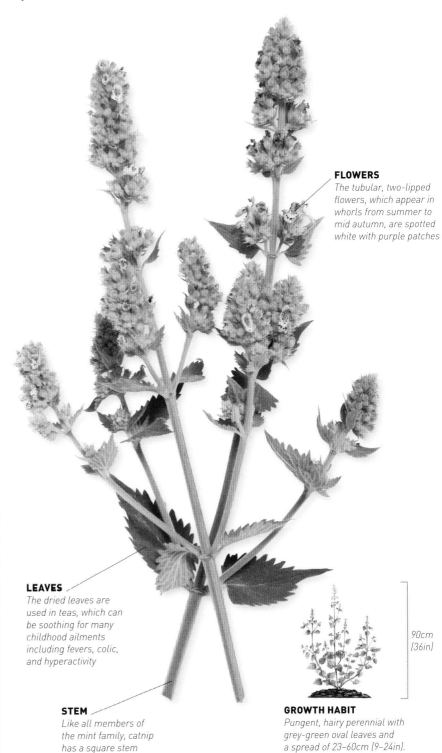

FLOWERS
The tubular, two-lipped flowers, which appear in whorls from summer to mid autumn, are spotted white with purple patches

LEAVES
The dried leaves are used in teas, which can be soothing for many childhood ailments including fevers, colic, and hyperactivity

STEM
Like all members of the mint family, catnip has a square stem

GROWTH HABIT
Pungent, hairy perennial with grey-green oval leaves and a spread of 23–60cm (9–24in).

90cm (36in)

Oenothera biennis **Evening primrose**

Native to North America, evening primrose is now grown worldwide both as a garden ornamental and as a commercial crop to supply a global trade in its seed oil, which is rich in essential fatty acids. The oil is marketed as a food supplement and remedy for a variety of ailments, including skin, arthritic, and menstrual disorders.

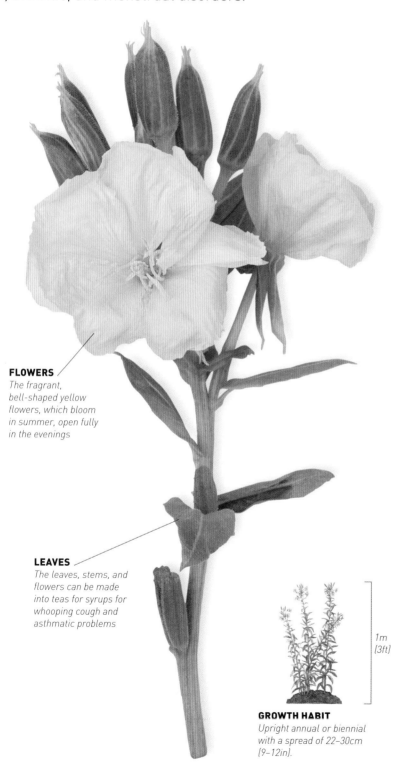

FLOWERS
The fragrant, bell-shaped yellow flowers, which bloom in summer, open fully in the evenings

LEAVES
The leaves, stems, and flowers can be made into teas for syrups for whooping cough and asthmatic problems

GROWTH HABIT
Upright annual or biennial with a spread of 22–30cm (9–12in).

1m
(3ft)

PARTS USED Seed oil, leaves, stems, flowers

MAIN CONSTITUENTS Seeds: rich in essential fatty acids, including gamma-linolenic acid – a precursor of prostaglandin E1

ACTIONS Whole plant: astringent, sedative. Seed oil: hypotensive, anticoagulant, hypolipidaemic

HOW TO USE

INFUSION Make a standard infusion (p.168) of the leaves and stems and take 1 cup 3 times daily for digestive upsets including poor appetite and diarrhoea.

SYRUP Combine 450g (1lb) of sugar or honey with 600ml (1 pint) of a strained standard infusion of the leaves and stems, bring to the boil, and simmer gently for 10 minutes; take in 5–10ml (1–2 tsp) doses as required for whooping cough.

CAPSULES Commercial capsules often contain vitamin E as a preservative; take 500mg daily or follow the directions on the pack. Generally used for menopausal problems, skin disorders including psoriasis and eczema, and rheumatoid arthritis. The oil is also combined with fish oils as an anti-ageing remedy. Follow the directions on the pack.

CREAM/SEED OIL Use 2–3 times daily on dry, scaling skin.

HOW TO SOURCE

GROW Prefers poor to moderately fertile, light, well-drained soil in full sun; tolerates dry periods. Sow seeds in a cold frame in late spring and transplant when established in summer, or sow directly in late summer to autumn.

FORAGE Naturalized in many parts of the world and often found in dry, stony, waste areas. Collect the leaves and stems in the second year when the flower stem appears.

HARVEST Collect the seeds when ripe.

CAUTION Do not take the oil if suffering from epilepsy.

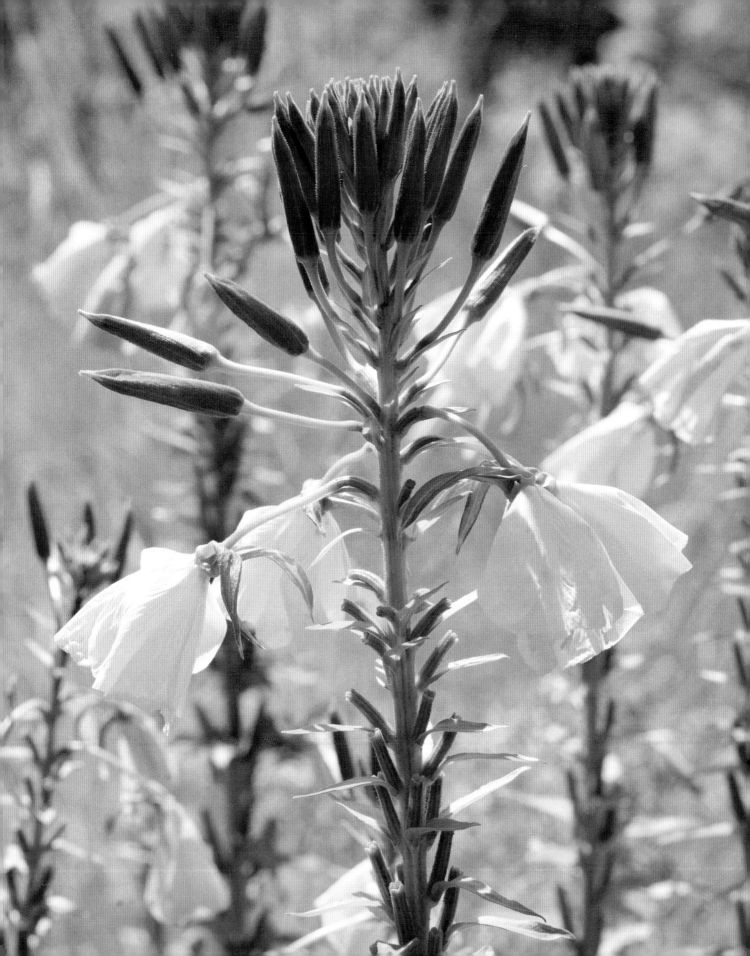

Panax japonicus **Japanese ginseng**

Found in mountainous woodland areas of Japan, Japanese ginseng is one of several related species used medicinally, and is largely used for coughs. The most popular is Korean ginseng (*Panax ginseng*) which, like American ginseng (*Panax quinquefolius*), is an important energy tonic. San qi ginseng (*Panax pseudo-ginseng*) is used to control bleeding.

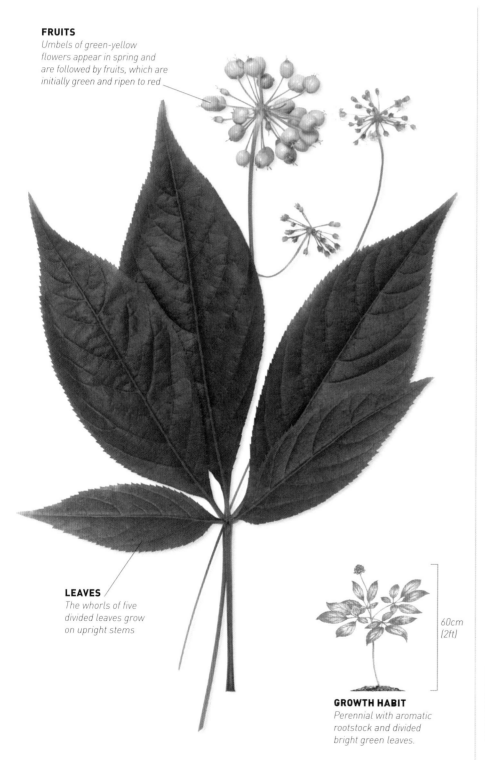

FRUITS
Umbels of green-yellow flowers appear in spring and are followed by fruits, which are initially green and ripen to red

LEAVES
The whorls of five divided leaves grow on upright stems

GROWTH HABIT
Perennial with aromatic rootstock and divided bright green leaves.

60cm
(2ft)

PARTS USED Root
MAIN CONSTITUENTS Saponins, steroidal glycosides, sterols, volatile oil
ACTIONS Expectorant, tonic, febrifuge

HOW TO USE

TABLETS/CAPSULES Available in Japan. Can be used as a substitute for Korean ginseng, although the tonic effect is significantly reduced. Take 600mg daily.
DECOCTION Recent research suggests that Japanese ginseng may have a mild stimulatory effect on the immune system. Take ½–1 cup of a decoction, made by heating 10g (¼oz) of root in 600ml (1 pint) of water for 20 minutes, 2–3 times daily for recurrent infections or as a general immune tonic. The decoction is used in Japanese folk medicine for non-insulin dependent diabetes and to combat obesity.
SYRUP Add 450g (1lb) of sugar to 600ml (1 pint) of a standard decoction, bring to the boil, and simmer for 5–10 minutes. Take in 5ml (1 tsp) doses for productive coughs.

HOW TO SOURCE

GROW Sow seeds in a shaded area in a cold frame as soon as they are ripe. Germination can be slow and erratic. Transplant to 7.5cm (3in) pots as soon as the seedlings are large enough to handle, and continue growing in a shady position in the greenhouse for at least the first winter. Plant into a permanent position in moist but well-drained soil in shade in late summer. Alternatively, propagate by root division in spring.
FORAGE Unlikely to be found outside its native habitat.
HARVEST The roots of plants that are at least four years old are dug in autumn.

CAUTION Avoid in pregnancy. Do not take with drinks containing caffeine. Japanese ginseng has been little researched and can be of poor quality.

Passiflora incarnata **Passionflower**

Native to woodlands in the eastern United States, passionflower, a species of which is shown below, is known locally as "maypop" and was used by many Native American people for swellings, fungal infections, and as a blood tonic. Today it is generally regarded as a sedative and used for problems ranging from hyperactivity in children to the tremors of Parkinson's disease.

PARTS USED Leaves and stems

MAIN CONSTITUENTS Flavonoids (incl. rutin and apigenin), cyanogenic glycosides, alkaloids, sapanarin

ACTIONS Analgesic, antispasmodic, bitter, cooling, hypotensive, sedative, heart tonic, relaxes blood vessels

HOW TO USE

INFUSION Take 1 cup of a standard infusion (p.168) made from equal amounts of passionflower and raspberry leaf 3 times daily for period pain. For insomnia, take $\frac{1}{2}$–1 cup of an infusion made from $\frac{1}{2}$ tsp of dried passionflower to 1 cup of boiling water infused for 15 minutes, at night. For period pain or tension headaches take 3 times daily; reduced doses are suitable for hyperactivity in children.

TINCTURE Take 2–4ml (40–80 drops) in water 3 times daily for nervous tension, high blood pressure associated with nervous stress, or to reduce the severity of attacks in Ménière's disease.

FLUID EXTRACT Take up to 2ml (40 drops) in water twice a day to ease the pain associated with shingles and toothache.

TABLETS/CAPSULES Take 1–2 x 200mg tablets or capsules night and morning for anxiety, tension, and nervous headaches.

HOW TO SOURCE

GROW Prefers poor, sandy soil that is slightly acid. Sow the seeds at 18–21°C (64–70°F) in trays in spring and transplant to 7.5cm (3in) pots when large enough. Plant in final growing positions when well established in summer. Alternatively, take semi-ripe cuttings in summer. Shelter the plants from cold, wet winds in winter.

FORAGE Unlikely to be found growing wild outside its native habitat. The fruits are edible and can be collected in summer, but are only suitable for jams or jellies.

HARVEST Collect aerial parts when flowering or in fruit.

CAUTION May cause drowsiness.

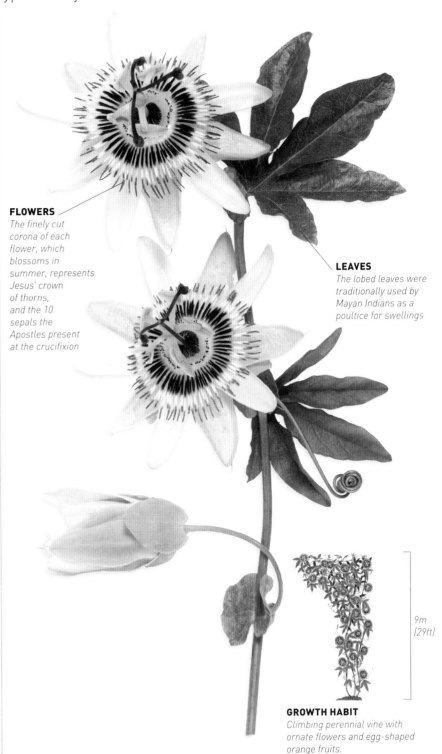

FLOWERS
The finely cut corona of each flower, which blossoms in summer, represents Jesus' crown of thorns, and the 10 sepals the Apostles present at the crucifixion

LEAVES
The lobed leaves were traditionally used by Mayan Indians as a poultice for swellings

9m (29ft)

GROWTH HABIT
Climbing perennial vine with ornate flowers and egg-shaped orange fruits.

Plantago lanceolata **Ribwort plantain**

Both ribwort plantain and its broad-leaved cousin common plantain (*Plantago major*) are among the most common European weeds likely to be found anywhere, from pavement cracks to hedgerows. The plants are also found in the temperate regions of Asia, and were introduced by settlers into North America and Australia. Both plantains are a first-aid standby in folk tradition.

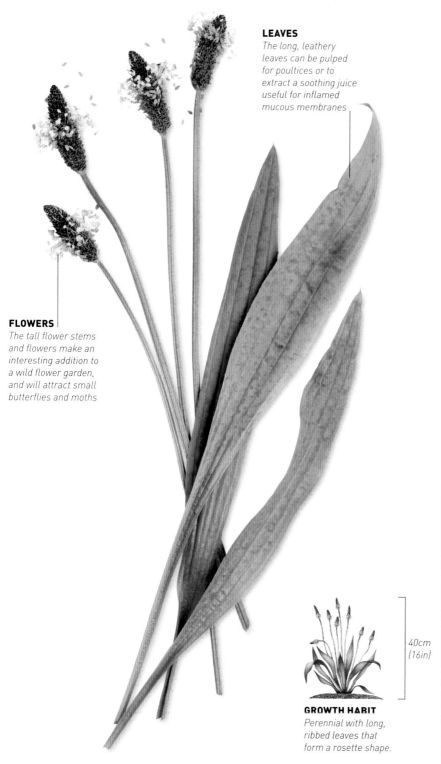

LEAVES
The long, leathery leaves can be pulped for poultices or to extract a soothing juice useful for inflamed mucous membranes

FLOWERS
The tall flower stems and flowers make an interesting addition to a wild flower garden, and will attract small butterflies and moths

40cm
(16in)

GROWTH HABIT
Perennial with long, ribbed leaves that form a rosette shape.

PARTS USED Leaves
MAIN CONSTITUENTS Flavonoids, iridoids, mucilage, tannins, minerals
ACTIONS Relaxing expectorant, tonifying to mucous membranes, anticatarrhal, antispasmodic, topically healing, haemostatic

HOW TO USE

TINCTURE Take 3–5ml (60 drops–1 tsp) 3 times daily for catarrhal conditions or digestive problems, including gastritis and irritable bowel syndrome.
JUICE Use fresh leaves to make a juice and take in 10ml (2 tsp) doses 3 times daily to soothe cystitis, diarrhoea, and lung infections. The juice can also be applied to wounds and sores.
INFUSION Take 1 cup of a standard infusion (p.168) 3 times daily for catarrhal conditions, or use as a gargle for sore throats.
SYRUP Add 225g (8oz) of honey to 300ml (10fl oz) of a standard infusion and take in 5ml (1 tsp) doses as required for sore throats or productive coughs.
POULTICE Use fresh leaves, mashed into a pulp, for slow-healing wounds and chronic ulcers, or apply the fresh leaves to insect bites and stings.

HOW TO SOURCE

GROW Prefers moist, poor to moderately fertile soil in sun, or partial shade. Usually found as a self-seeded garden weed, although seeds can be obtained from wild flower specialists. Sow seeds where you want them to grow in spring or in 7.5cm (3in) pots in a cold frame, and plant out when established. Flowers, usually produced in the second year, appear from early spring until first frosts. It is generally included in wild meadow plantings, but self-seeds enthusiastically and can easily become invasive.
FORAGE Easily found growing on wasteland, hedgerows, roadsides, and grassy areas. It is best to choose plants growing in uncultivated areas well away from traffic to reduce the risk of collecting contaminated specimens.
HARVEST Gather leaves in summer.

Plantago psyllium **Psyllium**

Both black psyllium seeds, and the pale beige ispaghula seeds from its near relative, *Plantago ovata*, are commonly used over-the-counter remedies for constipation. Psyllium originates in the Mediterranean region, while ispaghula is native to India and Pakistan. The seeds swell in water to produce a mucilaginous mass, which is used as a bulking laxative.

PARTS USED Seeds

MAIN CONSTITUENTS Mucilage, fixed oil (incl. linoleic, oleic, and palmitic acids), starch, vitamins, minerals

ACTIONS Demulcent, bulking laxative, antidiarrhoeal, anti-inflammatory

HOW TO USE

MACERATION Soak two rounded teaspoons of the seeds in a mug of warm water overnight. Take as a single dose in the morning for constipation. The mixture can be flavoured with fruit juice or mixed with porridge or yoghurt, which some people find more palatable. Drink a glass of water or fruit juice after taking the seeds.

POULTICE Mix 1 tsp of psyllium husks with ½ tsp of slippery elm powder, add a little water to make a paste, and apply to boils or abscesses.

POWDER The husks are generally sold in powdered form: stir ½ tsp into a cup of water and take 3 times daily for diarrhoea or to help reduce blood cholesterol levels.

HOW TO SOURCE

GROW Prefers well-drained soil in full sun. Sow seeds in spring in trays on the surface of compost; keep in a propagator at 15-21°C (59-70°F) and transplant to final growing positions in early summer when large enough to handle. The plant flowers about 60 days after planting and needs high temperatures to set seed.

FORAGE Likely to be found in southern Europe, North Africa, and western Asia in waste places and dry, scrubby ground. Both psyllium and ispaghula are widely cultivated commercially.

HARVEST Harvest the seeds when ripe in late summer or early autumn.

CAUTION Always take with plenty of water and do not exceed the stated dose. Although sometimes recommended for irritable bowel syndrome, psyllium can exacerbate symptoms in some cases, so use with caution. Take at least 1 hour before any other medication.

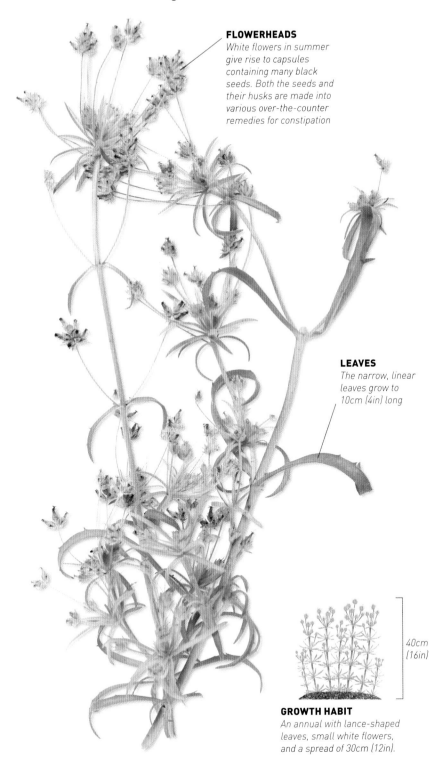

FLOWERHEADS
White flowers in summer give rise to capsules containing many black seeds. Both the seeds and their husks are made into various over-the-counter remedies for constipation

LEAVES
The narrow, linear leaves grow to 10cm (4in) long

40cm
(16in)

GROWTH HABIT
An annual with lance-shaped leaves, small white flowers, and a spread of 30cm (12in).

Platycodon grandiflorus **Chinese balloon flower**

Listed in the *Shen Nong Ben Cao Jing* – China's oldest herb book attributed to the legendary founder of herbal medicine, Shen Nong, who lived 5,000 years ago – the balloon flower, which is native to eastern Asia, is considered an important respiratory remedy in traditional Chinese medicine. In the West it is better known as a garden ornamental.

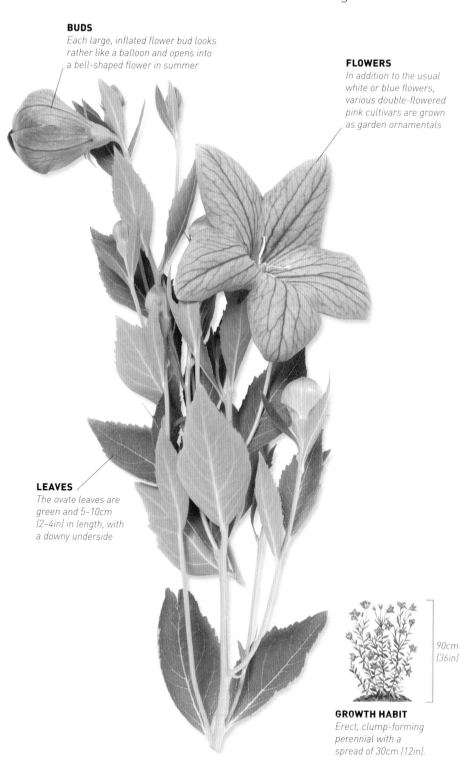

BUDS
Each large, inflated flower bud looks rather like a balloon and opens into a bell-shaped flower in summer

FLOWERS
In addition to the usual white or blue flowers, various double-flowered pink cultivars are grown as garden ornamentals

LEAVES
The ovate leaves are green and 5–10cm (2–4in) in length, with a downy underside

GROWTH HABIT
Erect, clump-forming perennial with a spread of 30cm (12in).

90cm
(36in)

PARTS USED Root
MAIN CONSTITUENTS Saponins, stigmasterol, inulin, platycodin
ACTIONS Antifungal, antibacterial, expectorant, hypoglycaemic, reduces cholesterol levels

HOW TO USE

DECOCTION Take 1 cup of a standard decoction of the root 3 times daily for productive coughs and sore throats associated with common colds.
SYRUP Combine 450g (1lb) of sugar or honey with 600ml (1pint) of strained standard root decoction, bring to the boil, and simmer gently for 10 minutes; take in 5–10ml (1–2 tsp) doses as required for bronchitis and other coughs producing profuse phlegm. Seek medical help if a productive cough does not improve after 2–3 days.
PATENT REMEDY Included in a number of commercially available pills and powders used in traditional Chinese medicine, including *sang ju yin* (a decoction of mulberry leaf with chrysanthemum), which is used for coughs, bronchitis, and the early stages of some feverish diseases.
GARGLE Use 1 cup of a standard decoction 2–3 times daily as a gargle for laryngitis and sore throats.

HOW TO SOURCE

GROW Prefers a well-drained site in sun or partial shade and forms in broad clumps 45cm (18in) in diameter when well established. Sow seeds in a seed tray in spring or early summer and transplant to 7.5cm (3in) pots when large enough to handle. Transplant to a permanent position when large enough to handle.
FORAGE Unlikely to be found naturalized outside China and Japan, although cultivated plants that self-seed may occur.
HARVEST Dig the root of established plants in autumn.

CAUTION Avoid this herb if there is blood in the phlegm.

Prunella vulgaris **Self-heal**

As with so many plants, the common name of this herb – self-heal – gives a good indication as to its use; it was once highly regarded as a wound remedy and cure-all. Native to Europe and Asia, self-heal is used as a wound healer and general tonic, and the flowers are a significant remedy in traditional Chinese medicine for soothing liver problems.

PARTS USED Aerial parts, flowers
MAIN CONSTITUENTS Flavonoids (incl. rutin), vitamins A, B1, C, K, fatty acids, volatile oil, bitter principle
ACTIONS Aerial parts: antibacterial, hypotensive, diuretic, astringent, haemostatic, wound herb
Flower spikes: liver stimulant, hypotensive, antibacterial, febrifuge

HOW TO USE

TINCTURE Best made from the freshly gathered leaves and stems. Take 5ml (1 tsp) 3 times daily for all sorts of bleeding, including heavy periods or traumatic injuries.
MOUTHWASH/GARGLE Use ½ tsp of dried herb to 1 cup of boiling water and allow to cool; use for bleeding gums and mouth inflammations or as a gargle for sore throats.
INFUSION Use a standard infusion (p.168) of flower spikes for liver problems linked to irritability and anger, over-excitability, high blood pressure, eye problems, headaches, or hyperactivity in children. (Consult a herbalist to treat children.) Often combined with Chinese chrysanthemum flowers, another herb used in Chinese medicine for liver problems.
POULTICE Use the fresh leaves on clean wounds.
CREAM/OINTMENT Use for bleeding piles.

HOW TO SOURCE

GROW Prefers moist, well-drained soil in full sun or partial shade, but will tolerate a wide range of conditions. Propagate from seeds sown in a cold frame in spring and transplant when established or by root division in spring or autumn. A prolific self-seeder that can become invasive.
FORAGE A common weed throughout Europe and many parts of Asia, it is found in grassland, roadsides, and sunny meadows. Collect the leaves and stems in early summer or harvest the flowers while in full bloom in mid- to late summer.
HARVEST In the West the leaves and young shoots are traditionally gathered before flowering.

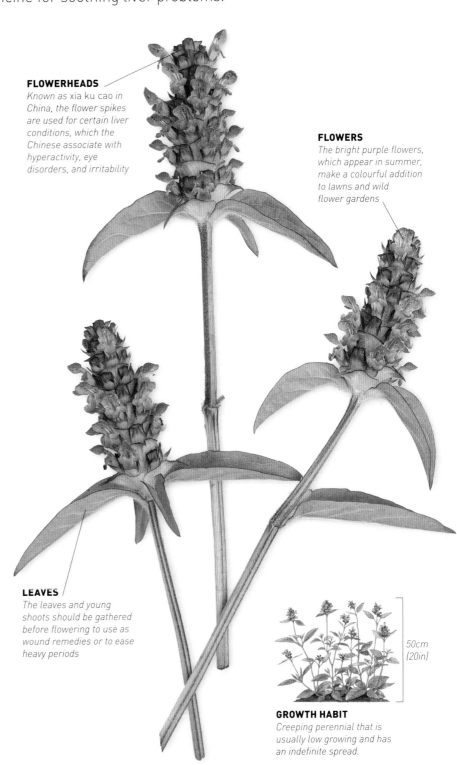

FLOWERHEADS
Known as xia ku cao in China, the flower spikes are used for certain liver conditions, which the Chinese associate with hyperactivity, eye disorders, and irritability

FLOWERS
The bright purple flowers, which appear in summer, make a colourful addition to lawns and wild flower gardens

LEAVES
The leaves and young shoots should be gathered before flowering to use as wound remedies or to ease heavy periods

50cm (20in)

GROWTH HABIT
Creeping perennial that is usually low growing and has an indefinite spread.

Ribes nigrum **Blackcurrant**

Native to temperate regions of Europe and Asia, blackcurrants are extensively cultivated for their juice and as a flavouring. Demand for the juice is so high that the fruits are rarely available in stores and should be grown in gardens for home use. While the fruits are rich in vitamin C, the leaves are largely used as a diuretic.

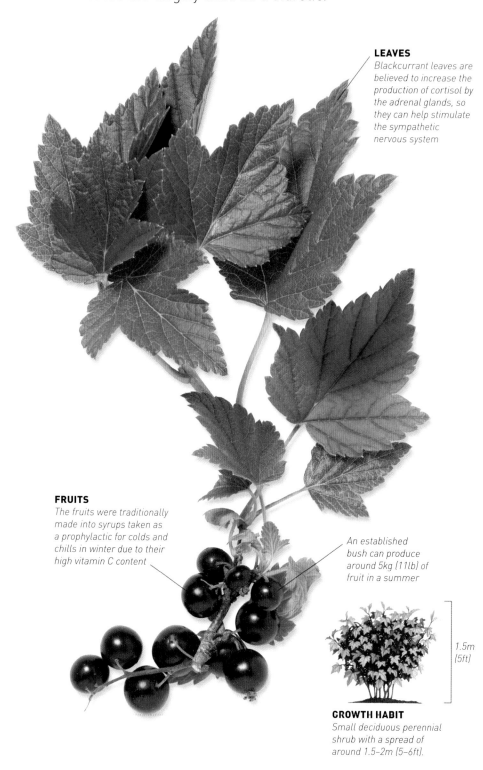

LEAVES
Blackcurrant leaves are believed to increase the production of cortisol by the adrenal glands, so they can help stimulate the sympathetic nervous system

FRUITS
The fruits were traditionally made into syrups taken as a prophylactic for colds and chills in winter due to their high vitamin C content

An established bush can produce around 5kg (11lb) of fruit in a summer

1.5m (5ft)

GROWTH HABIT
Small deciduous perennial shrub with a spread of around 1.5–2m (5–6ft).

PARTS USED Leaves, fruits, seed oil
MAIN CONSTITUENTS Leaves: volatile oil, tannins
Fruits: flavonoids, anthocyanosides, tannins, vitamin C, potassium
Seeds: Essential fatty acids incl. gamma-linolenic acid
ACTIONS Astringent, mild febrifuge, diuretic, antirheumatic; the fruits are a rich source of vitamin C

HOW TO USE

INFUSION Take ½–1 cup of a standard infusion (p.168) of the leaves as desired during the early stages of colds and feverish infections.
SEED OIL Rich in gamma-linolenic acid, blackcurrant seed oil capsules are available commercially as an alternative to evening primrose oil for treating eczema, menstrual irregularities, arthritis, etc. Follow dosage directions on the pack.
JUICE Take 10ml (2 tsp) 3 times daily (ideally as freshly made, unsweetened juice) for diarrhoea and digestive upsets; also provides additional vitamin C for infections such as flu or pneumonia.
GARGLE/MOUTHWASH Use 1 cup of a standard leaf infusion 2–3 times daily for sore throats and mouth ulcers.
TINCTURE Take 5ml (1tsp) of leaf tincture in a little water 3 times daily to increase elimination of fluids in high blood pressure.

HOW TO SOURCE

GROW Prefers full sun and rich, well-drained soil, but tolerates other conditions. Usually propagated by hardwood cuttings in autumn. Pot on until well established and plant in final positions in early winter or up to mid-March. Plant bushes 5cm (2in) deeper than the top of their pot; they produce stems from just below the surface: Water regularly and keep well weeded.
FORAGE Rarely found growing wild in Europe, although bushes may grow in hedgerows. Unlikely to be found growing wild in the US (it is host to a rust fungi and is therefore banned in some states).
HARVEST Pick fruits in midsummer when ripe and leaves through the growing season.

Rosa canina **Dog rose**

Native to Europe, western Asia, and north-west Africa, dog roses are now found throughout North America and New Zealand, where they are regarded as an invasive weed. The name reputedly derives from a Roman tradition that the root was, erroneously, a cure for rabies caused by dog bites. The hips are rich in vitamins, especially vitamin C, and can be made into syrups and jellies.

PARTS USED Fruits (hips), leaves
MAIN CONSTITUENTS Vitamins (A, B1, B2, B3, C, and K), flavonoids, tannins, polyphenols, carotenoids, volatile oil
ACTIONS Nutrient, astringent, diuretic, anti-inflammatory

HOW TO USE

SYRUP Popular form of nutritional supplement for young children. It is also used to flavour other medicines, and is added to cough mixtures. Add 225g (8oz) of honey to 300ml (10fl oz) of a strong decoction of hips (simmer a standard decoction gently until reduced in volume by half, then strain through a fine sieve or muslin cloth to remove the hairs from the seeds). Take 5ml (1 tsp) doses as required.
TINCTURE Take up to 5ml (1 tsp) of rose hip tincture 3 times daily for diarrhoea, gastritis, to relieve colicky pains, or as a mild diuretic.
FRESH HIPS The ripe hips can be eaten as a food supplement (remove the seeds before eating). They were traditionally baked in tarts or made into fruit jellies, often combined with apples.
INFUSION Once used as a substitute for tea, infused rose leaves can be made into a pleasant tisane for everyday drinking.

HOW TO SOURCE

GROW Usually grown from softwood cuttings in summer, it will self-seed freely once established. Often regarded as a weed by gardeners, dog rose is fast-growing and can be invasive. It will grow well in any well-drained moist soil in sun or partial shade, although it does not generally grow well in coastal areas. It is often grown as part of a mixed hedge.
FORAGE Found in hedgerows, roadside borders, and wasteland. The hips are best gathered in late autumn when they start to fall from the plant. If picked any earlier, they can be hard and will need to be cooked before use.
HARVEST Gather the bright red hips in autumn when ripe, and the leaves at any time for tea. Gather the rose petals in the summer to use in jam and jelly making.

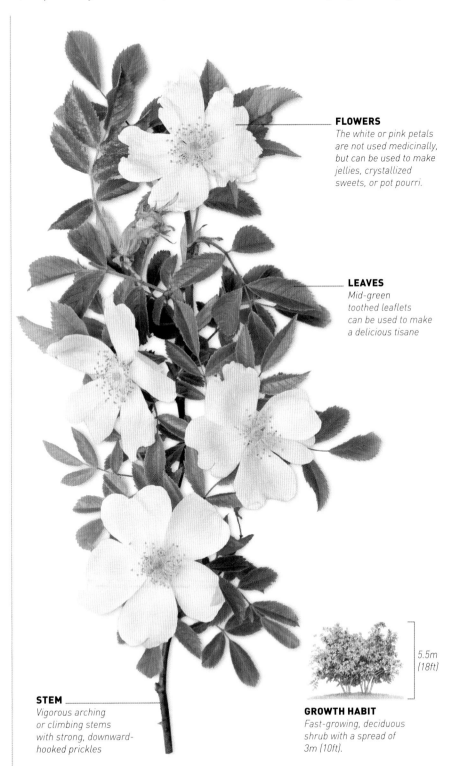

FLOWERS
The white or pink petals are not used medicinally, but can be used to make jellies, crystallized sweets, or pot pourri.

LEAVES
Mid-green toothed leaflets can be used to make a delicious tisane

STEM
Vigorous arching or climbing stems with strong, downward-hooked prickles

5.5m (18ft)

GROWTH HABIT
Fast-growing, deciduous shrub with a spread of 3m (10ft).

Rosa x damascena **Damask rose**

Damask roses originated in the near East and were introduced into Europe in the 13th century. Today, they are regarded as a cross between *Rose gallica* and *Rosa moschata*. The flowers vary in colour from pink to light red. Rose oil – known as rose otto – is extracted by steam distillation, mainly in Bulgaria and Turkey, and is said to be good for "the skin and the soul".

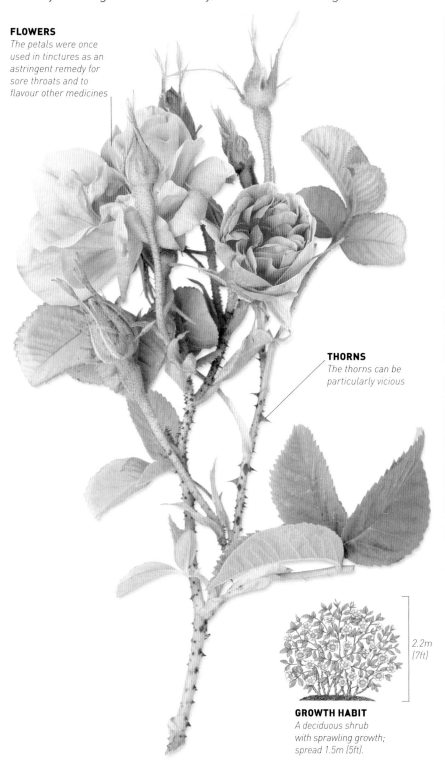

FLOWERS
The petals were once used in tinctures as an astringent remedy for sore throats and to flavour other medicines

THORNS
The thorns can be particularly vicious

GROWTH HABIT
A deciduous shrub with sprawling growth; spread 1.5m (5ft).

2.2m
(7ft)

PARTS USED Flowers, essential oil, hydrosol

MAIN CONSTITUENTS Geraniol, nerol, citronellol, geranic acid (rose oil contains around 300 chemicals, of which about 100 have been identified)

ACTIONS Sedative, antidepressant, anti-inflammatory, reduces cholesterol levels, astringent

HOW TO USE

MASSAGE OIL Use 1 drop of rose oil in 5ml (1 tsp) of almond oil to massage into the temples and neck for stress or exhaustion.

BATHS Add 2 drops of rose oil to bath water for depression, sorrows, or insomnia.

CREAM Made from the petals, or by adding a few drops of rose oil to a base cream. For dry or inflamed skin conditions.

LOTION Rosewater – the waste water from the steam distillation process (hydrosol) – can be used as the basis of various lotions: add 10% lady's mantle tincture for vaginal itching, or mix 50:50 with distilled witch hazel as a cooling lotion for skin prone to spots or acne.

TINCTURE Take 1–2 ml (20–40 drops) of a tincture made from the rose petals for nervous disorders, poor digestion, or to help reduce cholesterol levels.

HOW TO SOURCE

GROW Prefers fertile, moist but well-drained soil and needs at least 5 hours of sunlight a day during the growing season. Will tolerate temperate to sub-tropical temperatures. Usually propagated by hardwood cuttings in autumn.

FORAGE May be found growing wild, but more likely to be cultivated in hedges.

HARVEST Gather flowers in summer.

CAUTION Avoid during pregnancy. Do not take essential oils internally without professional advice. Rose oil is often adulterated or synthesized, so only buy from reputable sources.

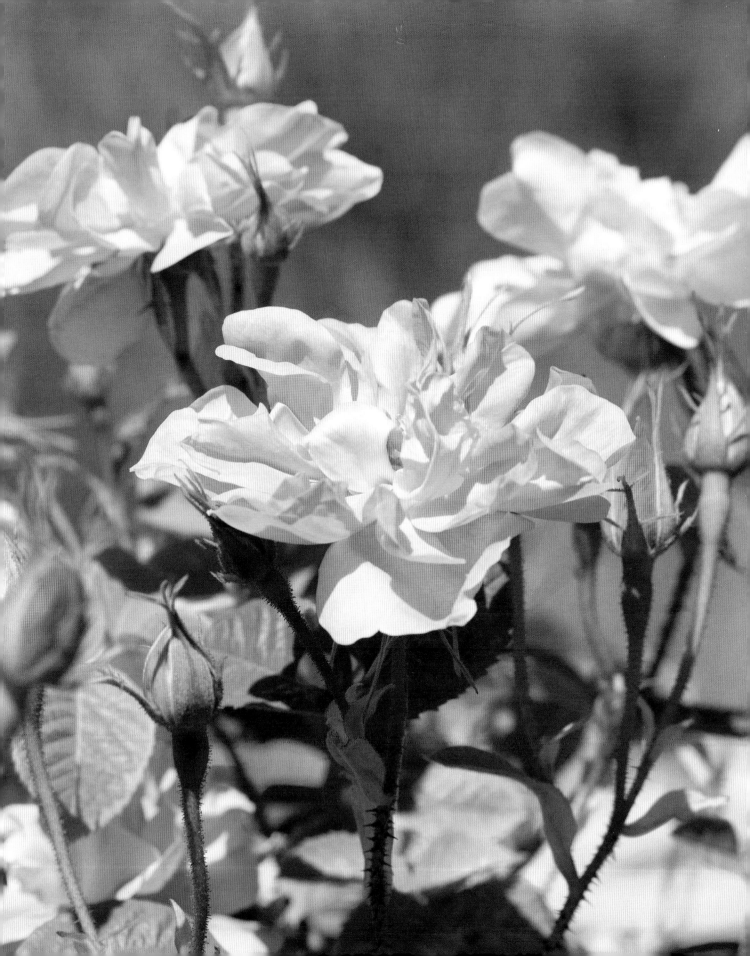

Rosmarinus officinalis **Rosemary**

Originally found in dry coastal areas around the Mediterranean region, rosemary is now cultivated worldwide and is grown both as a culinary herb and for its essential oil. Medicinally, the herb is largely used as a stimulating tonic and digestive remedy, while the oil is used for arthritic pains. It is an important ingredient in the cosmetics and fragrance market.

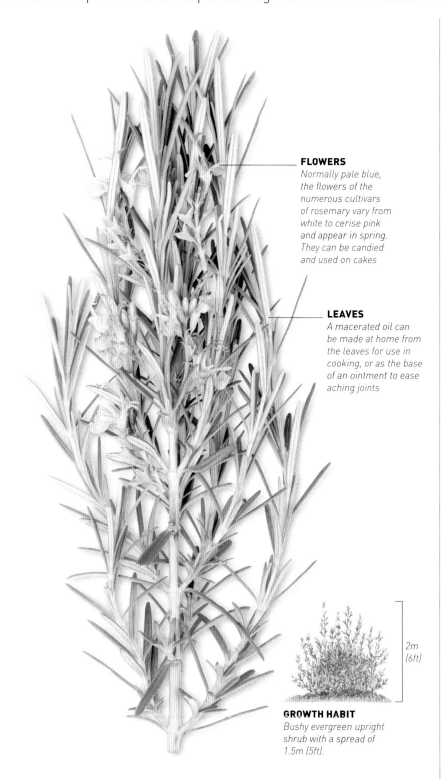

FLOWERS
Normally pale blue, the flowers of the numerous cultivars of rosemary vary from white to cerise pink and appear in spring. They can be candied and used on cakes

LEAVES
A macerated oil can be made at home from the leaves for use in cooking, or as the base of an ointment to ease aching joints

2m
(6ft)

GROWTH HABIT
Bushy evergreen upright shrub with a spread of 1.5m (5ft).

PARTS USED Leaves, flowers, essential oil
MAIN CONSTITUENTS Volatile oil (incl. borneol, camphene, cineole), flavonoids, rosmarinic acid, tannins
ACTIONS Astringent, nervine, carminative, antiseptic, diaphoretic, antidepressive, circulatory stimulant, antispasmodic, cholagogue, diuretic
ESSENTIAL OIL Topically rubefacient, analgesic

HOW TO USE

INFUSION A standard infusion (p.168) can taste unpleasant, so use a weaker mix; take 1 cup for tiredness and headaches, or after meals to improve digestion.
HAIR RINSE Use a standard infusion, strained, as a final rinse for dandruff.
INHALATION Inhaling a drop of essential oil from a tissue is an energising brain stimulant and concentration aid.
TINCTURE Take up to 2.5ml (50 drops/ ½ tsp) 3 times daily for tiredness and nervous exhaustion; combine with an equal amount of wild oat or vervain tincture for depression.
MASSAGE RUB Add ¼ml (5 drops) of the essential oil to 15ml (1 tbsp) of almond oil and massage aching joints and muscles. Massage also into the temples to ease tension headaches.
COMPRESS Use 1 cup of hot standard infusion in a compress to ease sprains. Alternating a very hot infusion with an ice pack every 2–3 minutes works best.

HOW TO SOURCE

GROW Can be grown from seed, although cultivars do not come true and must be propagated from semi-ripe cuttings. Prefers neutral to alkaline soil.
FORAGE Found in native areas – scrub and open woodland around the Mediterranean.
HARVEST Gather in spring and summer.

CAUTION Avoid therapeutic doses of the herb during pregnancy.

Rubus idaeus **Raspberry**

Familiar as a summer fruit, raspberry is native to Europe, Asia, and North America, and has been cultivated in kitchen gardens since at least the 16th century. The leaves are commonly taken in tea to strengthen the womb for childbirth, while the fruits can be made into vinegar to use in salad dressings or to add to cough mixtures.

PARTS USED Leaves, fruit
MAIN CONSTITUENTS Leaves: fragarine (uterine tonic), tannins, polypeptides
Fruit: vitamins A, B, C, and E, sugars, fruit acids, pectin
ACTIONS Astringent, prepares the womb for childbirth, stimulant, digestive remedy, increases urination, laxative

HOW TO USE

INFUSION 1 cup of a standard infusion (p.168) of the leaves can be taken daily in the last two months of pregnancy to help strengthen and prepare the womb for childbirth; drink the infusion as often as needed during labour. Take 1 cup 3 times daily to ease painful or heavy menstruation.
TINCTURE Take 3–5ml (60 drops–1 tsp) of the tincture 3 times daily for mild diarrhoea, or add to 100ml (3½fl oz) of warm water and use to bathe wounds, varicose veins, or skin inflammations. Put 2–5 drops into an eyebath of boiled, cooled water for conjunctivitis and eye inflammations.
MOUTHWASH/GARGLE Use 1 cup of an infusion for mouth ulcers or sore throats.
JUICE Take 10ml (2 tsp) 3–4 times daily of the juice (made from pulped berries) as a cooling remedy in mild fevers.

HOW TO SOURCE

GROW Prefers moist, slightly acidic soil. Propagate from rooted suckers, root division, or softwood cuttings, and plant out in winter/early spring; prune canes to 25cm (10in) above ground after planting. Cut fruited canes back to ground level after harvesting, and select and support young canes for the following year's crop.
FORAGE Found on scrubland and waste areas. Collect the leaves in early- to midsummer, and the berries when ripe.
HARVEST Gather the fruits in summer or autumn and the leaves in early summer.

CAUTION Therapeutic doses of raspberry leaf should only be taken in the last trimester of pregnancy, and avoided completely in the early stages.

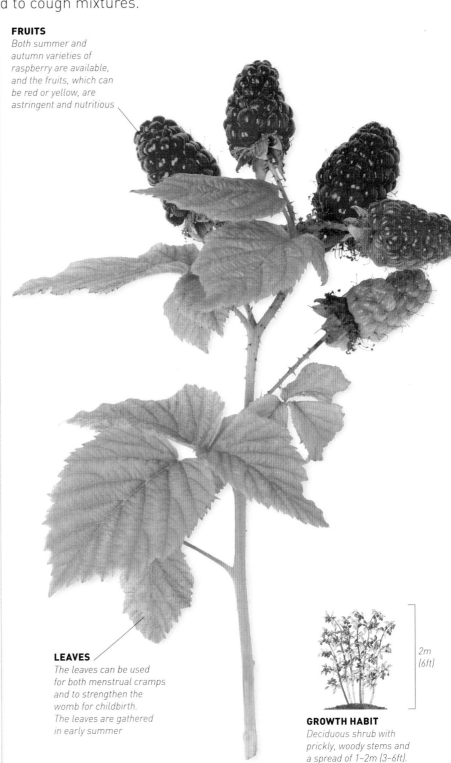

FRUITS
Both summer and autumn varieties of raspberry are available, and the fruits, which can be red or yellow, are astringent and nutritious

LEAVES
The leaves can be used for both menstrual cramps and to strengthen the womb for childbirth. The leaves are gathered in early summer

GROWTH HABIT
Deciduous shrub with prickly, woody stems and a spread of 1–2m (3–6ft).

2m (6ft)

Rumex crispus **Yellow dock**

Native throughout Europe and Africa, yellow dock is a common wayside plant and garden weed that thrives on scrubby waste ground and grass verges. Its main use today is as a detoxifying herb and as a mild laxative. It is often combined with other herbs, such as burdock root, in the treatment of chronic skin conditions.

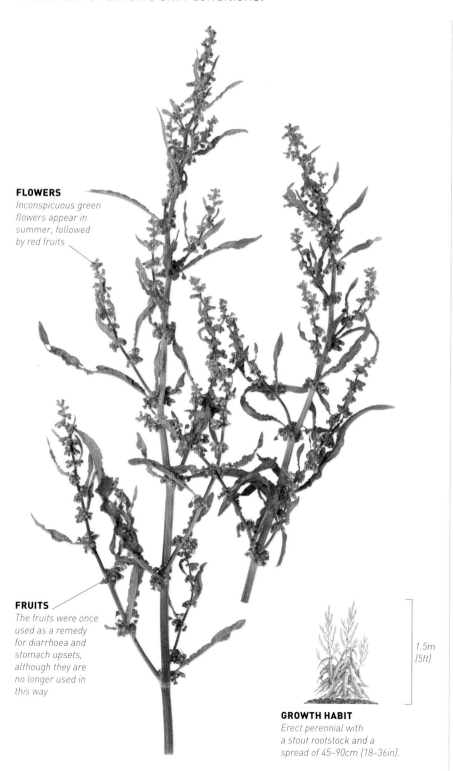

FLOWERS
Inconspicuous green flowers appear in summer, followed by red fruits

FRUITS
The fruits were once used as a remedy for diarrhoea and stomach upsets, although they are no longer used in this way

GROWTH HABIT
Erect perennial with a stout rootstock and a spread of 45–90cm (18–36in).

1.5m (5ft)

PARTS USED Root
MAIN CONSTITUENTS Anthraquinones (incl. emodin and chrysophanol), tannins, oxalates, volatile oil
ACTIONS Blood and lymphatic cleanser, bitter tonic, stimulates bile flow, laxative

HOW TO USE

DECOCTION Take ½–1 cup 3 times daily of a decoction made from 15g (½oz) of root to 550ml (17fl oz) of water simmered gently for 20 minutes for mild constipation, or to stimulate bile flow to improve the digestion and help clear toxins from the system.
TINCTURE Take 1–2ml (20–40 drops) of tincture 3 times daily as part of a cleansing regime for conditions such as irritant skin rashes and eczema, boils, acne, shingles, rheumatism, and osteoarthritis.
MOUTHWASH Use ½ cup of the decoction (made as above) diluted with an equal amount of warm water 2–3 times daily for mouth ulcers.
HOMOEOPATHIC EXTRACTS In homoeopathy, yellow dock root is used for coughs, sore throats, and hoarseness made worse by cold air and damp weather. Take 1–2 tablets up to 3 times daily.

HOW TO SOURCE

GROW A perennial weed that self-seeds enthusiastically, and which few people would want to cultivate in their gardens. Seeds can be gathered from hedgerows in autumn if required and scattered where you want them to grow. Once established, the plant can be difficult to eradicate thanks to its tough root. It will tolerate any soil and grows in both sun and shade.
FORAGE The roots are long and can be difficult to dig up unless the ground has been well wetted first. Gather in autumn.
HARVEST Dig up the roots in autumn, wash thoroughly, chop, and dry.

CAUTION Do not take in pregnancy or when breast-feeding. Use for occasional constipation; for chronic constipation, consult a herbalist.

Salix alba **White willow**

Originally found in temperate or cold regions in the northern hemisphere, white willow was classified as a cool and moist remedy due to its preference for growing near water. In 1828 the Bavarian pharmacist, Johann Buchner (1783–1852), extracted bitter-tasting crystals – which he named salicin – from the bark; these were synthesized as aspirin by Bayer in 1899.

PARTS USED Bark, leaves

MAIN CONSTITUENTS Salicin, salicylic acid, tannins, flavonoids

ACTIONS Antirheumatic, anti-inflammatory, febrifuge, antihidrotic (reduces sweating), analgesic, antiseptic, astringent, bitter digestive tonic

HOW TO USE

FLUID EXTRACT Take 1–2ml (20–40 drops) of the bark extract in water 3 times daily for rheumatic conditions, lumbago, sciatica, and neuralgia. Combine with an equal amount of rosemary tincture for headaches.

TINCTURE Use 5–10ml (1–2 tsp) doses of the bark tincture (p.168) 3 times daily for fevers: generally combined with other herbs such as boneset (*Eupatorium perfoliatum*) or elderflower. Add 20–40 drops to menopausal remedies to help reduce night sweats and hot flushes.

DECOCTION Take 1 cup of a standard decoction of the bark 3 times daily for feverish chills, headaches, or as part of arthritic treatments with herbs such as St John's wort and crampbark.

INFUSION Take 1 cup of a standard infusion (p.168) of the leaves after meals for indigestion.

HOW TO SOURCE

GROW Prefers moist but well-drained soil. Propagate from semi-ripe cuttings in summer or hardwood cuttings in winter, although it can be grown from seed.

FORAGE Often found growing near water such as rivers or canals. The leaves were once collected in summer and used in infusions as a fever remedy, for colicky pains, or for digestive problems, although they are no longer commercially harvested. The bark should not be stripped from wild trees.

HARVEST The bark is stripped in spring from branches of two- to five-year-old trees that have been pollarded.

CAUTION Avoid if allergic to aspirin or salicylates. Avoid during pregnancy.

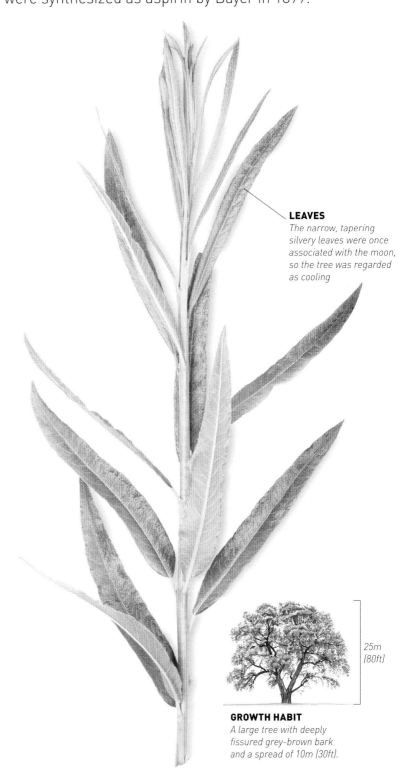

LEAVES
The narrow, tapering silvery leaves were once associated with the moon, so the tree was regarded as cooling

GROWTH HABIT
A large tree with deeply fissured grey-brown bark and a spread of 10m (30ft).

25m (80ft)

Salvia officinalis **Sage**

Saliva officinalis originates in Mediterranean regions, and is well known as a culinary and medicinal herb. It is largely used for digestive and menopausal problems, particularly hot flushes, and is traditionally associated with longevity: modern research has shown that it can slow the progress of Alzheimer's disease.

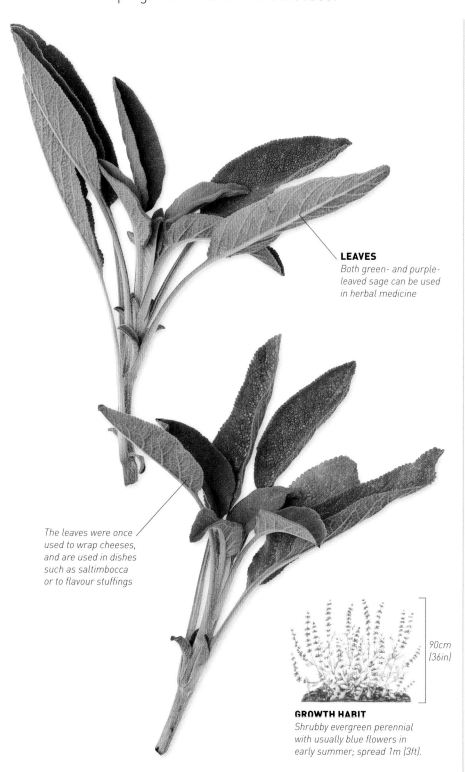

LEAVES
Both green- and purple-leaved sage can be used in herbal medicine

The leaves were once used to wrap cheeses, and are used in dishes such as saltimbocca or to flavour stuffings

90cm
(36in)

GROWTH HABIT
Shrubby evergreen perennial with usually blue flowers in early summer; spread 1m (3ft).

PARTS USED Leaves, essential oil
MAIN CONSTITUENTS Volatile oil (incl. thujone, linalool, and borneol), diterpene bitter, tannins, flavonoids, oestrogenic substances
ACTIONS Carminative, antispasmodic, astringent, antiseptic, reduces sweating, salivation, and lactation, uterine stimulant, stimulates bile flow

HOW TO USE

INFUSION Take 1 cup of a standard infusion (p.168) of the leaves 3 times daily for diarrhoea, to help improve digestive function in debility, or to ease menopausal symptoms, including night sweats. It can also help dry off milk at the weaning stage.
GARGLE/MOUTHWASH Use 1 cup of a standard infusion of the leaves as a gargle for sore throats, tonsillitis, quinsy, or as a mouthwash for mouth ulcers, gingivitis, etc.
TINCTURE Take 1–2ml (20–40 drops) of tincture 3 times daily for the menopause or as a tonic for digestive function.
HAIR RINSE Use 500ml (16fl oz) of a standard infusion as a final rinse to control dandruff or restore colour to greying hair.
CREAM/OINTMENT/LOTION Used as a household standby in many parts of Europe for treating minor cuts and grazes.

HOW TO SOURCE

GROW Prefers neutral to alkaline soil and full sun. Sow seeds in 7.5cm (3in) of compost in spring or summer and plant out the following year when sturdy, or propagate from softwood cuttings in summer. Prune after flowering and in early spring to stop the plant becoming too straggly.
FORAGE Found growing wild on dry, sunny hillsides in temperate regions.
HARVEST Cropped just before flowering in summer, or collect the leaves to use in cooking throughout the year.

CAUTION Due to its high thujone content, sage should not be taken in therapeutic doses by epileptics. Avoid therapeutic doses in pregnancy.

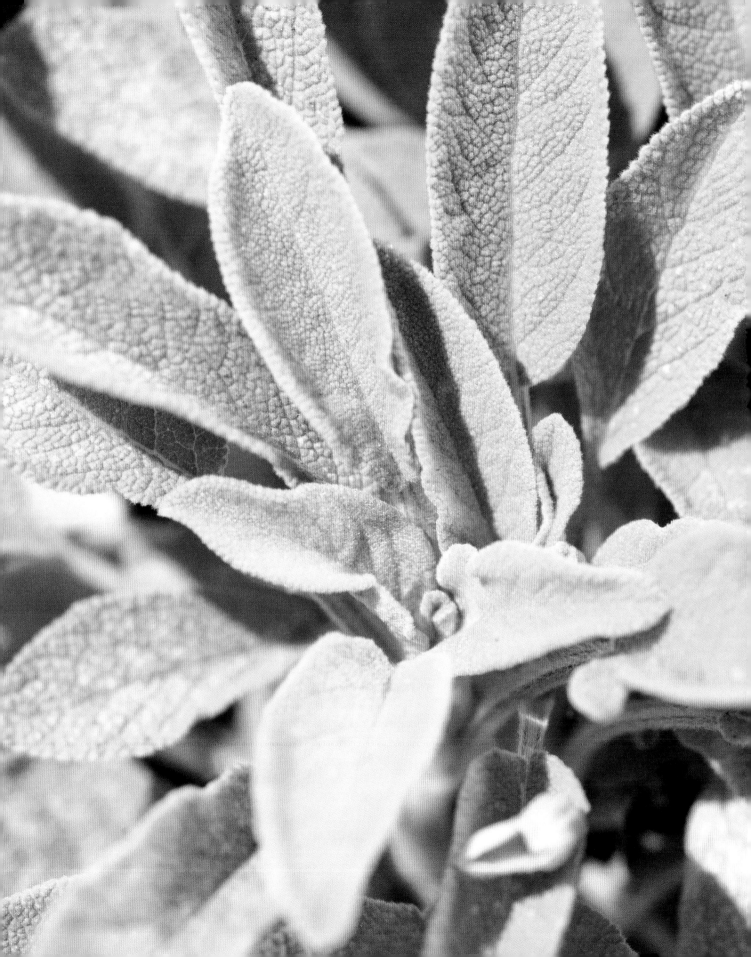

Sambucus nigra **Elder**

A common woodland tree throughout Europe, north Africa, and south-west Asia, elder was once regarded as a complete medicine chest: the root and bark made strong purgatives, while the leaves were made into a green ointment for use on bruises and sprains. Today, the flowers are most commonly used in refreshing elderflower cordials and medicinal brews.

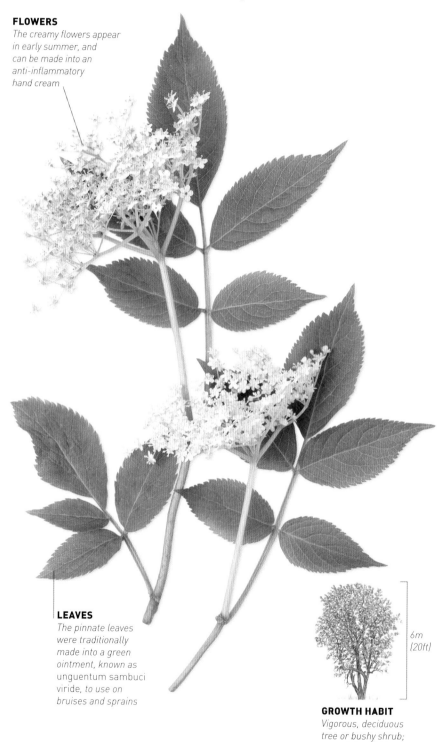

FLOWERS
The creamy flowers appear in early summer, and can be made into an anti-inflammatory hand cream

LEAVES
The pinnate leaves were traditionally made into a green ointment, known as unguentum sambuci viride, *to use on bruises and sprains*

GROWTH HABIT
Vigorous, deciduous tree or bushy shrub; spread 6m (20ft).

6m (20ft)

PARTS USED Leaves, flowers, fruits
MAIN CONSTITUENTS Volatile oil, flavonoids, mucilage, tannins, cyanogenic glycosides, viburnic acid, phenolic acid, sterols. Berries contain vitamins A and C.
ACTIONS Flowers: expectorant, anticatarrhal, circulatory stimulant, diaphoretic, antiviral, topically anti-inflammatory
Berries: diaphoretic, diuretic, laxative
Leaves: topically wound-healing

HOW TO USE

INFUSION Take 1 cup of a standard infusion (p.168) of the flowers 3 times daily for feverish and catarrhal conditions and coughs; combine with yarrow, boneset, and peppermint in equal proportions for seasonal colds.
MOUTHWASH/GARGLE Use 1 cup of a standard infusion of the flowers as a mouthwash and gargle for mouth ulcers, sore throats, or tonsillitis.
CREAM/OINTMENT Made from the flowers to soothe inflamed or chapped hands, or from the leaves for bruises, sprains, chilblains, or piles.
SYRUP Add 600ml (1 pint) of a standard decoction of berries to 450g (1lb) honey and take in 10ml (2 tsp) doses for colds and flu.
TINCTURE Take 2–4ml (40–80 drops) elderberry tincture three times a day for coughs, colds, and flu symptoms. Combines well with echinacea.

HOW TO SOURCE

GROW Tolerates almost any soil, but prefers a moist, well-drained site. Propagate from hardwood cuttings in winter or ripe seeds sown in a cold frame; it will also self-seed easily. Can be invasive.
FORAGE Collect from hedgerows away from busy roads to avoid pollutants.
HARVEST Gather flowers in early summer and berries in early autumn, removing them from the stalk before use.

CAUTION Excessive consumption of fresh berries can have a laxative effect.

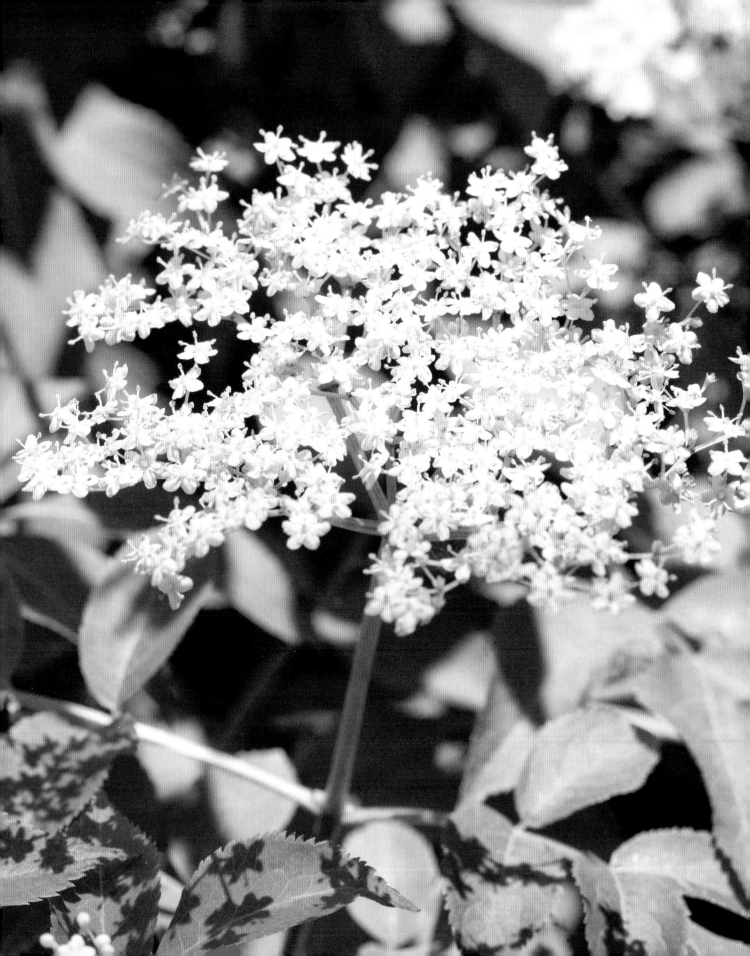

Scutellaria lateriflora **Virginian skullcap**

Native to North America, Virginian skullcap was once known as "mad dog herb" due to an erroneous belief that it could cure rabies. Today it is mainly used as a sedative. Its European relative, marsh, or hooded, skullcap (*Scutellaria galericulata*) has similar properties, while the root of the Chinese species (*Scutellaria baicalensis*), known as *huang qin*, is used in hot, feverish conditions.

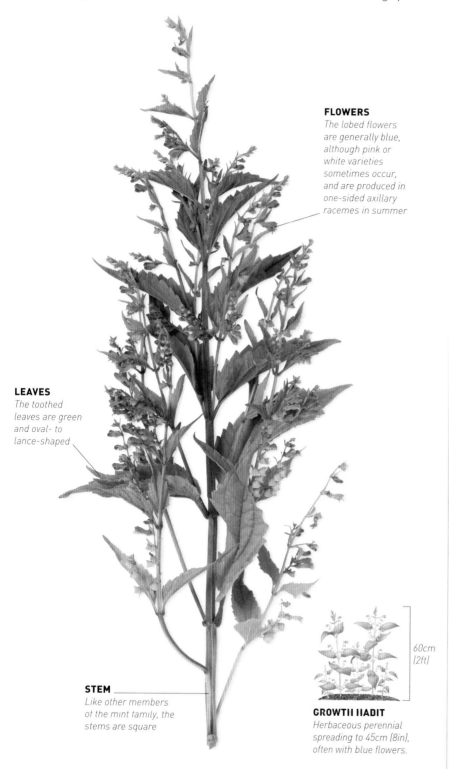

FLOWERS
The lobed flowers are generally blue, although pink or white varieties sometimes occur, and are produced in one-sided axillary racemes in summer

LEAVES
The toothed leaves are green and oval- to lance-shaped

STEM
Like other members of the mint family, the stems are square

GROWTH HABIT
Herbaceous perennial spreading to 45cm (8in), often with blue flowers.

60cm
(2ft)

PARTS USED Aerial parts
MAIN CONSTITUENTS Flavonoids, tannins, bitter iridoids, volatile oil, minerals
ACTIONS Relaxing and restorative nervine, sedative, antispasmodic, mild bitter

HOW TO USE

INFUSION Take ½–1 cup of a standard infusion (p.168) 3 times daily for nervous exhaustion, excitability, anxiety, or stress.
TEA Use 1 tsp of dried herb per cup, or 3–4 whole sprigs in a small teapot, to make a soothing tea to ease tensions at the end of the working day or to ease emotional upsets associated with premenstrual syndrome. A cup before bedtime can also help with insomnia.
TINCTURE Take 1–2ml (20–40 drops) in a little water 3 times daily for nervous tension, stress, anxiety, or associated headaches.
TABLETS/CAPSULES Commercially available, and often combining skullcap with passionflower. Follow dosage directions on the pack and use for anxiety and stress.

HOW TO SOURCE

GROW Prefers moist but well-drained soil in sun or partial shade. Sow seeds in autumn or spring in seed trays and transplant to 7.5cm (3in) pots when large enough to handle. Grow on until well established before planting in their final positions. Alternatively, divide plants in spring. Self-seeds enthusiastically and can become invasive.
FORAGE Found in hedgerows or riverbanks in the USA and Canada; likely elsewhere only in isolated groups that may have self-seeded in grass verges or hedgerows from neighbouring herb gardens. Common skullcap (*Scutellaria galericulata*) can be used in similar ways and is likely to be found along riverbanks or in fens.
HARVEST Cut while flowering and dry immediately; the aerial parts will contain both flowers and seed pods.

Senna alexandrina **Senna**

Native to Egypt, Sudan, Somalia, and Arabia, senna was used in the 9th century by Arabian physicians as a cathartic, or strong laxative. Its use soon spread, and both pods and leaves are still used as laxatives. The leaves are known as *fan xie ye* in traditional Chinese medicine, while their Indian name, *rajavriksha*, translates as "king of trees".

PARTS USED Leaves, pods

MAIN CONSTITUENTS Anthraquinone glycosides (incl. sennosides, dianthrone diglycosides) polysaccharides, mucilage, flavonoids (incl. kaempferol), salicylic acid

ACTIONS Stimulating laxative, antibacterial, anthelmintic, cooling

HOW TO USE

INFUSION For constipation, soak 3–6 pods (15–30mg) in 1 cup of warm water and drink last thing at night. Add a slice of fresh ginger root or 1 tsp of fennel seeds to combat griping pains caused by an increase in bowel movement. Use half the adult dose for children over 10 years.

FLUID EXTRACT Take ¼–½ml (5–10 drops) of senna leaf extract in a little water at night for constipation.

TINCTURE Take ½ml–1½ml (10–30 drops) in a little water at night for constipation.

TABLETS/POWDERS Take 1–2 tsp of granules or 2–4 tablets at night for occasional constipation.

HOW TO SOURCE

GROW Prefers rich, moist, sandy soil in full sun. Requires a minimum of 5°C (41°F) to grow, but can be grown in containers in cooler regions. Sow seeds in spring and transplant to containers or final growing positions when well established, or take semi-ripe cuttings in spring.

FORAGE Unlikely to be found growing wild outside its native habitat.

HARVEST Pick leaves before and during flowering; gather pods in autumn when ripe.

CAUTION Can cause abdominal cramps. Do not take in cases of inflammatory bowel disease (such as Crohn's disease or ulcerative colitis), or if pregnant or breast-feeding. Avoid in intestinal obstruction. Excessive use can cause diarrhoea and can damage the colon. Do not take leaf extracts or infusions for more than seven days at a time and take a break of at least two weeks before repeating the treatment.

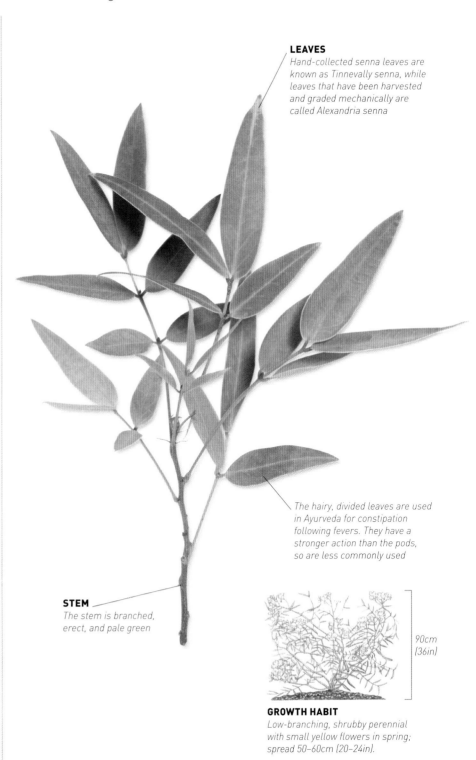

LEAVES
Hand-collected senna leaves are known as Tinnevally senna, while leaves that have been harvested and graded mechanically are called Alexandria senna

The hairy, divided leaves are used in Ayurveda for constipation following fevers. They have a stronger action than the pods, so are less commonly used

STEM
The stem is branched, erect, and pale green

90cm
(36in)

GROWTH HABIT
Low-branching, shrubby perennial with small yellow flowers in spring; spread 50–60cm (20–24in).

Silybum marianum **Milk thistle**

Native to stony areas in the Mediterranean region and south-west Asia, milk thistle is also known as Mary thistle, as the white veins on its leaves are reputedly due to splashes of the Virgin Mary's milk falling on them while she fed the Christ child. Although it encourages milk flow, it is probably now better known for its liver-protective qualities.

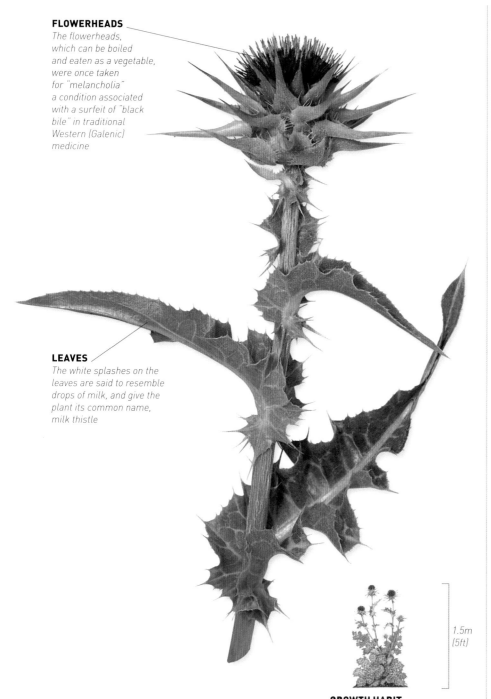

FLOWERHEADS
The flowerheads, which can be boiled and eaten as a vegetable, were once taken for "melancholia" a condition associated with a surfeit of "black bile" in traditional Western (Galenic) medicine

LEAVES
The white splashes on the leaves are said to resemble drops of milk, and give the plant its common name, milk thistle

1.5m
(5ft)

GROWTH HABIT
Biennial with spiny green leaves marbled with white; spread 60–90cm (24–36in).

PARTS USED Seeds, leaves, flowerheads
MAIN CONSTITUENTS Flavolignans (incl. silymarin), bitters, polyacetylenes
ACTIONS Bitter tonic, cholagogue, antiviral, choleretic, antidepressant, antioxidant, galactagogue, liver protector

HOW TO USE

TINCTURE Take 20–50 drops of the seed tincture with a little water 3 times daily for liver and gall bladder problems, or to stimulate the digestion. Take up to 5ml (1 tsp) daily in water as a preventative if you have a history of gallstones or liver disease. Treatment of gallstones requires professional advice.
CAPSULES Regular use of milk thistle capsules may help in the treatment of liver diseases.
INFUSION Drink 1–2 cups of a standard leaf infusion (p.168) daily to stimulate milk production when breast-feeding. The infusion can be used to stimulate a sluggish digestion.
DECOCTION Take ½ cup of a standard decoction (p.168) of the cracked seeds daily for liver disorders, including infections.

HOW TO SOURCE

GROW Prefers full sun in poor to moderately fertile soil that is well drained and neutral to alkaline. Sow seeds where you want to grow them in spring for annual growth or in late summer or early autumn for flowers the following year. Thin to at least 45cm (18in) between plants.
FORAGE May be found in hedgerows and waste areas in many parts of Europe, North and East Africa, and western Asia. The flowerheads can be cooked and eaten as a vegetable (rather like globe artichoke), the young leaves are used as a spinach substitute, and the root tastes rather like salsify.
HARVEST Collect the seeds in late summer; other parts of the plant can be gathered for culinary use during the summer.

Stellaria media **Chickweed**

Found throughout Europe and Asia, chickweed has long been used as a soothing and healing remedy for skin problems and wounds. Regarded by many as a weed, it is a favourite food for chickens – as the name implies – and other small birds: in the 16th century it was regularly fed to caged linnets.

PARTS USED Aerial parts
MAIN CONSTITUENTS Mucilage, saponins, coumarins, minerals, vitamins A, B, and C.
ACTIONS Astringent, antirheumatic, wound herb, demulcent, emollient, mild laxative

HOW TO USE

INFUSED OIL Fill a jar with fresh chickweed and cover completely with sunflower oil; steep for 2 weeks, then strain and use on eczema and irritant skin rashes – or add 25ml (5 tsp) to bath water for eczema sufferers.
CREAM/OINTMENT Use regularly on itching skin rashes and eczema. Can also soothe minor burns and be used to draw out thorns and splinters – put a little on the embedded splinter, cover with a sticking plaster, and leave overnight; the next morning the splinter can usually be found on the sticking plaster pad.
INFUSION Take 1 cup of a standard infusion (p.168) 3 times daily for muscular rheumatism, urinary tract inflammations, or whenever a cooling and cleansing remedy is required.
POULTICE Apply the crushed, fresh plant on gauze or in a muslin bag for boils, abscesses, skin sores, or gout.

HOW TO SOURCE

GROW Prefers moist soil and full sun, but will tolerate many conditions. Sow seeds directly at any time. Usually regarded as a weed, but worth growing as a useful source of food for domestic chickens.
FORAGE Generally found in hedgerows, ditches, waste areas, or grassy areas. Cut the aerial parts as required through the growing period. Chickweed can be sweated like spinach as a vegetable and served with butter.
HARVEST Can be cut throughout the growing period and used fresh or dried.

CAUTION If taken in excess, it may cause nausea and vomiting.

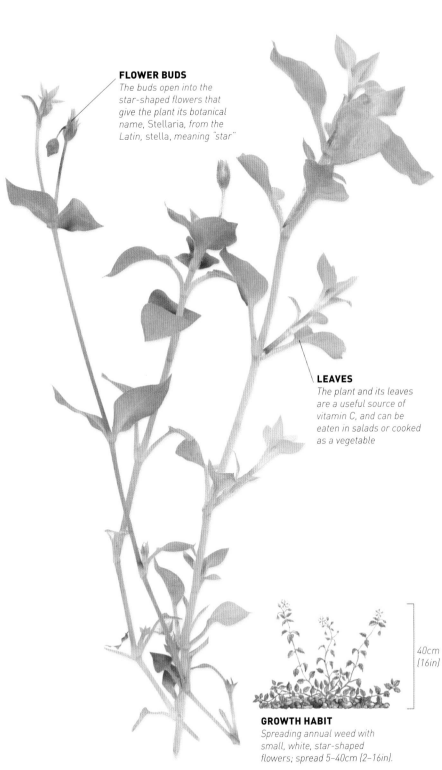

FLOWER BUDS
The buds open into the star-shaped flowers that give the plant its botanical name, Stellaria, *from the Latin,* stella, *meaning "star"*

LEAVES
The plant and its leaves are a useful source of vitamin C, and can be eaten in salads or cooked as a vegetable

40cm
(16in)

GROWTH HABIT
Spreading annual weed with small, white, star-shaped flowers; spread 5–40cm (2–16in).

Symphytum officinale **Comfrey**

Growing throughout Europe, comfrey has been used to heal broken bones since ancient times. In the 1970s it became popular as a remedy for arthritis when taken internally, which led to extensive animal studies using the plant and a realization that the alkaloids it contains may cause liver cancer. Since then it has been banned in a number of countries.

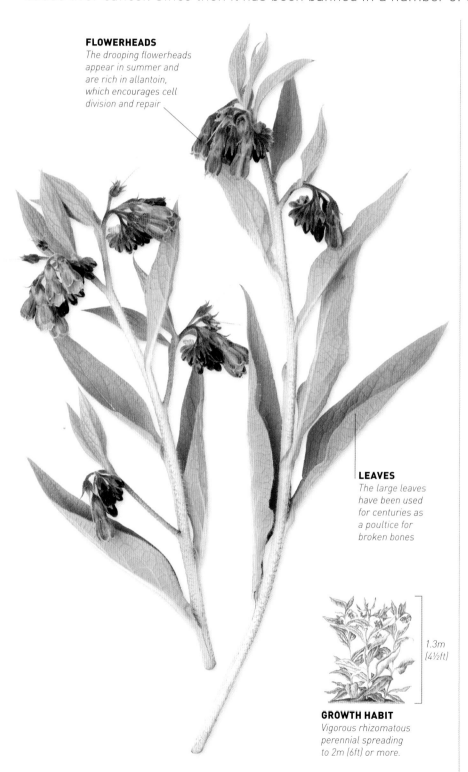

FLOWERHEADS
The drooping flowerheads appear in summer and are rich in allantoin, which encourages cell division and repair

LEAVES
The large leaves have been used for centuries as a poultice for broken bones

GROWTH HABIT
Vigorous rhizomatous perennial spreading to 2m (6ft) or more.

1.3m (4½ft)

PARTS USED Aerial parts, root
MAIN CONSTITUENTS Mucilage, steroidal saponins (root), allantoin, vitamin B12, tannin, pyrrolizidine alkaloids, rosmarinic acid
ACTIONS Cell proliferator, astringent, demulcent, anti-inflammatory, expectorant, wound herb

HOW TO USE

MACERATED OIL Use night and morning to massage arthritic joints, sprains, bruises, and other traumatic injuries.
OINTMENT: Use on clean cuts and grazes, or on skin sores such as nappy rash. Also useful for boils, acne, and psoriasis.
POULTICE Use puréed leaves as a poultice for minor breaks (broken toes, etc) not normally set in plaster. Make a paste with powdered root and a little water, and use on varicose ulcers, stubborn wounds, or bleeding piles.
COMPRESS Apply a pad soaked in a standard decoction of the root to bruises and sprains.

HOW TO SOURCE

GROW Prefers moist soil in a sunny or partially shaded site. Can be propagated from seed sown in autumn or spring, by root division in spring, or root cuttings in winter. Does not tolerate dry winters. Once established, it can be difficult to eradicate.
FORAGE Usually found in damp field borders or hedgerows. When not in flower, the plant can be confused with foxglove.
HARVEST Gather leaves and flowering tops in summer and roots in autumn.

CAUTION Avoid during pregnancy. Do not take comfrey internally; it contains compounds that may be carcinogenic when taken internally. Do not use on dirty wounds, as rapid healing may trap pus or dirt.

Tanacetum parthenium **Feverfew**

Found throughout northern temperate regions, feverfew is widely used today as a migraine remedy. Earlier herbalists thought of it as "a general strengthener of the womb" (Nicholas Culpeper, 1653). It has also traditionally been used to treat arthritis and rheumatism. Numerous cultivars have been developed as garden ornamentals.

PARTS USED Aerial parts

MAIN CONSTITUENTS Sesquiterpene lactones (parthenolide), volatile oil, pyrethrin, tannins, camphor

ACTIONS Anti-inflammatory, vasodilator, relaxant, digestive stimulant, emmenagogue, anthelmintic, bitter

HOW TO USE

TINCTURE Use 5–10 drops at 30-minute intervals at the onset of a migraine. It is most effective for preventing and treating "cold" type migraines involving vasoconstriction, which are eased by applying a hot towel to the head. For the acute stages of rheumatoid arthritis, add up to 2ml (40 drops) 3 times a day to herbal remedies such as celery seed, white willow, or devil's claw (*Harpagophytum procumbens*).

POULTICE Fry a handful of leaves in a little oil and apply to the abdomen as a poultice for colicky pains.

INFUSION Drink 1 or 2 cups of a weak infusion made from 15g (½oz) of the aerial parts to 600ml (1pint) of water after childbirth to encourage cleansing and tonifying of the womb; take 1 cup 3 times daily for period pain associated with sluggish flow and congestion.

HOW TO SOURCE

GROW Prefers full sun and well-drained soil, but tolerates a range of conditions. Sow seeds in a propagator at 10–18°C (50–64.4°F) in late winter or early spring, or take softwood cuttings in early summer. A prolific self-seeder that can be invasive.

FORAGE Often found in hedgerows and waste places. Easily confused with other daisy-like plants, look for its characteristic leaves, which have a very bitter taste.

HARVEST Collect the leaves as required throughout the growing period and the whole plant in summer while flowering.

CAUTION Mouth ulcers can occur after eating the fresh leaves. Avoid if taking anticoagulant drugs such as warfarin. Avoid during pregnancy.

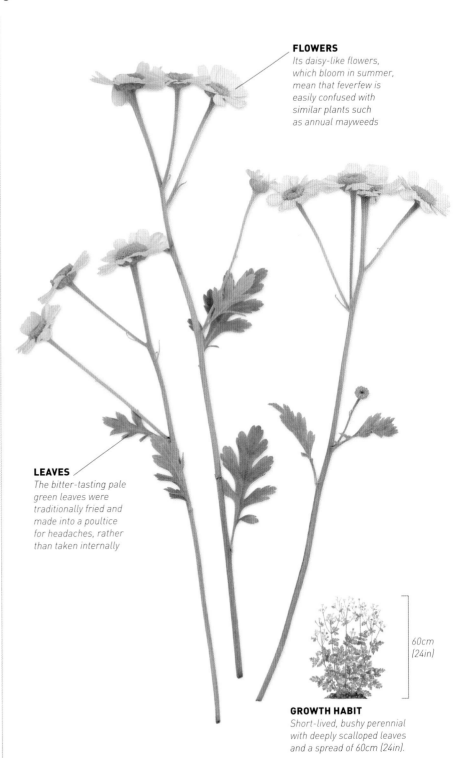

FLOWERS
Its daisy-like flowers, which bloom in summer, mean that feverfew is easily confused with similar plants such as annual mayweeds

LEAVES
The bitter-tasting pale green leaves were traditionally fried and made into a poultice for headaches, rather than taken internally

60cm
(24in)

GROWTH HABIT
Short-lived, bushy perennial with deeply scalloped leaves and a spread of 60cm (24in).

Taraxacum officinale **Dandelion**

Several species of dandelion are found throughout the temperate regions of Europe, Asia, and South America. The plant is a comparative newcomer to the medicinal repertoire, and was first mentioned in Arabic herbals in the 11th century, as a remedy to increase urination. The root, an effective liver tonic, was not used until much later.

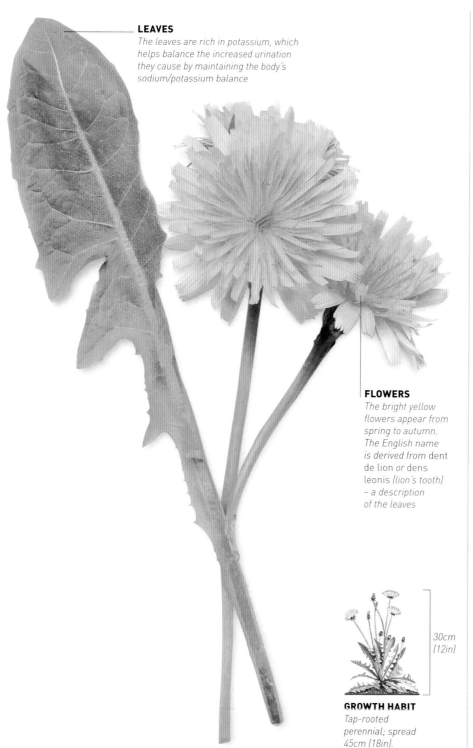

LEAVES
The leaves are rich in potassium, which helps balance the increased urination they cause by maintaining the body's sodium/potassium balance

FLOWERS
The bright yellow flowers appear from spring to autumn. The English name is derived from dent de lion *or* dens leonis *(lion's tooth) – a description of the leaves*

GROWTH HABIT
Tap-rooted perennial; spread 45cm (18in).

30cm (12in)

PARTS USED Leaves, root
MAIN CONSTITUENTS Sesquiterpene lactones, vitamins A, B, C, D, choline, minerals (incl. potassium)
Leaf only: coumarins, carotenoids.
Root only: taraxacoside, phenolic acids.
ACTIONS Diuretic, liver and digestive tonic, cholagogue, stimulates pancreas and bile duct, mild laxative (root only)

HOW TO USE

DECOCTION Take 1 cup of a standard decoction of the root 3 times daily for any condition – such as osteoarthritis, gout, rheumatism, acne, psoriasis, and eczema – where liver stimulation and detoxification may help.
INFUSION Take 1 cup of a standard infusion (p.168) of the leaves 3 times daily to encourage urination in conditions such as cystitis, fluid retention, or high blood pressure.
JUICE Process the leaves in a juicer and take up to 20ml (4 tsp) 3 times daily as a stronger alternative to the infusion.
TINCTURE Take 2–5ml (40 drops–1 tsp) of combined root and leaf tincture 3 times daily to stimulate bile flow, act as a mild laxative, or help dissolve small gallstones.

HOW TO SOURCE

GROW Tolerates a wide range of soils and will grow in full sun or partial shade. Sow the seeds in spring. It self-seeds enthusiastically. The plant is also cultivated for salad leaves in parts of Europe.
FORAGE Found in many parts of the world growing in hedgerows, field borders, waste areas, and even in city pavement cracks. Avoid collecting plants where traffic pollution may be a problem.
HARVEST Gather young leaves for salads in the spring, and the larger leaves in summer for medicinal use. The two-year-old roots are collected in autumn.

CAUTION If suffering from gallstones, only use dandelion root under professional supervision.

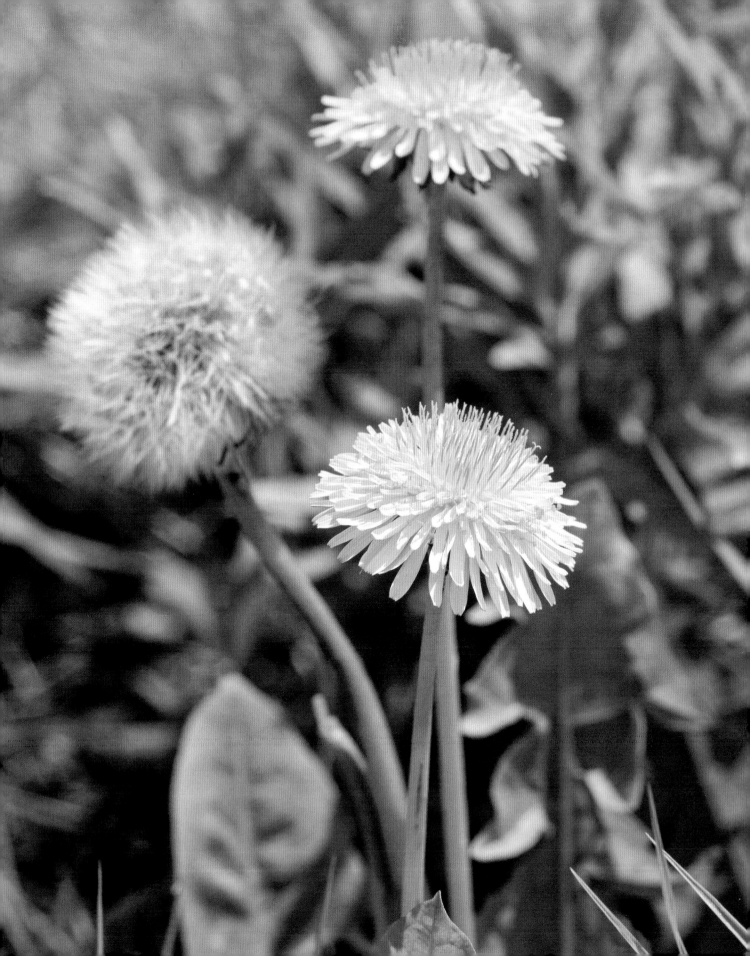

Thymus vulgaris **Common thyme**

Originating from the dry, grassy areas of southern Europe, thyme is now widely grown worldwide as a culinary herb. It is mainly used as an expectorant and antiseptic for the lungs to clear productive coughs and infections, while the essential oil is used in aromatherapy. Research in the 1990s also suggested antioxidant and anti-ageing properties.

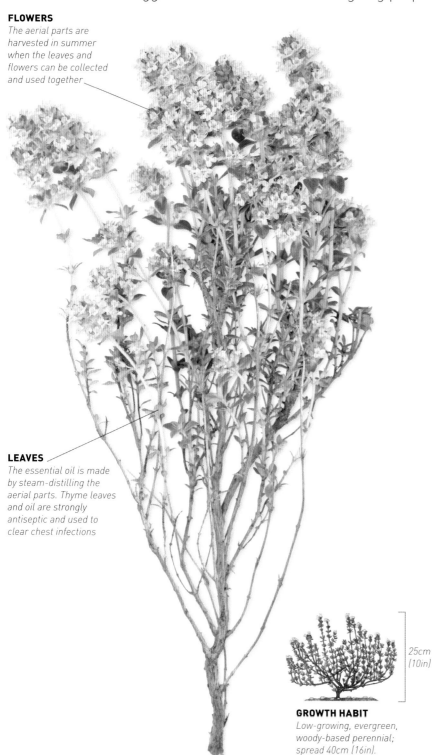

FLOWERS
The aerial parts are harvested in summer when the leaves and flowers can be collected and used together

LEAVES
The essential oil is made by steam-distilling the aerial parts. Thyme leaves and oil are strongly antiseptic and used to clear chest infections

25cm
(10in)

GROWTH HABIT
Low-growing, evergreen, woody-based perennial; spread 40cm (16in).

PARTS USED Aerial parts, essential oil
MAIN CONSTITUENTS Volatile oil (incl. thymol, cineole and borneol), flavonoids, bitter, tannins, saponins
ACTIONS Antiseptic expectorant, antispasmodic, antiseptic, astringent, antimicrobial, diuretic, antitussive, antibiotic, wound herb, topically rubefacient

HOW TO USE

INFUSION Take 1 cup of a standard infusion (p.168) 3 times daily for seasonal colds, chest infections, mild asthma, hayfever, stomach chills, or irritable bowel syndrome.
SYRUP Add 450g (1lb) of honey to 600ml (1 pint) of strained infusion to make a syrup for coughs and chest infections and take in 5ml (1 tsp) doses as required.
MOUTHWASH/GARGLE Use 1 cup of standard infusion morning and night for gum disease and sore throats.
CHEST RUB/MASSAGE OIL Use 10 drops of thyme oil in 25ml (5 tsp) of almond oil as a chest rub for bronchitis and infections. Use with an equal amount of lavender oil for rheumatic pains and strained muscles.
LOTION Dilute 1ml (20 drops) of thyme oil in 60ml (2fl oz) of water and use for insect bites and infected wounds.

HOW TO SOURCE

GROWS Prefers dry alkaline soil in full sun. Sow seeds in trays in a greenhouse or cold frame in spring, potted into 7.5cm (3in) pots when large enough to handle, and planted out when well established. Alternatively, take softwood cuttings in summer as flowering starts.
FORAGE Found in scrubby, rocky wasteland or dry grassland throughout Europe and Asia.
HARVEST Gather aerial parts in mid- to late summer, and sprigs for cooking throughout the growing period.

CAUTION Avoid therapeutic doses in pregnancy. Do not take the essential oil internally, and always use well diluted.

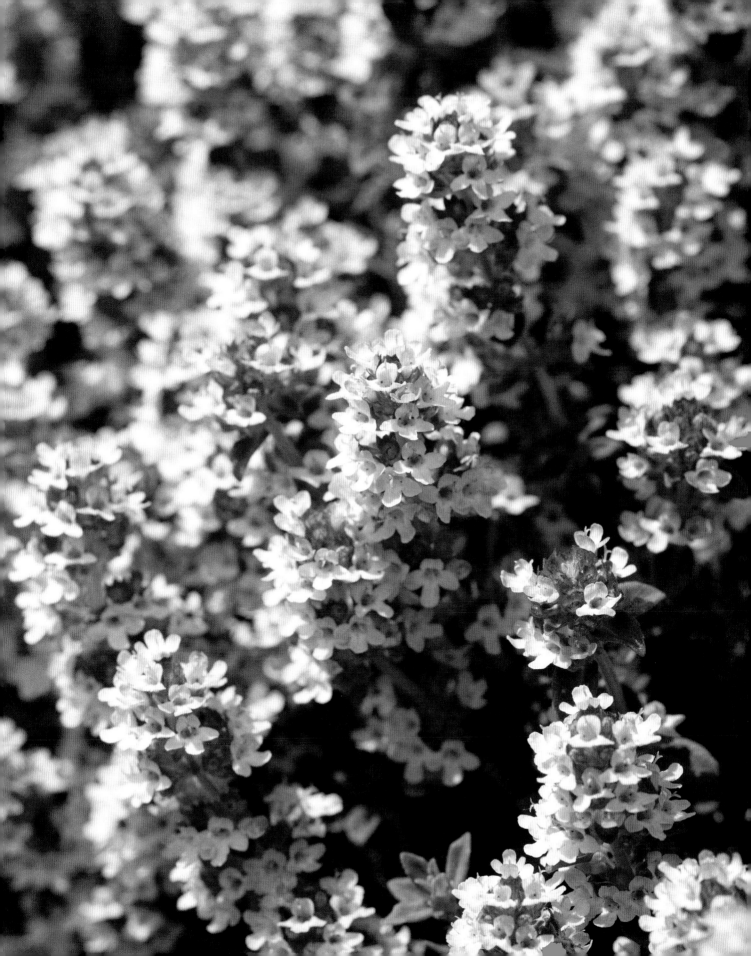

Tilia cordata **Lime flowers**

Native to central and eastern Europe, the lime, or linden tree, is popular in urban street plantings in many countries – perhaps most notably in the iconic avenue, the *Unter den Linden*, leading to the Brandenburg Gate in Berlin. The flowers are mainly used in sedative mixtures, although they can also be used in soothing lotions.

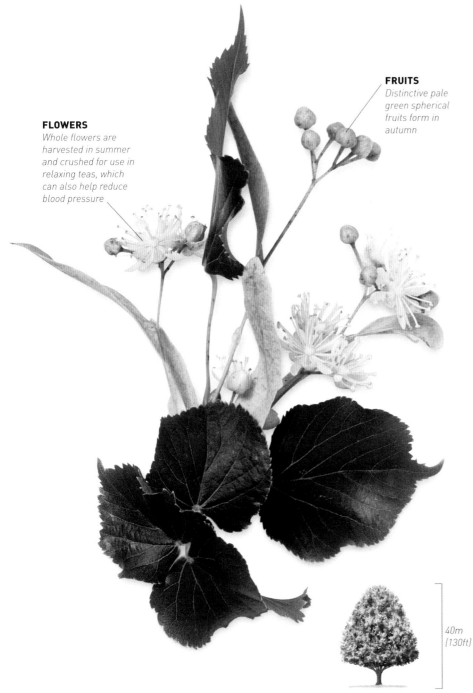

FLOWERS
Whole flowers are harvested in summer and crushed for use in relaxing teas, which can also help reduce blood pressure

FRUITS
Distinctive pale green spherical fruits form in autumn

GROWTH HABIT
Medium-large columnar tree; spread 10-30m (30–100ft).

40m
(130ft)

PARTS USED Flowers
MAIN CONSTITUENTS Flavonoids (incl. quercetin and kaempferol), caffeic acid, mucilage, tannins, volatile oil
ACTIONS Antispasmodic, diaphoretic, diuretic, sedative, hypotensive, anticoagulant

HOW TO USE

INFUSION Take 1 cup of a standard infusion (p.168) up to 3 times daily to soothe tension, stress or nervous headaches, or to relieve colds, flu, and nasal catarrh. Commercial teabags often combine lime with chamomile, or mix the dried flowers with equal amounts of lemon balm and chamomile and use 1–2 tsp of the dried mix in a cup of boiling water for a relaxing and calming tea.
TINCTURE Take 5ml (1 tsp) of the tincture in water 3 times daily, for high blood pressure associated with stress and anxiety or arteriosclerosis. Usually used in combination with other herbs such as valerian or hawthorn.
OINTMENT/LOTION Use as required for itching skin caused by rashes or insect bites.
CHILDREN'S TEA Can be used as a soothing remedy in the early stages of childhood infections such as flu, seasonal colds, or chicken pox. Consult a herbalist for advice on dosage.

HOW TO SOURCE

GROW Prefers fertile, moist but well-drained soil that is neutral to alkaline. The seeds need to be stratified over winter and planted in a seed bed outside in the spring, but it can be slow to germinate. It is a large tree, so is not suitable for small or congested gardens.
FORAGE Limes are found throughout Europe and in many other temperate zones, often as part of a street-planting scheme. The flowers can be collected in early to mid-summer, but it is best to avoid trees in high traffic areas to minimize pollution.
HARVEST Gather the flowers in midsummer. They can be collected with the sepals and crushed when dry.

Trifolium pratense **Red clover**

Native to temperate regions of Europe and Asia, red clover is now naturalized in many parts of North America and Australia. The plant was known as "honey stalk", as children sucked the sweet sap from its stems. In the 1930s it became popular for treating breast cancer. Today it is mainly used for coughs, skin problems and menopausal symptoms.

PARTS USED Flowerheads

MAIN CONSTITUENTS Flavonoids, salicylates, coumarins, phenolic glycosides, cyanogenic glycosides, volatile oil (incl. methyl salicylate and benzyl alcohol), sitosterol

ACTIONS Antispasmodic, diuretic, lymphatic cleanser, possible oestrogenic activity, expectorant

HOW TO USE

INFUSION Take 1 cup of a standard infusion (p.168) 3 times daily for coughs, menopausal problems, or as part of a cleansing regime for skin problems.

SYRUP Make a standard infusion and use 600ml (1 pint) to make a syrup with 450g (1lb) of honey. Take in 5ml (1 tsp) doses as required for stubborn coughs, especially whooping cough or bronchitis.

MOUTHWASH/GARGLE Use 1 cup of a standard infusion for mouth ulcers and sore throats.

TINCTURE Take 5–10ml (1–2 tsp) 3 times daily for eczema, psoriasis, and old sores that are slow to heal. Combines well with heartsease for childhood eczema.

CREAM/OINTMENT Use frequently for lymphatic swellings.

FRESH HERB Use the crushed flowers directly on insect bites and stings.

HOW TO SOURCE

GROW Prefers moderate summer temperatures and adequate moisture throughout the growing period. Scatter seeds where you want them to grow in late winter or early spring, and then cover with a light dusting of good compost.

FORAGE Widely cultivated as a fodder crop and as part of a crop-rotation programme, red clover can be found growing in many parts of the world. Look for it growing in hedgerows and meadows and collect the flowerheads when they are newly opened.

HARVEST Gather throughout the summer, choosing newly opened flowerheads.

CAUTION Avoid during pregnancy.

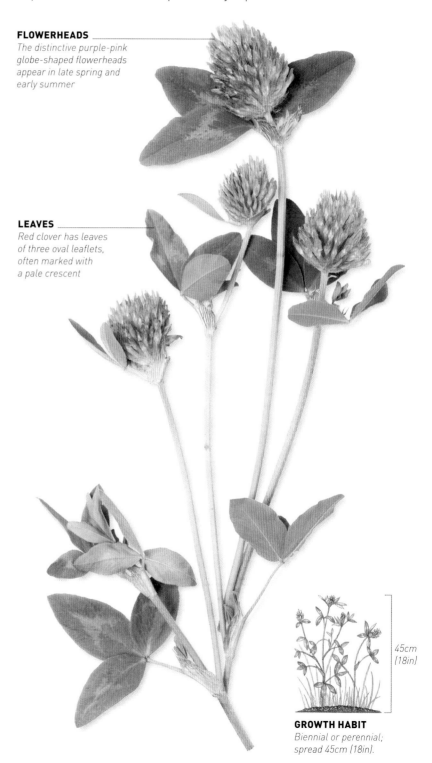

FLOWERHEADS
The distinctive purple-pink globe-shaped flowerheads appear in late spring and early summer

LEAVES
Red clover has leaves of three oval leaflets, often marked with a pale crescent

45cm (18in)

GROWTH HABIT
Biennial or perennial; spread 45cm (18in).

Tropaeolum majus **Nasturtium**

Originally found in the Andes from Bolivia to Colombia, nasturtiums have now spread worldwide as a popular and easy-to-grow garden ornamental. They naturalize readily and are classified as an invasive weed in New Zealand and other areas. Valued both as an antiseptic and respiratory remedy, the flowers and seeds also have many culinary uses.

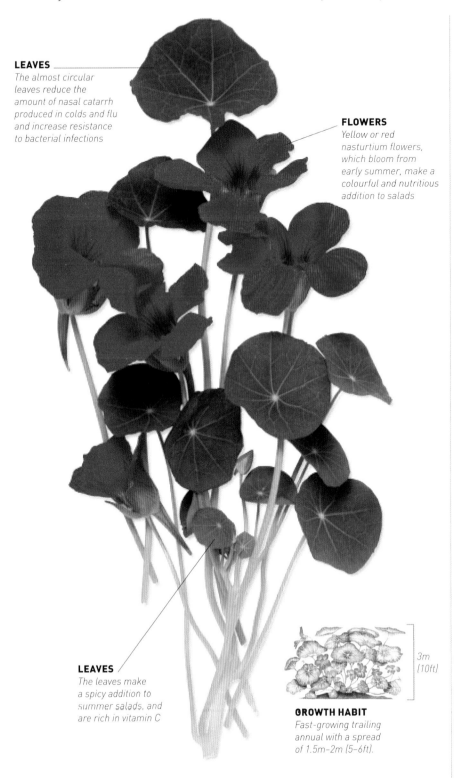

LEAVES
The almost circular leaves reduce the amount of nasal catarrh produced in colds and flu and increase resistance to bacterial infections

FLOWERS
Yellow or red nasturtium flowers, which bloom from early summer, make a colourful and nutritious addition to salads

LEAVES
The leaves make a spicy addition to summer salads, and are rich in vitamin C

GROWTH HABIT
Fast-growing trailing annual with a spread of 1.5m–2m (5–6ft).

3m
(10ft)

PARTS USED Flowers, leaves, seeds
MAIN CONSTITUENTS Glucocyanates, spilanthol, myrosin, mineral salts (incl. iodine, iron, and phosphates), oxalic acid, vitamin C
ACTIONS Antibiotic, antitussive, diuretic, expectorant

HOW TO USE

INFUSION Take 1 cup of a standard infusion (p.168) of the leaves 3 times daily to increase resistance to bacterial infection; also effective for clearing catarrh due to colds and flu.
TINCTURE Take 5–10ml (1–2 tsp) of a leaf tincture 3 times daily for colds, influenza, and dry coughs.
JUICE Pulp the whole plant in a food processor or juicer and take 20ml (4 tsp) 3 times daily in a little milk for chronic lung conditions such as emphysema; the juice rubbed into the scalp is said to stimulate hair growth in alopecia.
LOTION Use 1 cup of a standard infusion of the leaves as an antiseptic wash for cuts and grazes.
FRESH LEAVES AND FLOWERS Add both to salads – the leaves have a spicy flavour and are rich in vitamin C.

HOW TO SOURCE

GROW Nasturtiums will grow almost anywhere, but prefer well-drained soil and a sunny site. A rich soil encourages leaf growth rather than flowers. Sow the seeds where you want to grow them in early summer, or plant in trays in mid-spring at 13–16°C (55–61°F) and transplant when all danger of frost has passed.
FORAGE An invasive weed in some parts of the world, in temperate zones they may be found in urban areas outside gardens as self-seeded plants. Gather the flowers as required and the whole plant in late summer for use in tinctures.
HARVEST Gather leaves and flowers as required for salads, or the whole plant in summer for drying.

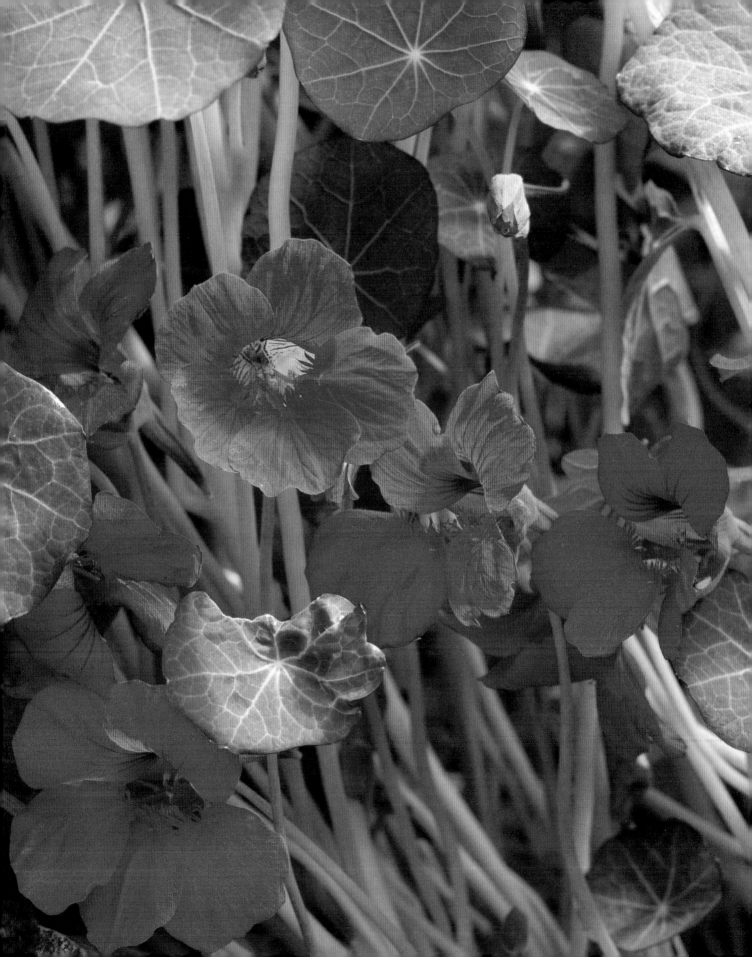

Tussilago farfara **Coltsfoot**

Once a remedy for coughs, as the botanical name suggests (from *tussis*, the Latin for "cough"), coltsfoot has fallen from favour in recent years since pyrrolizidine alkaloids, which are carcinogenic and have been linked to liver cancer, were identified in the plant. Found throughout Europe, western Asia, and North Africa, the plant is an invasive weed. It is restricted in some countries.

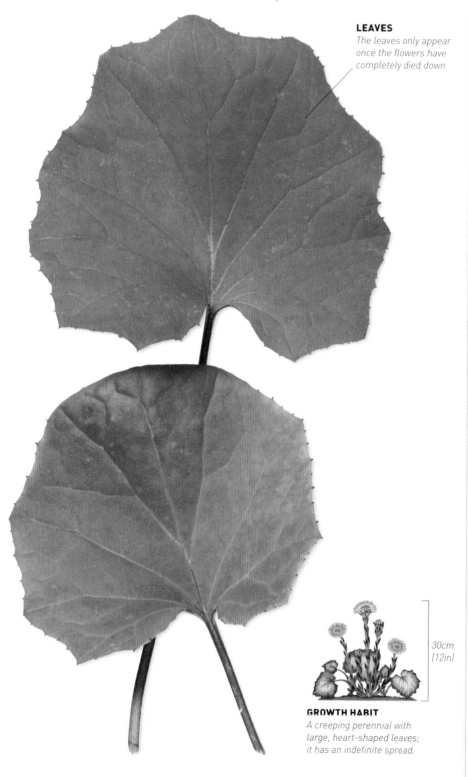

LEAVES
The leaves only appear once the flowers have completely died down

GROWTH HABIT
A creeping perennial with large, heart-shaped leaves; it has an indefinite spread.

30cm (12in)

PARTS USED Leaves, flowers
MAIN CONSTITUENTS Mucilage, tannins, pyrollizidine alkaloids, inulin, zinc, bitter principle, sterols, flavonoids (incl. rutin), potassium, calcium
ACTIONS Relaxing expectorant, anticatarrhal, demulcent

HOW TO USE

NB: Do not take internally without professional guidance
POULTICE Chop fresh leaves in a blender or food processor, spread on gauze, and use as a poultice for ulcers, sores, and other slow-healing wounds.
SYRUP Add 450g (1lb) of honey or sugar to 600ml (1 pint) of a strained standard leaf infusion (p.168), bring to the boil, and simmer gently for 5–10 minutes to form a syrup. Use in 5ml (1 tsp) doses for dry, unproductive, irritating coughs or asthma.
TINCTURE Use 2–5 ml (40 drops–1 tsp) of leaf tincture 3 times daily for whooping cough or bronchitis.
DECOCTION Simmer 15g (½oz) of dried flowers in 600ml (1 pint) of water for 15 minutes and take ½–1 cup 3 times daily for asthma, bronchitis, or persistent coughs.

HOW TO SOURCE

GROW Prefers moist neutral to alkaline soil in sun or partial shade. Sow seeds in spring in a prepared seed bed, or divide clumps after the flowers, which appear before the leaves, fade, or in autumn as the leaves die down. Extremely invasive.
FORAGE Found in hedges and waste ground.
HARVEST Gather the flowers as soon as they open and use fresh or dried; collect the leaves when fully grown in summer.

CAUTION Contains pyrrolizidine alkaloids; do not take internally without professional guidance. Do not use it pregnant or if breast-feeding.

Ulmus rubra **Slippery elm**

One of the most widely used herbal remedies, slippery elm is native to eastern areas of North America from Quebec to Mexico. It is used to heal and soothe damaged tissues – both external wounds and internal mucous membranes – and is also extremely nutritive, so is used as a food in debility and convalescence.

PARTS USED Inner bark
MAIN CONSTITUENTS Mucilage, starch, tannins
ACTIONS Soothing demulcent, emollient, laxative, expectorant, antitussive, nutritive

HOW TO USE

FOOD SUPPLEMENT Use as a food in debility or for infants. Mix ¼–1 level tsp of the powder with a little water to make a paste and add boiling water or hot milk, stirring constantly, to make up to 1 cup of thin gruel. Alternatively, sprinkle the powder on porridge or muesli.

OINTMENT Use to "draw" pus, thorns, or splinters; often combined with marshmallow powder.

POULTICE Mix 1 tsp of powder with a little water or calendula infusion to form a paste, spread on gauze, and apply to boils, abscesses, varicose ulcers, or suppurating wounds.

CAPSULES/TABLETS Take 200mg 3 times daily for gastric or oesophageal inflammation or ulceration or chronic indigestion. Take 1 tablet or capsule before a journey to allay travel sickness.

HOW TO SOURCE

GROW Prefers moist, deep soil in full sun. Usually propagated by seed sown in autumn, from suckers, or from semi-ripe cuttings in summer. Not generally grown in gardens. Susceptible to pests, fungal infections, and Dutch elm disease.

FORAGE Planted as a street tree in parts of the USA, but rarely cultivated elsewhere, and unlikely to be found in the wild outside its native habitat. Stocks have been depleted by elm leaf beetle and Dutch elm disease, so great care needs to be taken when gathering the bark to avoid damaging trees further.

HARVEST Strip the inner bark from the trunks and branches of mature trees in spring.

CAUTION Availability of the whole bark is restricted in some countries.

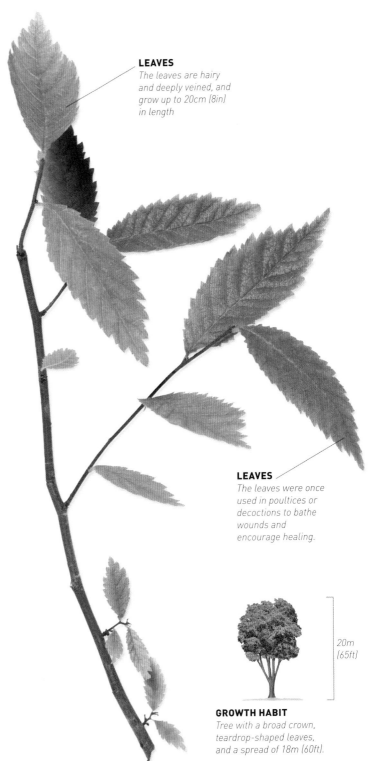

LEAVES
The leaves are hairy and deeply veined, and grow up to 20cm (8in) in length

LEAVES
The leaves were once used in poultices or decoctions to bathe wounds and encourage healing.

20m
(65ft)

GROWTH HABIT
Tree with a broad crown, teardrop-shaped leaves, and a spread of 18m (60ft).

Urtica dioica **Nettle**

Found throughout the temperate regions of Europe and Asia, the stinging nettle is an all-too-familiar weed that thrives in the rich soil of cultivated land. The "sting" is caused by hairs on the plant that contain histamine and formic acid. Nettles are said to rob the soil of its minerals and vitamins by absorbing them and concentrating them in its leaves, so becoming highly nutritious.

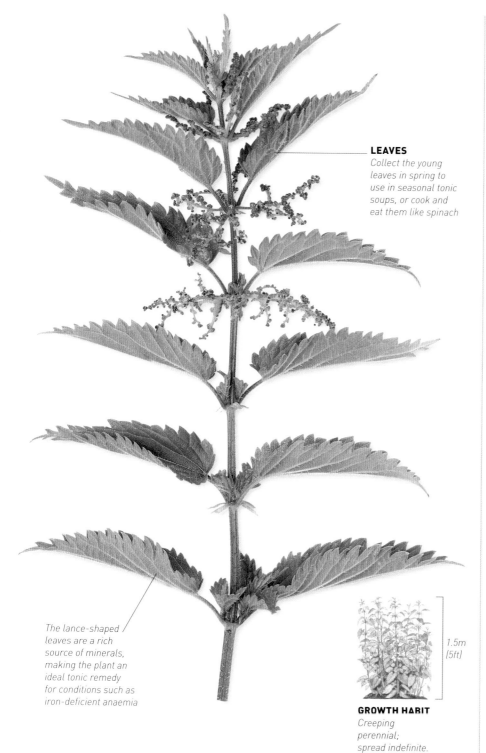

LEAVES
Collect the young leaves in spring to use in seasonal tonic soups, or cook and eat them like spinach

The lance-shaped leaves are a rich source of minerals, making the plant an ideal tonic remedy for conditions such as iron-deficient anaemia

GROWTH HABIT
Creeping perennial; spread indefinite.

1.5m (5ft)

PARTS USED Aerial parts, root
MAIN CONSTITUENTS Amines (histamine, acetylcholine, choline, serotonin), flavonoids, formic acid, glucoquinones, minerals (incl. silica and iron), vitamins A, B, and C, tannins
ACTIONS Astringent, diuretic, tonic, nutritive, haemostatic, circulatory stimulant, galactogogue, hypotensive, antiscorbutic, anti-allergenic

HOW TO USE

JUICE Pulverize or process the whole fresh plant to obtain juice. Take in 10ml (2 tsp) doses 3 times daily as a tonic for debilitated conditions and anaemia.
INFUSION Take 1 cup of standard infusion (p.168) of leaves 3 times daily as part of a cleansing regime in arthritis, rheumatism, gout, and eczema, or use as a final hair rinse for dandruff.
CREAM/OINTMENT Use for minor cuts and grazes, skin rashes including eczema, or piles.
FRESH LEAVES AND STEMS Lashing arthritic joints (urtication) is an uncomfortable but traditional remedy with some recent studies showing its efficacy.
COMPRESS Use a pad soaked in a strong infusion or diluted tincture of leaves to relieve pain in arthritis, gout, neuralgia, sprains, tendonitis, and sciatica.
TINCTURE Take 2–4ml (40–80 drops) of the leaf tincture 3 times daily for allergic skin conditions and hay fever. Take 2–4ml (40–80 drops) of the root tincture 3 times daily for benign prostatic hypertrophy.

HOW TO SOURCE

GROW It is not usually necessary to cultivate nettles, as they grow freely in the wild.
FORAGE Found growing in hedgerows, waste areas, and scrub.
HARVEST Gather aerial parts when in flower. Dig up roots in autumn, and young leaves in spring.

CAUTION Wear rubber gloves when harvesting the plant.

Vaccinium myrtillus **Bilberry**

Native to temperate regions of Europe and Asia, bilberry is closely related to the North American blueberry. It has become renowned as a "superfood" thanks to the potent antioxidant proanthocyanidins contained in the fruit. Bilberry jam was eaten by fighter pilots during World War II as it was believed to improve night vision.

PARTS USED Fruit, leaves
MAIN CONSTITUENTS Tannins, sugars, fruit acids, anthocyanosides, glucoquinone, glycosides, vitamin A
ACTIONS Astringent, hypoglycaemic, tonic, antiseptic, anti-emetic, anti-inflammatory, diuretic, venous tonic

HOW TO USE

MOUTHWASH Use 1 cup of a standard infusion (p.168) of the leaves as a gargle or mouthwash for mouth ulcers and throat inflammations; 10ml (2 tsp) of the fresh berry juice diluted in 120ml (4fl oz) of water can be used in the same way.
LOTION Mix 30ml (1fl oz) of unsweetened berry juice with 30ml (1fl oz) of distilled witch hazel and use as a cooling lotion for sunburn and other skin inflammations.
DECOCTION Use 1 cup of a standard dried berry decoction daily for chronic diarrhoea.
FRESH RAW BERRIES Eat a large bowl of fresh berries with sugar and milk or cream for constipation.
INFUSION Take 1 cup of a standard infusion (p.168) of the leaves 3 times daily to support dietary control in late-onset, non-insulin dependent diabetes mellitus.

HOW TO SOURCE

GROW Prefers moist, very acid soil (pH5.5 or less) in sun or partial shade and water, as it is shallow-rooted. Sow seeds in a cold frame in autumn and transplant to final growing positions when large enough. Or propagate by semi-ripe cuttings in summer. Prune in spring to encourage bushy growth. Grow in a sheltered position. Best grown in large containers in alkaline soil areas.
FORAGE Grows wild in acidic, poor soil such as peat bogs, moors, and similar areas in temperate and sub-arctic regions.
HARVEST Gather the leaves in spring and the fruits when ripe in late summer.

CAUTION Insulin-dependent diabetics should not use bilberry leaf teas without professional guidance. Do not use the leaves for more than four weeks.

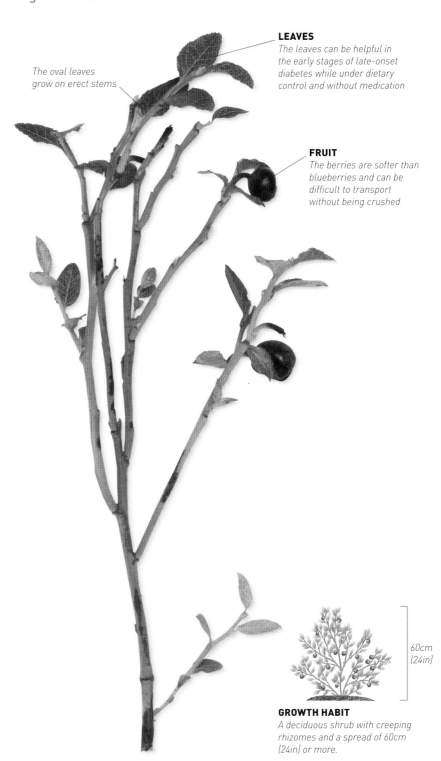

The oval leaves grow on erect stems

LEAVES
The leaves can be helpful in the early stages of late-onset diabetes while under dietary control and without medication

FRUIT
The berries are softer than blueberries and can be difficult to transport without being crushed

60cm (24in)

GROWTH HABIT
A deciduous shrub with creeping rhizomes and a spread of 60cm (24in) or more.

Verbena officinalis **Vervain**

Once regarded as a cure-all, and sacred to the ancient Greeks, Romans, and Druids, vervain – which grows throughout much of Europe, Asia, and North Africa – is associated with a wealth of folklore and was once used in fortune-telling. Today it is a favourite after-dinner "tisane" to stimulate the digestion, and is also used to ease headaches, nervous tension, and depression.

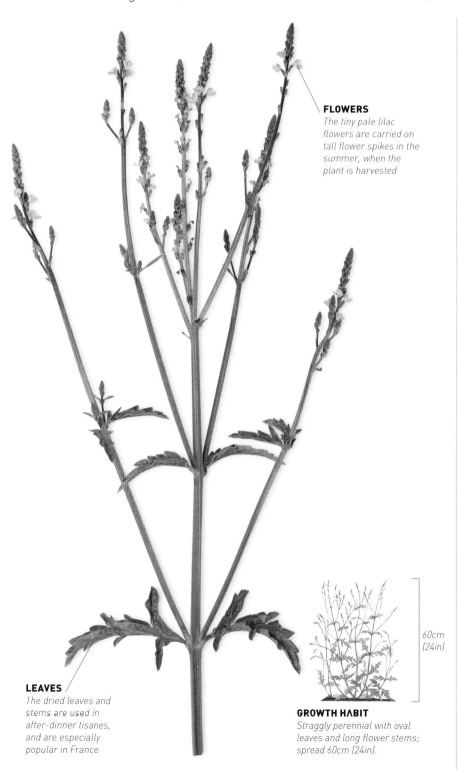

FLOWERS
The tiny pale lilac flowers are carried on tall flower spikes in the summer, when the plant is harvested

LEAVES
The dried leaves and stems are used in after-dinner tisanes, and are especially popular in France

GROWTH HABIT
Straggly perennial with oval leaves and long flower stems; spread 60cm (24in).

60cm (24in)

PARTS USED Aerial parts
MAIN CONSTITUENTS Volatile oil (incl. citral), bitter iridoids (incl. verbenin and verbenalin), alkaloids, tannins
ACTIONS Relaxant tonic, galactagogue, diaphoretic, nervine, sedative, antispasmodic, hepatic restorative, laxative, uterine stimulant, cholagogue

HOW TO USE

TINCTURE Take 2–4ml (40–80 drops) 3 times daily for nervous exhaustion, stress, anxiety, or depression; as a liver stimulant for sluggish digestion, toxic conditions, or jaundice; and with other urinary herbs for stones and excess uric acid.
INFUSION Take 1 cup of a standard infusion (p.168) of the aerial parts 3 times daily as a digestive stimulant, or in feverish conditions; take 1 cup at night for insomnia.
CREAM/OINTMENT Use on eczema, wounds, and running sores or for painful neuralgia.
FLOWER REMEDY Dilute 2 drops in 10ml (2 tsp) of water in a dropper bottle and take in drop doses as required for mental stress and over exertion with related insomnia and an inability to relax.

HOW TO SOURCE

GROW Prefers a sunny site in well-drained soil, but tolerates other conditions. Sow the seeds in a seed bed in spring or autumn and transplant (60cm/24in apart) when established, or propagate by division in late spring. Self-seeds in the right conditions.
FORAGE An inconspicuous plant that is easily missed, it can be found growing wild, mainly in hedgerows and dry grassy areas, throughout its native region and elsewhere. Collect the aerial parts while flowering in summer.
HARVEST Traditionally collected when the plant is in flower.

CAUTION Avoid in pregnancy. May cause vomiting if taken in excess.

Viburnum opulus **Crampbark**

As with many plants, the common name of this herb aptly describes its properties. It is effective at treating cramping and spasmodic pains affecting both smooth and skeletal muscles – so, for example, it is a useful treatment for colic as well as for leg cramps. Native to Europe, northern Asia, and North America, the shrub is an attractive and popular garden plant.

PARTS USED Bark
MAIN CONSTITUENTS Bitter (viburnin), valerianic acid, tannins, coumarins, saponins
ACTIONS Antispasmodic, sedative, astringent, muscle relaxant, cardiac tonic, sedative, anti-inflammatory

HOW TO USE

TINCTURE Take 5ml (1 tsp) 3 times daily as a relaxant for nervous or muscular tension, or for colicky pains affecting the digestive tract or urinary system. Add 1ml (20 drops) to remedies for IBS or combine with rhubarb root for constipation.
DECOCTION Take ½–1 cup of a standard decoction (p.168) every 3–4 hours for period pain or colic. Can also be used with other remedies for excessive menstrual bleeding associated with the menopause.
CREAM/LOTION Use regularly for muscle cramps, including night cramps in the legs, or for shoulder tension.
MASSAGE RUB Use the macerated oil as a basis for massage rubs for muscular aches and pains associated with cramps and spasm. Add 10 drops of lavender, thyme, or rosemary essential oil to 5ml (1 tsp) of the macerated oil.

HOW TO SOURCE

GROW Prefers moist yet well-drained soil in sun or dappled shade, and can be a useful addition to a hedge or woodland garden. Propagate by softwood cuttings in summer, or plant seed as soon as it is ripe and over-winter in a cold frame or unheated greenhouse.
FORAGE May be found growing in woodlands in Europe or North America. As always when collecting bark, it is important not to damage the bush. Only harvest a small amount from each shrub.
HARVEST Bark from the branches is collected in spring and summer when the plant is flowering.

CAUTION Avoid during pregnancy except under professional supervision.

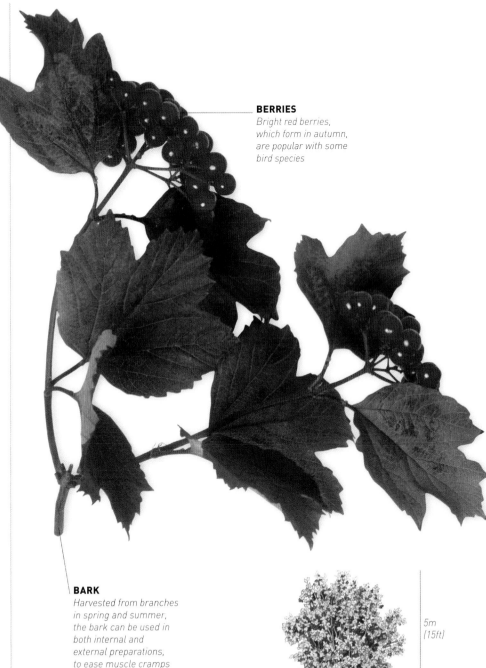

BERRIES
Bright red berries, which form in autumn, are popular with some bird species

BARK
Harvested from branches in spring and summer, the bark can be used in both internal and external preparations, to ease muscle cramps

5m (15ft)

GROWTH HABIT
Vigorous, bushy shrub with lace-capped white flowers in spring; spread 4m (12ft).

Viola tricolor **Heartsease**

The name "heartsease" is reputedly derived from its use in medieval love potions, although it was also once used for heart problems. Also known as wild pansy, the herb is native to Europe, North Africa, and temperate regions of Asia. Today it is mainly used for skin disorders and coughs, as well as making an attractive garnish in cooking.

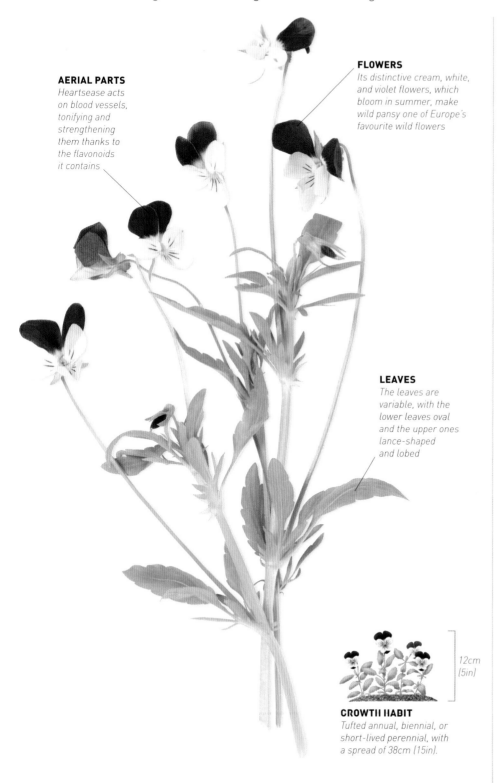

AERIAL PARTS
Heartsease acts on blood vessels, tonifying and strengthening them thanks to the flavonoids it contains

FLOWERS
Its distinctive cream, white, and violet flowers, which bloom in summer, make wild pansy one of Europe's favourite wild flowers

LEAVES
The leaves are variable, with the lower leaves oval and the upper ones lance-shaped and lobed

GROWTH HABIT
Tufted annual, biennial, or short-lived perennial, with a spread of 38cm (15in).

12cm (5in)

PARTS USED Aerial parts
MAIN CONSTITUENTS Saponin, salicylates, flavonoids (incl. rutin), volatile oil, mucilage
ACTIONS Expectorant, anti-inflammatory, diuretic, antirheumatic, laxative, stabilizes capillary membranes

HOW TO USE

CREAM/OINTMENT Use regularly for skin rashes, eczema, nappy rash, or cradle cap.
INFUSION Take 1 cup of a standard infusion (p.168) 3 times daily as a cleansing remedy for toxic conditions, or as a gentle stimulant for the circulation and immune system in rheumatic disorders, chronic skin conditions, urinary infections, and chronic infections.
WASH Use 1 cup of a standard, well-strained infusion (p.168) to bathe nappy rash, cradle cap, weeping sores, varicose ulcers, or oozing insect bites.
SYRUP Add 450g (1lb) of honey or sugar to 600ml (1 pint) of strained infusion, bring to the boil, and simmer gently for 5–10 minutes to form a syrup. Use in 5ml (1 tsp) doses to soothe bronchitis and asthma.
TINCTURE Take 5ml (1 tsp) in a little water 3 times daily for capillary fragility, urinary disorders, or skin disorders

HOW TO SOURCE

GROW Prefers moist but well-drained soil in full sun or dappled shade. Sow seeds in seed trays in a cold frame in summer or in spring when ripe; transplant to final positions when large enough to handle. Alternatively, take basal cuttings in spring or divide established clumps in autumn.
FORAGE Found in grassy places, such as meadows and waste ground. Gather in summer while flowering. The flowers are edible and can be added to salads or used to garnish pasta dishes.
HARVEST Collect all the aerial parts in summer.

CAUTION Very high doses may cause nausea due to the saponin content.

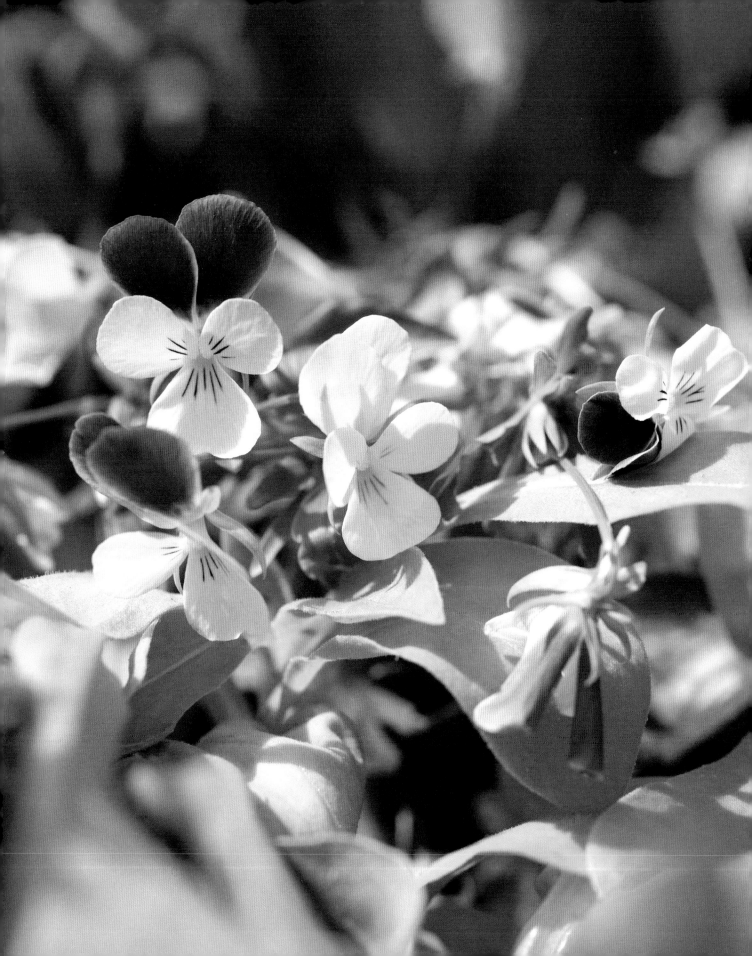

Viscum album **Mistletoe**

Traditionally associated with fertility rites, and significant in Norse legend as the only plant capable of killing the Norse god Baldur, mistletoe has been used as a cancer treatment since the days of the Druids. Some modern research has confirmed this action, although its most common use is to lower high blood pressure. It is native to Europe and northern Asia.

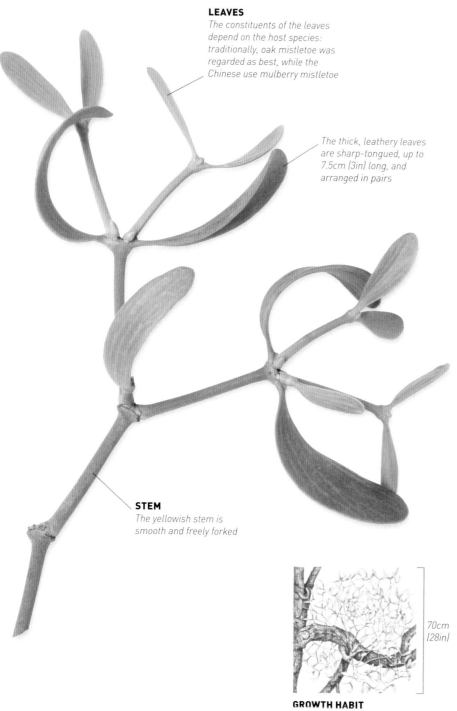

LEAVES
The constituents of the leaves depend on the host species: traditionally, oak mistletoe was regarded as best, while the Chinese use mulberry mistletoe

The thick, leathery leaves are sharp-tongued, up to 7.5cm (3in) long, and arranged in pairs

STEM
The yellowish stem is smooth and freely forked

70cm
(28in)

GROWTH HABIT
Bushy parasitic that grows on various trees; flowers appear in autumn and fruits in winter.

PARTS USED Leaves, branches, berries
MAIN CONSTITUENTS Alkaloids, glycoproteins, viscotoxin, flavonoids, acetylcholine, polysaccharides (berries)
ACTIONS Hypotensive, sedative, anti-inflammatory, diuretic, immune tonic

HOW TO USE

NB Use only under medical supervision
INFUSION Take ½–1 cup of a standard leaf infusion (p.168) 3 times daily for high blood pressure, petit mal, or to assist with withdrawal in benzodiazepine addiction. Combine with skullcap, valerian, or betony (*Stachys officinalis*) for nervous disorders. Take ½ cup of a half-strength infusion 3 times daily for panic attacks or headaches.
TINCTURE Best made from the fresh plant; take 10 drops 3 times a day to lower blood pressure.
FLUID EXTRACT Consult a herbalist for usage to strengthen the immune system during treatments for cancer, including after surgery and during radiotherapy.
BERRY EXTRACTS Used in anthroposophical medicine to treat cancer.

HOW TO SOURCE

GROW Encourage mistletoe to grow on garden trees by making a small incision in the bark and crushing freshly gathered ripe berries into the cut. The berries are ripe in late winter/early spring. Collect berries only from the same type of tree (i.e. mistletoe berries from an oak tree will usually only grow on another oak). Once established, the plant is spread to other parts of the tree by birds.
FORAGE Often found growing high up on deciduous trees, it can easily be seen in winter; use secateurs on an extendable pole to cut the stems in autumn.
HARVEST Gather leaves and branches in late autumn and ripe berries in late winter.

CAUTION Avoid during pregnancy. Can be toxic (especially the berries); take only under professional supervision.

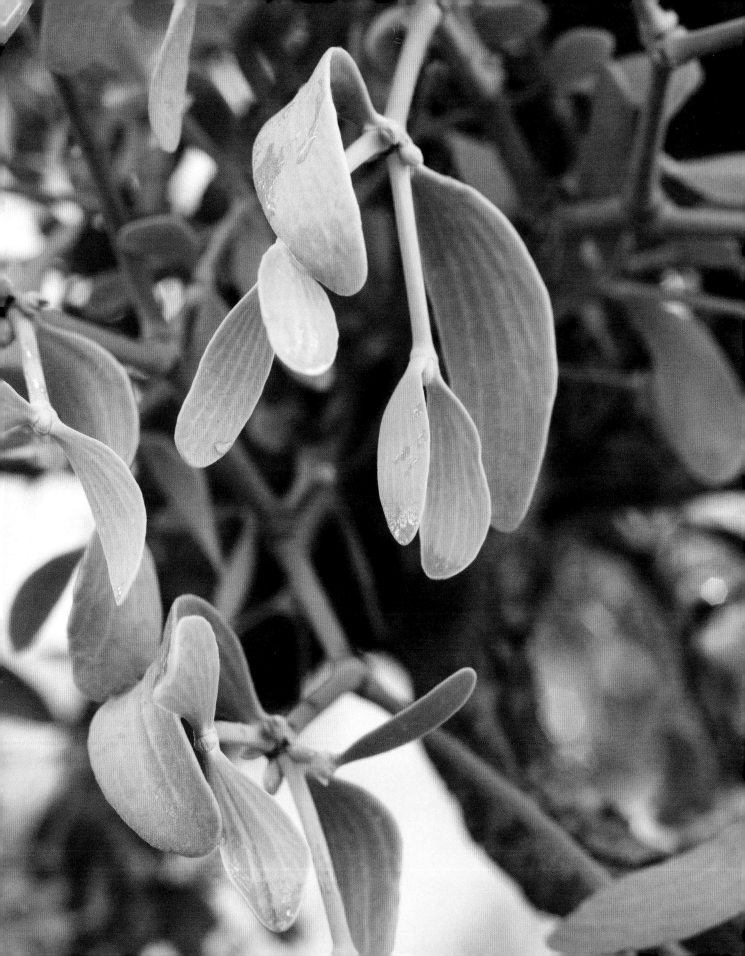

Vitex agnus-castus **Agnus castus**

Native to the Mediterranean region, agnus castus was known as the "chaste tree", while its berries were called "monk's pepper" – a reference to their medieval use as an anaphrodisiac to reduce the libido of celibate monks. The herb has the opposite effect on women, stimulating the production of female hormones, and is used for a wide range of gynaecological problems.

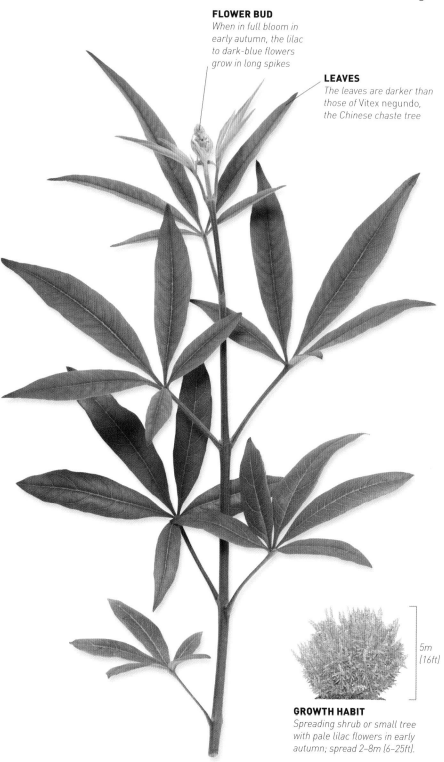

FLOWER BUD
When in full bloom in early autumn, the lilac to dark-blue flowers grow in long spikes

LEAVES
The leaves are darker than those of Vitex negundo, the Chinese chaste tree

5m (16ft)

GROWTH HABIT
Spreading shrub or small tree with pale lilac flowers in early autumn; spread 2–8m (6–25ft).

PARTS USED Fruit
MAIN CONSTITUENTS Iridoid glycosides (incl. aucubin and agnuside), volatile oil (incl. cineol), flavonoids, alkaloids (incl. viticine), bitter, fatty acids
ACTIONS Hormone regulator, progesterogenic, galactagogue

HOW TO USE

TINCTURE Take up to 2ml (40 drops) first thing in the morning during the second half of a menstrual cycle to stimulate hormone production in irregular menstrual cycles or PMS. It is easy to overdose, so start with a low dose and gradually increase the amount if there are no side effects (see Caution). It will also ease migraine or acne related to the menstrual cycle.
TABLETS/ CAPSULES Readily available commercially; follow the dosage directions on the pack and take to ease PMS.

HOW TO SOURCE

GROW Prefers well-drained soil in full sun and a warm site. Sow seeds in a cold frame in autumn or spring; transplant to 10cm (4in) pots when large enough to handle. Alternatively, take semi-ripe cuttings in summer. Grow on until well established before planting in permanent positions. Protect from cold, dry winds and severe winters. Prune in spring while still dormant.
FORAGE Generally cultivated, but can be found growing wild in southern Europe and naturalized in other sub-tropical regions. Can be confused with *Vitex negundo* (Chinese chaste tree), which has paler leaves and flowers and is native to India, Taiwan, and China. Does not always set seed to form berries in cooler climates.
HARVEST Gather ripe berries in autumn.

CAUTION Excess can cause formication – a sensation like ants crawling over the skin. Do not use if taking progesterone drugs. Avoid during pregnancy except under professional supervision.

Withania somnifera **Ashwagandha**

Also known as Indian ginseng, ashwagandha is found in the drier regions of India and the Middle East. The name translates as "that which has the smell of a horse" and the plant is traditionally associated with the strength and sexual energy of a stallion. Traditionally used as a tonic, modern research has shown it to have significant antitumour activity.

PARTS USED Root, leaves
MAIN CONSTITUENTS Alkaloids (incl. anaferine and isopelietierine), steroidal lactones (incl. withanolides and withaferins), saponins, iron
ACTIONS Tonic, nervine, sedative, adaptogen, anti-inflammatory, antitumour

HOW TO USE

POWDER/CAPSULES Take 250mg–1g of powdered root or capsule equivalent 3 times daily as a restorative tonic for over-work, exhaustion, sleep problems, and debility caused by chronic disease. Regular use can also help in degenerative disorders such as arthritis.
FLUID EXTRACT Take 2–4ml (40–80 drops) in water 3 times daily as an energy tonic, a calming remedy for insomnia, to nourish the blood in anaemia, or for stress or debility.
DECOCTION Take 1/2–1 cup of a decoction made from 1 tsp of dried root and 120ml (4fl oz) of milk or water simmered for 15 minutes for stress or exhaustion.

HOW TO SOURCE

GROW Prefers dry, stony soil in full sun. Sow seeds in spring in seed trays and transplant to 7.5cm (3in) pots when the seedlings are large enough to handle. Alternatively, propagate by heeled greenwood cuttings in late spring. Rarely seen cultivated in the West.
FORAGE Unlikely to be found growing wild outside its native region.
HARVEST The leaves are collected in spring and the root is dug in autumn.

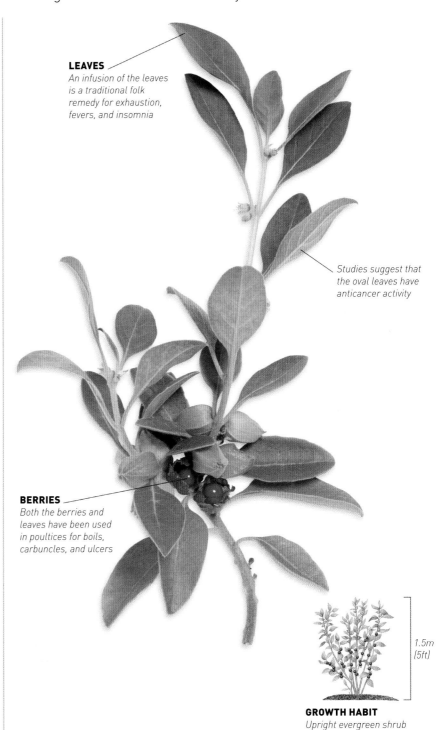

LEAVES
An infusion of the leaves is a traditional folk remedy for exhaustion, fevers, and insomnia

Studies suggest that the oval leaves have anticancer activity

BERRIES
Both the berries and leaves have been used in poultices for boils, carbuncles, and ulcers

1.5m (5ft)

GROWTH HABIT
Upright evergreen shrub with inconspicuous yellow flowers; spread 1m (3ft).

CAUTION Avoid during pregnancy.

Zea mays **Cornsilk**

Cultivated for 4,000 years both as a cereal crop and for fodder, maize was originally grown by the Aztecs and Mayans in South America and is now the continent's most widely grown crop. Cornsilk, used medicinally, consists of the brown whiskery parts of the styles and stigmas that can be seen at the top of the cobs, and is mainly used for urinary disorders.

FLOWER
The male inflorescence is called a tassel and is made up of many small flowers, while the female forms the cob and only the silky stigma can be seen

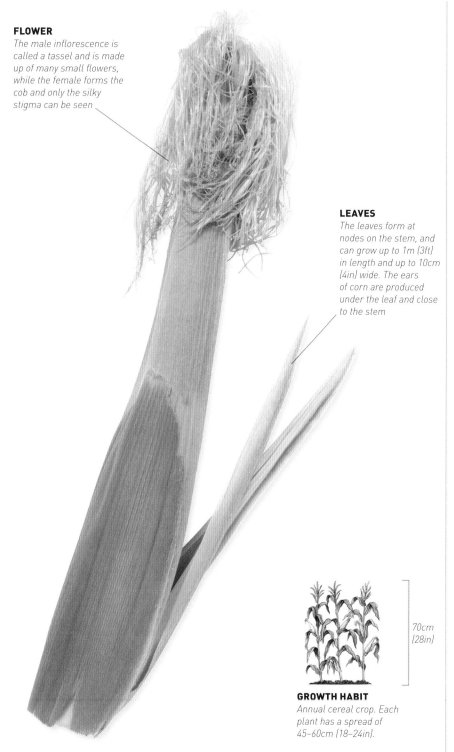

LEAVES
The leaves form at nodes on the stem, and can grow up to 1m (3ft) in length and up to 10cm (4in) wide. The ears of corn are produced under the leaf and close to the stem

70cm (28in)

GROWTH HABIT
Annual cereal crop. Each plant has a spread of 45–60cm (18–24in).

PARTS USED Styles and stigmas (cornsilk), maize meal
MAIN CONSTITUENTS Allantoin, saponins, flavonoids, mucilage, volatile oil, vitamins C and K, potassium
ACTIONS Diuretic, urinary demulcent, mild stimulant

HOW TO USE

INFUSION Generally regarded as more effective than the tincture. Take 1 cup of a standard infusion (p.168) up to 6 times daily for cystitis, urethritis, benign prostate gland enlargement, urinary retention, or urinary gravel.
TEA Combine 1 tsp each of dried cornsilk and agrimony with 1 cup of boiling water, infuse for 15 minutes, and strain. Give to children with bed-wetting problems; consult a herbalist for advice on dosage.
TINCTURE Take 5–10ml (1–2 tsp) 3 times daily for acute or chronic inflammation of the urinary system.
POULTICE Mix 2 tsp of powdered maize meal with a little water into a paste, spread on gauze, and use as a poultice for ulcers and boils.

HOW TO SOURCE

GROW Prefers moist but well-drained soil in full sun. Sow seeds directly in spring when the ground is not too wet. Can be grown in kitchen gardens and allotments with the ripe cobs used as a food.
FORAGE Maize is widely cultivated worldwide and cornsilk can be gleaned from standing crops just before harvest, as long as landowners do not object. Snip the brown whiskery parts of the styles and stigmas from the cob with scissors.
HARVEST The cornsilk is harvested with the ripe cobs in summer, then separated and dried.

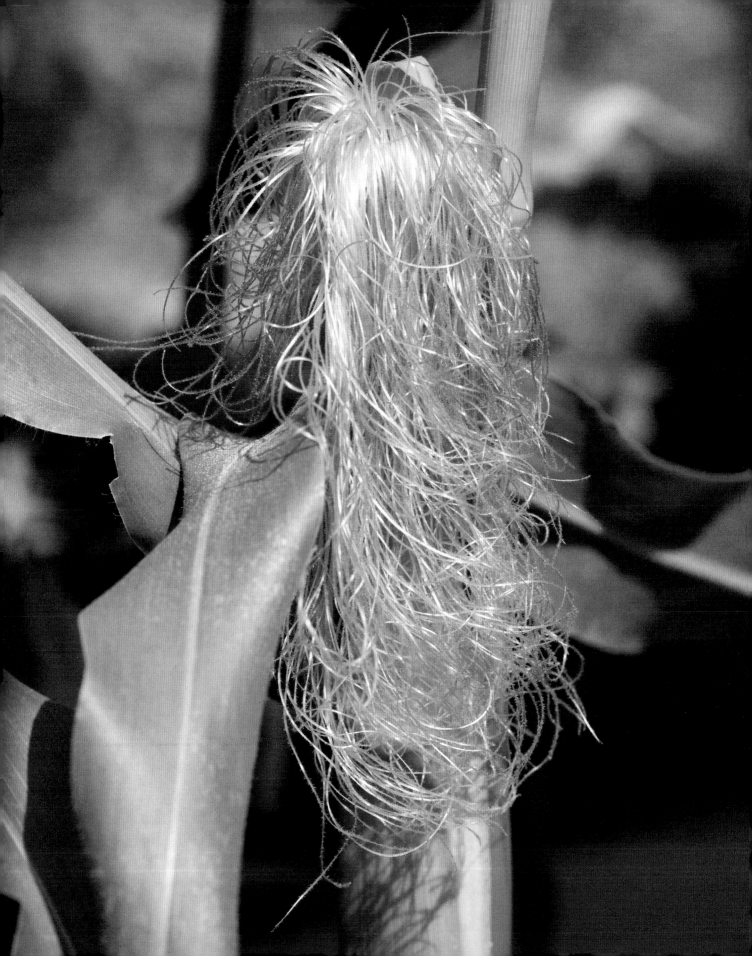

Use
Herbs

Learn how to use herbs to help treat **ten common health concerns.** For soothing skin complaints, settling digestion, combatting colds, and more, **discover how home-made herbal remedies** can help to heal **body and mind.**

✋ Healthy skin and hair

Our skin may form a wonderfully protective barrier against the outside world, but it is also a mirror of our inner health. Effective cleansing and care can maintain skin and hair health from the outside, but most skin problems require both internal and external remedies to effectively relieve and treat symptoms such as rashes, spots, and itching. This chart is not comprehensive, but it does contain the key herbs for skin health.

Herb	Action
Calendula *Calendula officinalis* (p.36)	A soothing herb that also stimulates healing of the skin. Take an infusion of the herb or dilute the tincture for abrasions, wounds, ulcers, or as a mouthwash. Use as a cream or macerated oil to relieve eczema, rashes, or sore skin.
Oats *Avena sativa* (p.33)	Cleansing and soothing, oats make a good alternative to soap or detergents for very sensitive skin. Grind oats to a powder and add to the bath water, or mix with a little water or oil to make a soothing mask or cleanser.
Chamomile *Matricaria recutita* (p.78)	Soothing and anti-inflammatory. Use cooled chamomile tea as a lotion to relieve any hot, inflamed skin condition (e.g. sunburn, hives, or rashes). Drink the tea, with its calming and anti-allergenic properties, to alleviate eczema, rashes, and so on.
Chickweed *Stellaria media* (p.107)	A wonderfully cooling and soothing herb for the skin, chickweed will relieve any irritation such as eczema, psoriasis, hives, or ulcers. Mash the fresh plant, adding a little boiling water, wrap in a muslin cloth, and apply once cold as a poultice to the skin.
Burdock root *Arctium lappa* (p.28)	One of the most effective cleansing herbs, which is used internally to treat chronic skin problems such as psoriasis, eczema, acne, persistent boils, ulcers, and so on. Combine with dandelion and make a decoction of the root, or take the tincture.
Lavender *Lavandula angustifolia* (p.72)	The soothing, anti-inflammatory, and antiseptic properties of lavender make it a very versatile herb. Use the essential oil or a cooled infusion to calm rashes, redness, eczema, sunburn, thrush, and so on.
Dandelion leaf *Taraxacum officinale* (p.110)	One of the best-known cleansing herbs, dandelion leaf can be combined with burdock and red clover and taken as an infusion three times a day for several weeks to help clear acne, eczema, psoriasis or problem skin.
Nettle *Urtica dioica* (p.120)	Taken internally as an infusion, nettles help to reduce inflammation and have an anti-allergenic action. Combine with chamomile for urticaria (hives) or any itchy rash. Allow the infusion to cool and use as an excellent final rinse for dandruff or psoriasis of the scalp.
Thyme *Thymus vulgaris* (p.112)	An effective antiseptic and antifungal herb. Dilute the essential oil in a base oil to treat fungal infections such as ringworm, thrush, and athlete's foot. Make a strong infusion to use as a lotion to prevent infection, for example in wounds, ulcers, or gum disease.
Red clover *Trifolium pratense* (p.115)	A cleansing herb that promotes healing of the skin. Combine with dandelion and burdock and drink as an infusion or as tinctures to help clear eczema, psoriasis, recurrent boils, or any chronic skin disease.

Recipes

▪ Aloe and elderflower body scrub
(see page 381)

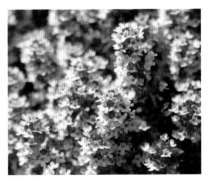

Thyme *Thymus vulgaris*

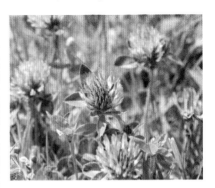

Red clover *Trifolium pratense*

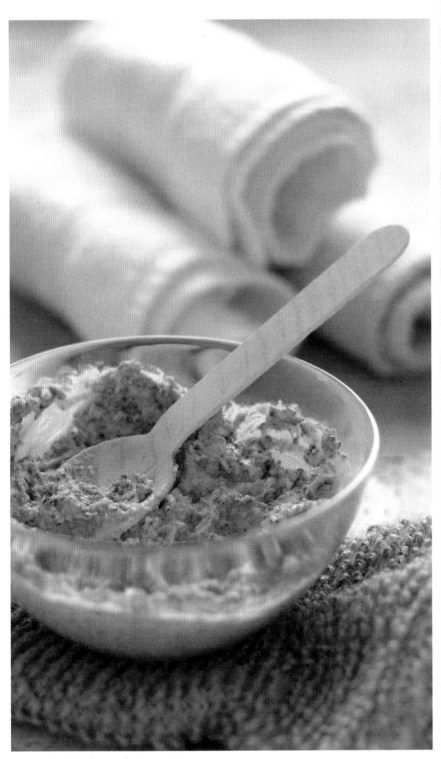

Aloe and elderflower body scrub

Digestion

Careless eating habits, drugs, emotional upsets, and stress can all trigger a variety of symptoms, so keeping the digestive system in good working order is essential to our well-being and is the foundation of good health. If any symptoms worsen or are persistent, seek professional advice, as they may mask a more serious underlying complaint. This chart is not comprehensive, but it does contain the key herbs for digestive health.

Herb	Action
Fennel *Foeniculum vulgare* (p.57)	A gentle digestive stimulant suitable for delicate stomachs. Chew a few seeds or make an infusion to dispel wind, griping pains, and colic.
Peppermint *Mentha x piperita* (p.82)	A versatile herb for the effective relief of a range of digestive complaints. Drink as an infusion for symptoms of indigestion, flatulence, travel sickness, colic, nausea, and vomiting. Essential oil capsules are used to treat IBS.
Chamomile *Matricaria recutita* (p.78)	A gentle herb that calms digestive problems. Drink an infusion or use the tincture to relieve indigestion, gastrointestinal spasm, and "nervous" tummy. This herb is a favourite remedy for babies and children.
Meadowsweet *Filipendula ulmaria* (p.56)	A natural antacid that will relieve the symptoms of a range of gastrointestinal problems associated with flatulence or hyperacidity. Drink an infusion to treat wind, peptic ulcers, reflux, mild diarrhoea, and gastritis.
Lemon balm *Melissa officinalis* (p.81)	A wonderfully soothing and gentle herb for an overwrought digestive system in both adults and children. Drink an infusion to relieve colic, flatulence, stomach cramps, and any stress-related digestive symptoms.
Liquorice *Glycyrrhiza glabra* (p.62)	Soothing to the digestive tract and mildly laxative. Combine with chamomile and meadowsweet and take as an infusion for symptoms of indigestion, acidity, and gastritis, or combine with senna to relieve constipation.
Marshmallow *Althaea officinalis* (p.23)	Soothes inflammation of the entire digestive tract. Combine with chamomile and drink as an infusion to relieve symptoms of acidity or discomfort or irritation of the mouth, stomach, or duodenum.
Slippery elm *Ulmus rubra* (p.119)	Adds a protective and healing coating to the digestive tract. Mix the herb with a little water and drink the resulting paste to relieve symptoms of acidity, reflux, gastritis, gastroenteritis, and diarrhoea.
Ginger *Zingiber officinale*	Acts as an antispasmodic and anti-emetic: use to relieve symptoms of flatulence, colic, nausea, irritable bowel, hiccups, and vomiting. It is also anti-inflammatory and antiseptic, so is beneficial for gastrointestinal infections.
Senna *Senna alexandrina* (p.105)	A stimulant laxative that will relieve occasional constipation. Make an infusion to drink at bedtime that will stimulate a bowel motion the following morning. Adding a little liquorice or ginger powder will help prevent any griping pain.

Recipes

▨ Peppermint and thyme tincture
(see page 373)

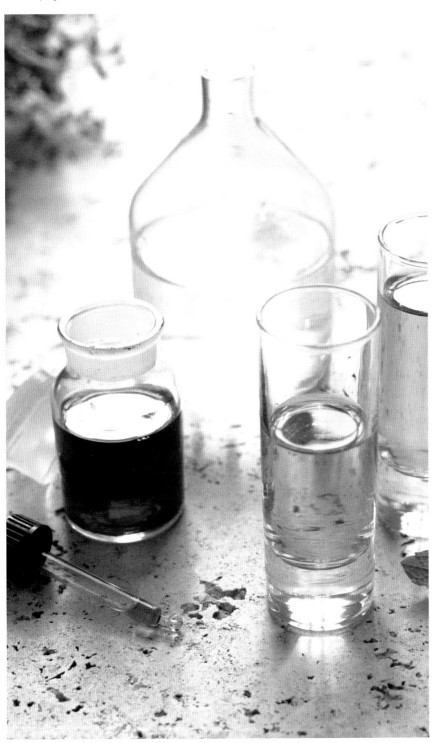

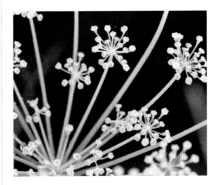

Fennel *Foeniculum vulgare*

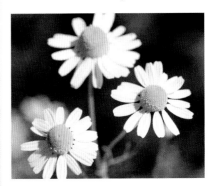

Chamomile *Matricaria recutita*

Peppermint and thyme tinture

● Circulation

Cardiovascular disease is caused by lack of exercise, obesity, diets that are rich in saturated fats, smoking, and excessive stress. Improving your diet and regular exercise helps, as can simple herbal remedies to reduce cholesterol levels and alleviate stress. If you take medication, seek medical advice first. This chart is not comprehensive, but it does contain the key herbs for improving circulation.

Herb	Action
Nettle *Urtica dioica (p.120)*	Nettle tea is an excellent iron tonic in the treatment of anaemia. It helps to lower blood pressure when combined with hawthorn and lime flowers, and is a traditional remedy for varicose veins when combined with motherwort and melilot.
Ginger *Zingiber officinale*	An effective circulatory stimulant and vasodilator that has an anti-cholesterol action. Add powdered ginger to hot water, or take the tincture or capsules, to relieve cold hands and feet and to support the treatment of atherosclerosis.
Hawthorn *Crataegus laevigata (p.44)*	Traditionally used as a restorative for the heart and circulation, hawthorn helps to regulate heartbeat and high blood pressure. Take it as an infusion, tincture, or as capsules.
Yarrow *Achillea millefolium (p.12)*	Combined with lime flowers and hawthorn as a tea or tincture, yarrow will reduce high blood pressure and treat arteriosclerosis. Soak a cotton wool pad in the diluted tincture or cooled tea to stop a nosebleed.
Lime flowers *Tilia cordata (p.114)*	Helps to relieve the stress and tension associated with high blood pressure, and also used to treat hardening of the arteries and relieve headaches associated with high blood pressure. Often combined with hawthorn and taken as an infusion or tincture.
Garlic *Allium sativum (p.19)*	Helps prevent the build-up of cholesterol and has an anticoagulant action that is beneficial in thrombosis and arteriosclerosis. Eat garlic raw or take the juice or capsules.
Rosemary *Rosmarinus officinalis (p.96)*	A circulatory tonic traditionally used to strengthen the heart, improve varicose veins, and help prevent arteriosclerosis. Combine with lime flowers as an infusion to relieve headaches associated with high blood pressure.
Ginkgo *Ginkgo biloba (p.61)*	A circulatory stimulant and peripheral vasodilator. Combine with hawthorn to treat coronary artery disease. Combine with yarrow to treat varicose veins. Combine with ginger to treat cold extremities, intermittent claudication, and chilblains.
Goji *Lycium barbarum (p.77)*	A traditional Chinese tonic, believed to promote long life. The berries, now thought of as a "superfood" in the West, are a tonic for the circulatory system and blood, and can relieve dizziness and tinnitus. The root relaxes the artery muscles and lowers blood pressure.
Witch hazel *Hamamelis virginiana (p.63)*	Soak a cotton wool pad in distilled witch hazel and apply locally to relieve the heat, inflammation, and itching of varicose veins, piles (haemorrhoids), phlebitis, and chilblains.

Recipes

- Lime flower and hawthorn berry tincture
  (see page 375)

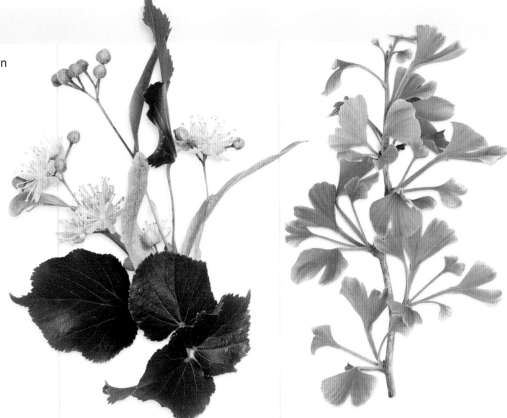

Lime flower *Tilia cordata*

Ginkgo *Ginkgo biloba*

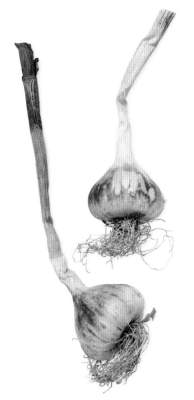

Garlic *Allium sativum*

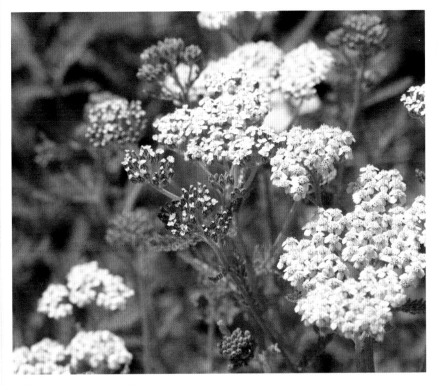

Yarrow *Achillea millefolium*

⚲ Women's health

Herbs can help treat a range of problems associated with menstruation (such as painful or heavy periods), premenstrual syndrome, boosting fertility, vaginal infections, and menopausal symptoms. For persistent problems, consult an experienced herbalist. This chart is not comprehensive, but it does contain the key herbs for women's health. Do not use the herbs listed during pregnancy without checking their appropriateness.

Herb	Action
Lady's mantle *Alchemilla xanthochlora (p.18)*	An astringent herb that is a menstrual regulator. Use to relieve heavy and painful periods: combine with shepherd's purse and raspberry leaf and drink as an infusion three times a day. Or use a cooled infusion as a douche for vaginal inflammation, thrush, or pruritis.
Chamomile *Matricaria recutita (p.78)*	A soothing and antispasmodic herb with a multitude of uses. As an infusion or tincture, it can help to relieve painful periods and alleviate stress. A cooled infusion or diluted essential oil can be used externally to relieve vaginal itching or irritation.
Raspberry leaf *Rubus idaeus (p.97)*	An astringent and toning herb with a special affinity for the uterus. Drink as an infusion to relieve heavy or painful periods.
Chaste berry *Vitex agnus-castus (p.128)*	A hormonal regulator used in the treatment of an irregular menstrual cycle, symptoms of premenstrual syndrome, and to relieve symptoms of the menopause. It is often used in the treatment of polycystic ovary syndrome (PCOS). Most often used as a tincture.
St John's wort *Hypericum perforatum (p.68)*	An effective antidepressant herb, proven to relieve symptoms of mild or moderate depression. Also important for anxiety and stress, it can be helpful for premenstrual syndrome and emotional problems arising during the menopause.
Rose *Rosa x damascena (p.94)*	A soothing, uplifting, and balancing herb and essential oil. Take as an infusion combined with motherwort for stress or headaches associated with premenstrual syndrome or the menopause. Use a cooled infusion or essential oil to soothe vaginal dryness and irritation.
Chinese angelica *Angelica sinensis*	An essential women's tonic herb of traditional Chinese medicine, Chinese angelica is taken to increase vitality and libido, treat infertility, regulate periods, and for anaemia due to blood loss. Take as a tincture or add to soups.
Schisandra *Schisandra chinensis*	An excellent Chinese tonic herb and restorative. It is helpful for night sweats and as a tonic to support the body through menopause. It also helps to improve stamina, fatigue, and physical stress. Best taken as a tincture.
Black cohosh *Actaea racemosa (p.14)*	A North American herb traditionally used for gynaecological complaints. It helps to relieve pain and is used for painful periods and the bloating and discomfort associated with premenstrual syndrome. Combine with sage to relieve menopausal symptoms.
Vervain *Verbena officinalis (p.122)*	An antispasmodic herb that helps to relieve pain, stress, and tension. Use for headaches associated with periods or during the menopause, premenstrual syndrome, scanty periods, and nervous exhaustion. Best taken as an infusion or tincture.

Recipes

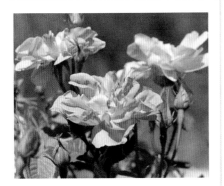

Damask rose *Rosa* x *damascena*

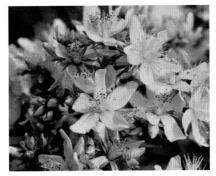

St John's wort *Hypericum perforatum*

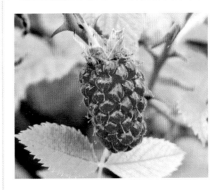

Raspberry *Rubus idaeus*

- Jasmine and lemon grass tea
  (see page 366)
- Goji berry and damiana tea
  (see page 366)
- Rose petal syrup
  (see page 370)

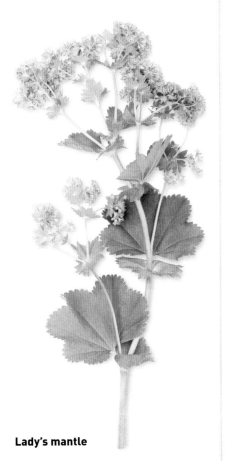

Lady's mantle

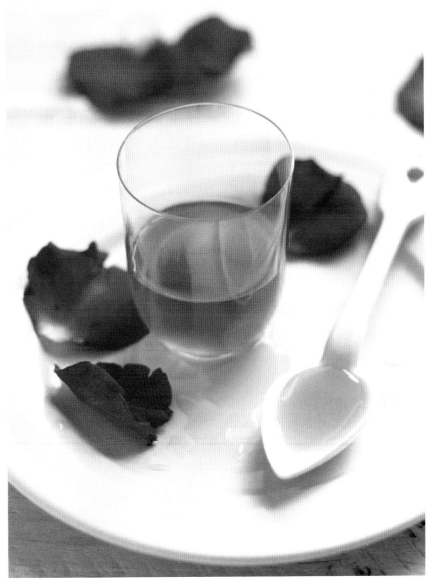

Rose petal syrup

⚲ Men's health

In the West we tend to look to herbs to treat specific problems (unlike traditional Chinese medicine, where herbs are recognized for their virtues as energy tonics), and modern research is backing up the benefits of certain herbs to deal with prostate health, infertility, erectile dysfunction, and stress. If any symptoms worsen or are persistent, seek medical advice. This chart is not comprehensive, but it does contain the key herbs for men's health.

Herb	Action
Saw palmetto *Serenoa repens*	Proven to relieve the symptoms of an enlarged prostate by reducing elevated testosterone levels. It acts as an antiseptic diuretic in the treatment of cystitis or urethritis. Traditionally used as a male aphrodisiac, and to treat infertility. Best taken as a tincture or capsules.
Ginkgo *Ginkgo biloba (p.61)*	Proven to stimulate peripheral circulation. It has a direct effect on the blood flow to the penile arteries and veins, and is used in the treatment of erectile dysfunction and impotence. Combine with cinnamon in an infusion, or drink the tincture regularly for a few months.
Damiana *Turnera diffusa*	Acts as an antidepressant and energy tonic and helps to combat chronic exhaustion and anxiety. It is also used to treat premature ejaculation, impotence, and a loss of interest in sex. Take in combination with other appropriate herbs as an infusion or tinctures.
Ashwagandha *Withania somnifera* *(p.129)*	A traditional energy tonic from the Ayurvedic tradition, this herb is used to combat stress and as an aphrodisiac. Used in the treatment of chronic stress, anaemia, impotence, and infertility. Best taken as a tincture or capsules.
Ginseng *Panax ginseng (p.86)*	The most famous of all energy or "chi" tonics from the Chinese tradition, ginseng has a long tradition as an aphrodisiac and to generally improve stamina and boost natural immunity and resistance to stress. Best taken as capsules, a tincture, or in soups.
Goji berries *Lycium barbarum* *(p.77)*	Goji berries have established a reputation in the West as a "superfood", and are used in traditional Chinese medicine as a blood tonic and to promote longevity. Eat the berries or combine the tincture with damiana as an energy tonic and as an aphrodisiac.
Schisandra *Schisandra chinensis*	A major tonic herb that acts to protect the liver, it is also frequently used as a sexual tonic and aphrodisiac. Combine with ginkgo to improve concentration, or with damiana to treat stress, erectile dysfunction, or loss of interest in sex. Best taken as a tincture.
Gotu kola *Centella asiatica* *(p.40)*	A herb from the Ayurvedic tradition that is used as a tonic and to revitalize. Combine with ginkgo to improve memory and concentration and help erectile dysfunction, or with other aphrodisiac herbs to improve libido and general energy levels. Take as an infusion or tincture.
Nettle root *Urtica dioica (p.120)*	Several studies have shown the root of this versatile herb to be of value in the relief of benign prostate hypertrophy (enlargement). Combine with saw palmetto and take as a decoction or tinctures.
Pumpkin seeds *Cucurbita* spp.	Pumpkin seeds are a rich source of zinc, which is essential for reproductive health and for a healthy prostate and bladder in particular. Eat a few of the seeds every day, or take the cold-pressed oil, which is also an excellent source of omega fatty acids.

Recipes

- Jasmine and lemon grass tea
  (see page 366)

- Goji berry and damiana tea
  (see page 366)

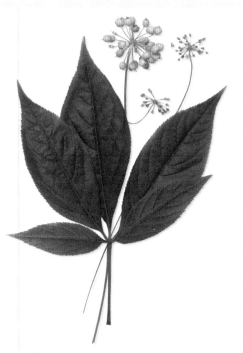

Ginseng *Panax ginseng*

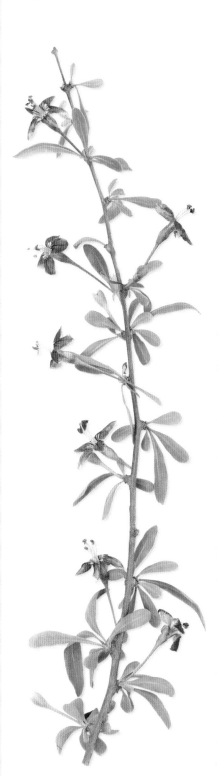

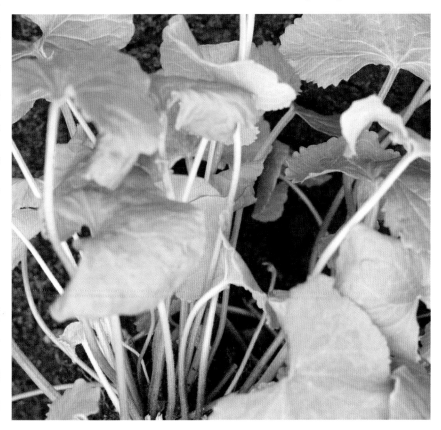

Gotu kola *Centella asiatica*

Goji *Lycium barbarum*

🖌 Coughs and colds

Early treatment is the key to preventing coughs, colds, and flu from becoming too serious or developing complications. This chart is not comprehensive, but it does contain key herbs that help to combat a fever, reduce catarrh or inflammation, and boost natural immunity. They work best if you take the opportunity to rest and reduce excess stress in your life. If symptoms become serious or do not clear up in a couple of days, seek medical advice.

Herb	Action
Garlic *Allium sativum (p.19)*	An excellent respiratory antiseptic and anticatarrhal. Take for all types of chest infections, bronchitis, colds, flu, ear infections, and for excess catarrh. Add to food or take capsules or make a cough syrup.
Mullein *Verbascum thapsus*	A soothing expectorant for irritating coughs, tracheitis, and bronchitis. Helps to dispel excess catarrh. Combine with coltsfoot and take as an infusion. The macerated oil is a traditional remedy for earache: place on cotton wool and position in the outer ear.
Yarrow *Achillea millefolium (p.12)*	Reduces the fever of colds and flu by promoting sweating, and also boosts natural immunity. It can be made into a traditional cold and flu tea when combined with elderflower and peppermint; drink three times a day. Avoid during pregnancy.
Echinacea *Echinacea purpurea (p.50)*	A natural antibiotic and immune booster, echinacea has been proven to shorten the duration of colds and flu. Best taken as a tincture, and combines well with elderberry. Use for coughs, colds, flu, earache, sore throats, and any infection or viruses.
Eucalyptus *Eucalyptus globulus (p.53)*	A native Australian tree renowned for its antibacterial, decongestant, and immune-boosting properties. Add the leaves to hot water or use the essential oil and use as a steam inhalation or chest salve for colds, flu, catarrh, sinusitis, coughs, bronchitis, asthma, and throat infections.
Elecampane *Inula helenium*	An important herb for chest complaints, as it clears mucus off the chest and has a warming and tonic effect on the lungs. It is also antibacterial, so is great for lung infections. Use to treat any chest infection, bronchitis, asthma, or chronic cough. Take as a decoction or tincture.
Liquorice *Glycyrrhiza glabra (p.62)*	An anti-inflammatory and expectorant herb, liquorice is well loved in Chinese and European medicine. Add liquorice powder or tincture to combinations of other appropriate herbs for coughs, catarrh, respiratory infections, and bronchitis.
Thyme *Thymus vulgaris (p.112)*	A highly effective respiratory antiseptic and expectorant herb useful for infections that involve coughing. Used to treat throat and chest infections, bronchitis, pleurisy, and whooping cough. Take as an infusion or combine the tincture with other appropriate herbs.
Sage *Salvia officinalis (p.100)*	An astringent and tonic herb that is excellent for the relief of sore throats. Use as an infusion or tincture to drink or gargle for sore throats, tonsillitis, laryngitis, and mouth or gum problems. Avoid during pregnancy.
Elderberry *Sambucus nigra (p.102)*	A traditional remedy for both adults and children in the prevention and treatment of colds, coughs, and sore throats. Has an antiviral and immune-boosting action and is proven to shorten the duration of colds and flu. Take as a decoction, syrup, or tincture.

Recipes

- Chrysanthemum and elderflower tea
  (see page 367)

- Blackberry and lime cordial
  (see page 369)

- Elderberry and liquorice tincture
  (see page 374)

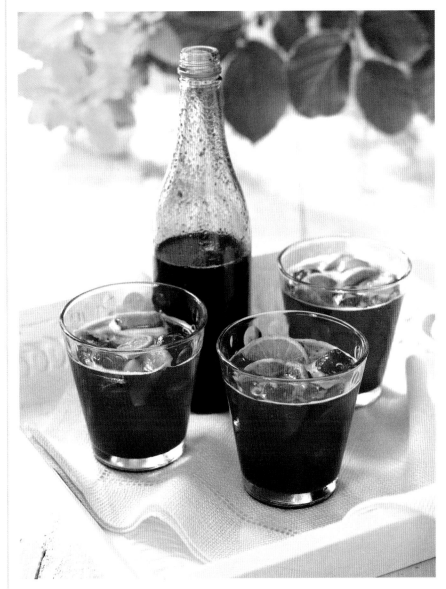

Blackberry and lime cordial

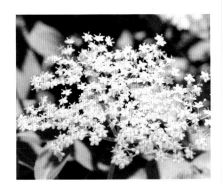

Elder *Sambucus nigra*

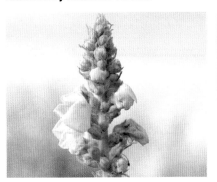

Mullein *Verbascum thapus*

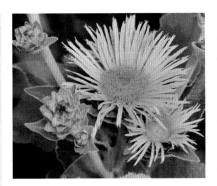

Elecampane *Inula helenium*

✚ First Aid

Every home should have a few simple herbal remedies to hand in addition to a first-aid kit. Many situations that need a first-aid solution – such as minor accidents and injuries, insect bites and stings, abrasions, and minor burns and scalds – will also benefit from the healing properties of a herbal remedy. If you are in any doubt, seek urgent medical advice first. This chart is not comprehensive, but it does contain the key herbs for emergency aid.

Herb	Action
Aloe vera *Aloe vera (p.20)*	Highly effective soothing and cooling properties. Break off a leaf from a fresh plant, split it open, and use the fresh gel to soothe rashes, minor burns, scalds, or sunburn. Alternatively, buy aloe vera juice.
Calendula *Calendula officinalis (p.36)*	An antiseptic and healing herb. Combine the tincture with St John's wort and dab neat onto spots, or dilute 1 teaspoon in half a cup of boiled water to use as an antiseptic and cleansing lotion for abrasions, or use as a healing cream.
Chamomile *Matricaria recutita (p.78)*	Soothing and calming. Sip the tea to ease fevers, insomnia, and nausea, or sweeten with honey to relieve shock. The cooled tea can be used as a cooling and soothing lotion for inflamed skin and rashes.
Comfrey *Symphytum officinale (p.108)*	Traditionally known as "knitbone" because of its healing properties. Pound the fresh leaves into a pulp and apply as a poultice for sprains, bruises, and ulcers. Alternatively, apply as a macerated oil or cream.
Echinacea *Echinacea purpurea (p.50)*	Known as "nature's antibiotic'", echinacea should be used whenever necessary to prevent an infection. Dilute the tincture and use as a lotion for wounds, insect or animal bites, and stings. Also take internally to boost immunity.
Garlic *Allium sativum (p.19)*	A pungent but effective kitchen herb with antiseptic and anticatarrhal properties. Eat a raw clove twice daily to alleviate congestion and help prevent infections. A fresh clove rubbed onto an infected spot or boil is also effective.
Lavender *Lavandula angustifolia (p.72)*	Healing, calming and anti-inflammatory, this versatile essential oil can be dabbed onto the skin to relieve insect bites, sunburn or minor burns, and scalds. Inhaling the oil can relieve shock, or dab a little on the temples to alleviate tension headaches or insomnia.
Plantain *Plantago lanceolata (p.88)*	A naturally soothing herb with an antihistamine action. Bruise the fresh leaves and apply to rashes, insect bites, and stings to calm the irritation. Combine the tincture with calendula as a healing mouthwash or for cuts and abrasions.
Slippery elm *Ulmus rubra (p.119)*	Lines the stomach and reduces inflammation: mix with water and drink to relieve indigestion, gastritis and stomach upsets. Mix a little water into a paste to make a poultice to draw out splinters, boils, and abscesses.
Witch hazel *Hamamelis virginiana (p.63)*	This plant is well known as an instantly cooling and soothing herb. Soak some cotton wool in distilled witch hazel and apply liberally to relieve discomfort from insect bites, bruising, minor burns, sunburn, and piles (haemorrhoids).

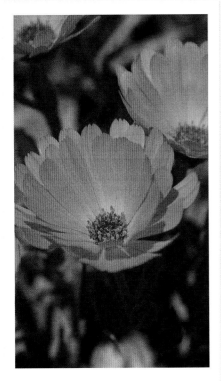

Calendula *Calendula officinalis*

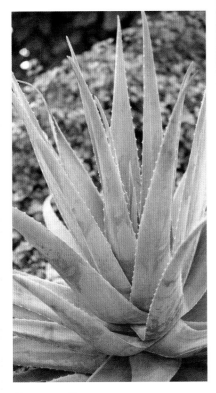

Aloe vera *Aloe vera*

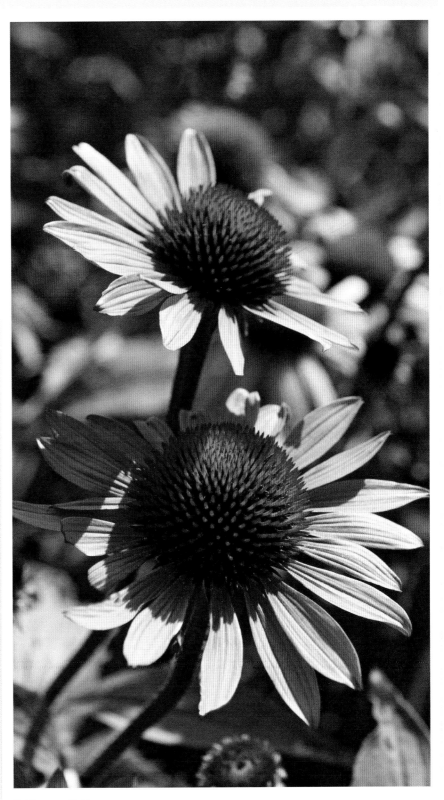

Echinacea *Echinacea purpurea*

⚡ Muscles and joints

The key to healthy muscles and joints is to balance a strong structure with flexibility; this can become a challenge as we grow older. If you do have long-standing problems with muscles or joints, a combination of manipulation, diet, lifestyle changes, and herbal remedies to detoxify and reduce inflammation will all help. This chart is not comprehensive, but it does contain key herbs that help to prevent pain and inflammation.

Herb	Action
Arnica *Arnica montana*	The first remedy to think of following any injury to muscles or joints such as bruising, sprains, or strains. Can also be used to relieve backache and the pain of arthritis and rheumatism. Apply locally as a cream, macerated oil, or salve.
Comfrey *Symphytum officinale* (p.108)	Traditionally known as "knitbone" because of its remarkable healing properties. The fresh leaves can be pulverised to make a poultice for sprains, strains, aches and pains, and arthritis. Alternatively, use the cream or macerated oil.
Celery *Apium graveolens* (p.26)	Detoxifying and anti-inflammatory, celery seeds are an important remedy in the treatment of gout, rheumatism, and arthritis. Combine with white willow and drink three times a day for several weeks as a decoction, or use the tinctures.
Meadowsweet *Filipendula ulmaria* (p.56)	With its anti-inflammatory and antirheumatic properties, meadowsweet is helpful in relieving the pain and inflammation of rheumatism and arthritis. Take as an infusion or tincture three times daily.
Rosemary *Rosmarinus officinalis* (p.96)	Stimulates the circulation and brings a feeling of warmth and comfort to aching muscles and joints. Dilute the essential oil in a massage base and rub into painful areas. Excellent for sports injuries such as pulled muscles; rub into the muscle before and after any exertion.
St John's wort *Hypericum perforatum* (p.68)	With its analgesic and anti-inflammatory properties, St John's wort is particularly appropriate for treating areas rich in nerves. Massage the macerated oil into the skin to treat backache, sciatica, and neuralgia.
Juniper *Juniperus communis* (p.71)	A diuretic, detoxifying, and antirheumatic essential oil. Make a compress using the essential oil to relieve gout. Combine with ginger essential oil in a vegetable base oil to relieve muscular aches and pains.
Crampbark *Viburnum opulus* (p.123)	An effective antispasmodic and sedative herb. Use to relieve the pain of backache (combine with white willow) and muscular cramp. Best used as a tincture. Combine with devil's claw (*Harpagophytum procumbens*) for swollen joints and arthritis.
Devil's claw *Harpagophytum procumbens*	An effective anti-inflammatory herb useful in the treatment of swollen joints and arthritis. Take as a tincture or capsules. Works well combined with crampbark or white willow.
White willow *Salix alba* (p.99)	Analgesic and anti-inflammatory, white willow relieves pain in a similar way to aspirin. Helpful in the treatment of painful joints and muscles, arthritis, neuralgia, and sciatica. Take as a decoction or tincture in combination with other appropriate herbs.

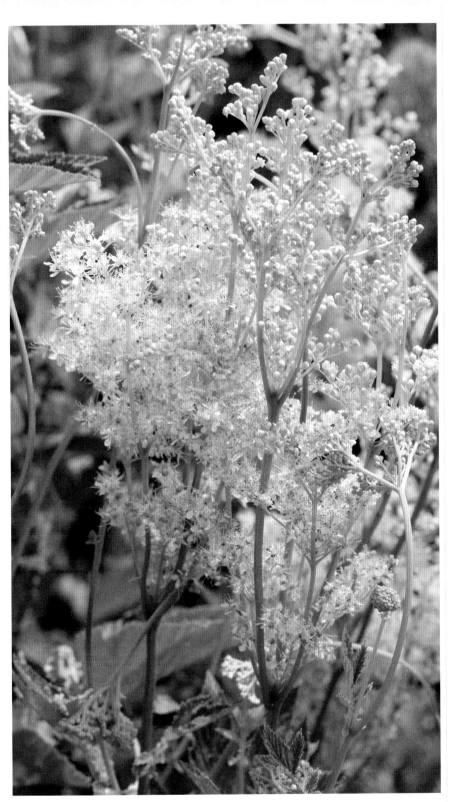

Meadowsweet *Filipendula ulmaria*

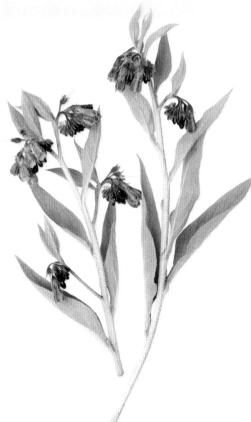

Comfrey *Symphytum officinale*

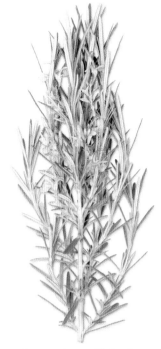

Rosemary *Rosmarinus officinalis*

Mind and emotions

Modern life can be stressful. Herbs can help us to cope better with stress and relieve symptoms of depression, exhaustion, and tension, but to bring about lasting benefits, we must change our lifestyles and use remedies to support us during that change. Refer any severe or long-standing complaints to a medical practitioner for professional help. This chart is not comprehensive, but it does contain the key herbs for emotional and mental well-being.

Herb	Action
Oats *Avena sativa (p.33)*	An excellent tonic for the nervous system, oats help to improve nervousness, exhaustion, anxiety, and decrease stress. Eat as porridge every morning or use the tincture in combination with other appropriate herbs.
St John's wort *Hypericum perforatum (p.68)*	Proven to relieve the symptoms of mild to moderate depression, and also helpful in cases of SAD, anxiety, and exhaustion. Take as an infusion, tincture, or capsules. Not to be used in conjunction with any other medication without medical advice.
Lemon balm *Melissa officinalis (p.81)*	An uplifting antidepressant and calming remedy. It lifts the spirits and calms anxiety, nervousness, and panic attacks. Also good for treating insomnia and headaches. This very safe, pleasant-tasting herb is suitable for everyone. Best taken as an infusion or tincture.
Vervain *Verbena officinalis (p122)*	A tonic herb that is strengthening for the nervous system and useful for the relief of tension, headaches, depression, exhaustion, and stress. Combines well with lemon balm and skullcap. Take as an infusion or as tincture.
Skullcap *Scutellaria lateriflora (p.104)*	An important nervine tonic with antispasmodic action that has mild sedative qualities. Useful in the treatment of stress, anxiety, overwork, migraine, and following an emotional shock. Combines well with lemon balm and chamomile. Use as an infusion or tincture.
Lavender *Lavandula angustifolia (p.72)*	With its calming and sedative properties, lavender is useful in the treatment of restlessness, shock, and stress. Drink as an infusion combined with lemon balm to relieve tension headaches. Use the essential oil to relieve insomnia.
Passionflower *Passiflora incarnata (p.87)*	A mild sedative herb that is excellent in the treatment of sleeplessness and anxiety. Combines well with chamomile to make an infusion for the relief of insomnia.
Ashwagandha *Withania somnifera (p.129)*	A herb from the Ayurvedic tradition that is known as an adaptogen – helping the body to cope with the effects of long-term stress. Helps to restore energy and vitality to those suffering from exhaustion. Best taken as a tincture or powder.
Damiana *Turnera diffusa*	An effective antidepressant herb that helps to restore an enthusiasm and vitality for life. Use to relieve symptoms of anxiety and depression. Take as an infusion or tinctures combined with other appropriate herbs such as lemon balm.
Borage *Borago officinalis (p.34)*	The phrase "borage for courage" indicates its use in strengthening the adrenal glands of those fatigued by long-term stress. Used for stress, depression, and exhaustion, but only for short periods of time and only under the advice of a qualified herbalist.

Recipes

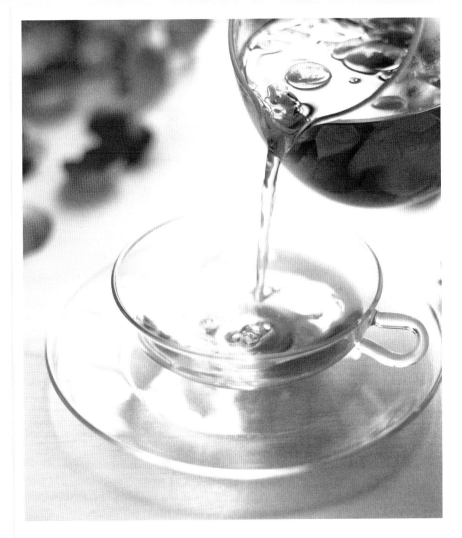

Lemon balm and rose tea

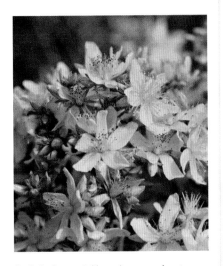

St John's wort *Hypericum perforatum*

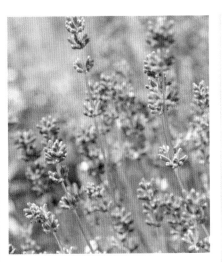

Lavender *Lavandula angustifolia*

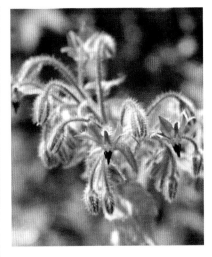

Borage *Borago officinalis*

Pregnancy and childbirth

No medicinal herb other than those known to be safe as everyday foods should be taken during early pregnancy or while breast-feeding without the advice of a qualified herbalist. However, some dietary plants and external lotions can relieve common ailments such as morning sickness or varicose veins, and heal the body after childbirth. This chart contains the key herbs that are beneficial for pre- and postnatal mothers.

Herb	Action
Ginger *Zingiber officinale*	A highly effective anti-emetic that helps to relieve the symptoms of nausea and morning sickness. Add a couple of slices of fresh ginger root to a cupful of hot water and sip as required.
Chamomile *Matricaria recutita* *(p.78)*	A versatile and gentle everyday herb that is calming and soothing to the nerves and digestion. Drink a cupful of infusion to relieve morning sickness, stress and tension, to aid relaxation before going to sleep, and as an aid to the digestion.
Witch hazel *Hamamelis virginiana* *(p.63)*	A cooling and astringent herb that benefits veins. Soak a pad of cotton wool in distilled witch hazel and apply to aching legs, varicose veins, or haemorrhoids.
Lavender *Lavandula* *angustifolia (p.72)*	A calming and anti-inflammatory essential oil that promotes healing after childbirth. Add 4–5 drops of lavender oil to the bath water. To relieve mastitis, add 3–4 drops of essential oil to warm water and apply using a clean facecloth as a compress.
Linseed *Linum usitassimum*	Acts as a gentle laxative and bowel lubricant, and is also very rich in omega fatty acids – particularly essential during pregnancy. Add a tablespoon to breakfast cereal or muesli and increase your fluids to help prevent constipation.
Calendula *Calendula officinalis* *(p.36)*	Highly nourishing and healing to the skin. Combine the tincture with St John's wort and dilute to use as a lotion to bathe any tearing or stitches after childbirth. Massage the macerated oil into the skin during pregnancy to help prevent stretch marks.
St John's wort *Hypericum* *perforatum (p.68)*	Has effective antiseptic and pain-relieving properties. Combine the tincture with calendula and dilute to use as a lotion to heal tearing or stitches after childbirth; also use to bathe cracked nipples, although rinse with clear water before breast-feeding.
Raspberry leaf *Rubus idaeus (p.97)*	A uterine tonic that helps to prepare the body for childbirth. Drink the infusion daily during the last trimester of pregnancy (not suitable during early pregnancy). Continue drinking it for two to three weeks after the birth to help contract the muscles and promote breast milk.
Dill *Anethum graveolens*	The seeds make an excellent infusion to drink during breast-feeding, as dill helps to promote the breast milk and also relieves any colic or wind in the baby. May be combined with fennel seeds.
Jasmine *Jasminum officinale* *(p.70)*	A delightfully fragrant essential oil that is traditionally used during labour for its relaxing properties and to help instil feelings of calmness and confidence. Dilute in a base oil and ask your partner to massage it into your lower back.

Herbs to avoid in pregnancy

This list of herbs should not be used internally in pregnancy unless prescribed by a qualified medical herbalist trained in the appropriate use of these substances. Please note that this list is not exhaustive. Culinary herbs marked with an asterisk are acceptable, but avoid them in large therapeutic doses.

- *Achillea millefolium* **Yarrow**
- *Actaea racemosa* **Black cohosh**
- *Agastache rugosa* **Purple giant hyssop***
- *Aloe vera* **Aloe vera**
- *Angelica archangelica* **Angelica root**
- *Apium graveolens* **Celery seed**
- *Aralia racemosa* **American spikenard**
- *Arctostaphylos uva-ursi* **Bearberry**
- *Artemisia absinthium* **Wormwood**
- *Borago officinalis* **Borage**
- *Calendula officinalis* **Calendula**
- *Curcuma longa* **Turmeric***
- *Cymbopogon citratus* **Lemon grass***
- *Eupatorium cannabinum* **Hemp agrimony**
- *Eupatorium purpureum* **Gravel root**
- *Filipendula ulmaria* **Meadowsweet**
- *Glycyrrhiza glabra* **Liquorice root***
- *Hydrastis canadensis* **Golden seal**

- *Hypericum perforatum* **St. John's wort**
- *Hyssopus officinalis* **Hyssop**
- *Inula helenium* **Elecampane**
- *Juniperus communis* **Juniper**
- *Leonurus cardiaca* **Motherwort**
- *Levisticum officinale* **Lovage**
- *Lycium barbarum* **Goji***
- *Nepeta cataria* **Catnip**
- *Panax japonicus* **Japanese ginseng**
- *Rosa x damascena* **Damask rose**
- *Rosmarinus officinalis* **Rosemary***
- *Rumex crispus* **Yellow dock**
- *Salix alba* **White willow**
- *Salvia officinalis* **Common sage**
- *Saussurea costus* **Costus**
- *Schisandra chinensis* **Schisandra**
- *Senna alexandrina* **Senna**
- *Symphytum officinale* **Comfrey**
- *Tanacetum parthenium* **Feverfew**
- *Thymus vulgaris* **Thyme***

- *Trifolium pratense* **Red clover**
- *Tussilago farfara* **Coltsfoot**
- *Verbena officinalis* **Vervain**
- *Viburnum opulus* **Crampbark**
- *Viscum album* **Mistletoe**
- *Vitex agnus castus* **Agnus castus/ Chaste berry**
- *Withania somnifera* **Ashwaghanda**

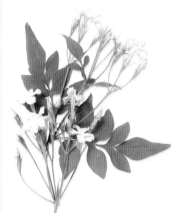

Jasmine *Jasminum officinale* In labour, a few drops of jasmine essential oil added to a massage oil can help.

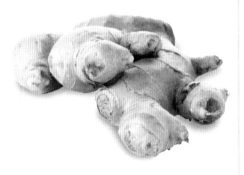

Ginger *Zingiber officinale*

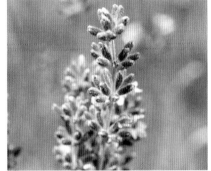

Lavender *Lavandula angustifolia*

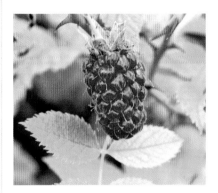

Raspberry *Rubus idaeus*

Source
Herbs

Find out how to **grow medicinal herbs** for yourself, whether in a **garden** or in a **windowbox**, and discover how to **forage for herbs** in the wild or buy the best fresh or dried herbs to **make your own remedies.**

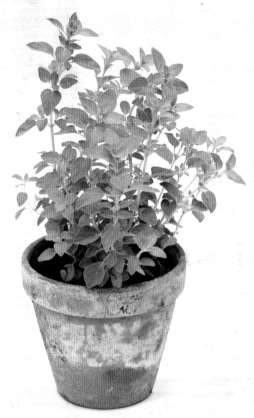

Planning your herb garden

Choosing your favourite herb plants and growing them is a great way to start your own herb garden. Select herbs that will flourish in your climate, and take some time to choose which plot – or in what containers – to grow your herbs. Be mindful of how much sun your herbs need and position them appropriately in your garden.

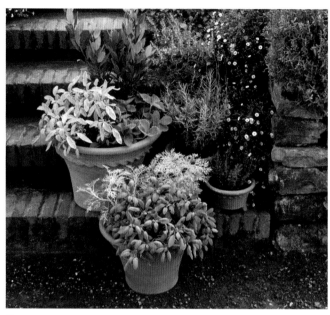

Use your space Position pots against a south-facing wall in a sheltered spot to give them the best of the sun.

Pots

• Most culinary herbs take well to pot culture, and the advantage of planting herbs in different pots is that you can move the plants around the garden for more sun or shade depending on the month, or move any frost-tender herb plants indoors during the winter months.

• Alternatively, window boxes allow you to grow a good selection of herbs in one space, and can be conveniently positioned by a kitchen window to make picking them at the last moment for cooking or garnishing dishes even easier.

• Plant herbs in generous containers with drainage holes in the bottom. Use fine soil mixed in equal quantities with vermiculite for Mediterranean herbs, and 100 per-cent potting soil for delicate herbs.

• Potted herbs require frequent watering, and daily watering in the summer.

Beds and borders

• If you have a vegetable garden or ornamental beds or borders, plant culinary and medicinal herbs in between existing plants. Position sun-loving herbs where they will get lots of light, and tuck shade-lovers around taller ornamentals.

• A small, informal, dedicated herb garden packed with herbs can occupy as little as 1.5 x 3.5m (5 x 11½ft). If possible, position it where you can see it.

• A formal arrangement is possible even in the tiniest of gardens: plant low-growing herbs such as thyme or chamomile between paths made of crushed rocks, bricks, or flagstones.

• Sketch out your dream garden on graph paper before you dig it. Then mark out planting areas in geometric or soft, curving patterns.

• If you add trellises, arbors, arches, pillars, water features, and statues you can give it a formal look. If you have a sloping garden, terraces make a beautiful addition to the design.

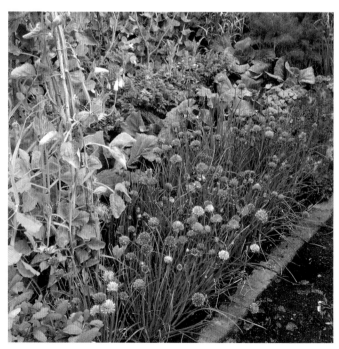

Sharing space Many herbs make pretty and practical additions to vegetable beds.

Testing the soil

Try this simple test before you plant herbs. The best soil is loam (a mix of clay and sand). Clay needs sand and compost to improve aeration; sandy soil retains water and nutrients only when you add compost to it.

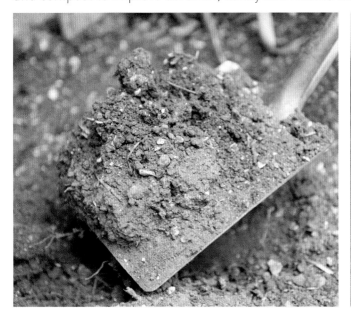

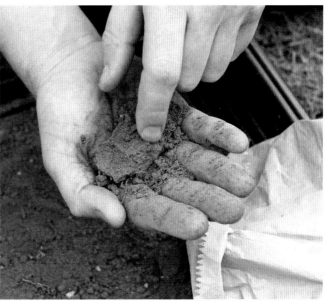

1 *Remove any grass,* *weeds, or plants from the surface and lift out a clod of earth with a spade. Repeat in two other places in your garden patch.*

2 *Mix the samples* *well, squeeze some mixed soil in your palm, and thump it with a finger. If it falls apart, it is loam; if gritty, it is sandy; if it forms a lump, it is clay.*

Making your own compost

Add grass clippings, leaves, uncooked vegetable waste, and dead (but not diseased) plants to a compost bin that is 1.5m (5ft) square and 90cm (3ft) high. Do not add weeds or grasses that have set seed.

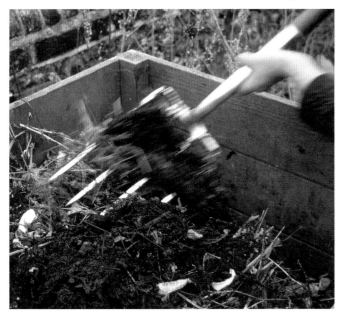

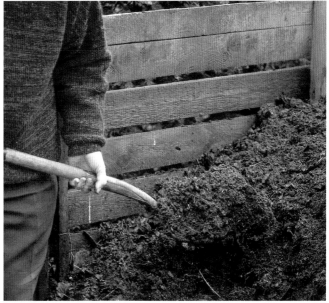

1 *Collect your compostable material* *in the bin. Keep the heap moist and turn it every two weeks, using a fork or shovel, until the material starts to break down.*

2 *You can use* *your compost when it has turned dark brown in colour, is crumbling in texture, and looks and smells like soil.*

Growing herbs

There are many advantages to growing herbs from seed. Home-sown herbs are cheaper than those bought from a nursery, and home-grown seedlings have healthy, garden-ready root balls when the time comes to plant them out. Some herbs are best propagated in other ways, though (p.160).

Growing from seed

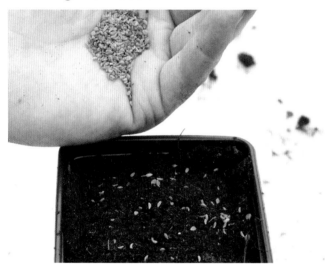

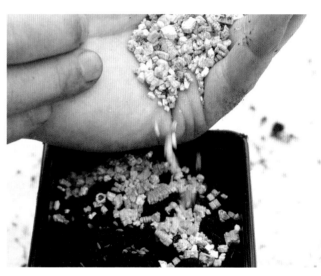

1 Fill a pot with fine soil and gently firm down. Water the soil and let it drain. Sow seed in dents or on the soil surface (according to the packet instructions).

2 Lightly cover the seed with vermiculite or more potting soil. Water again. Set the tray in a warm place and never let the soil dry out.

Transplanting

As seedlings develop they need more space to grow. Transplant them into individual or bigger pots when they have formed four or more true leaves above the seed leaves.

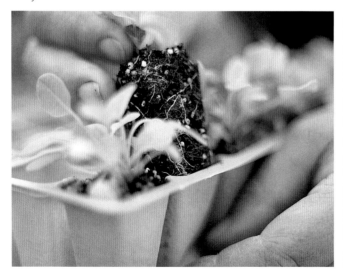

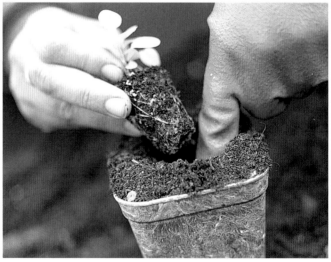

1 Remove the seedlings from their pot, gently pulling them out by their true leaves, not by the stem, and squeezing the base of the pot or tray.

2 Make a hole in a pot of soil and lower in the seedling. Fill with more soil, firm down gently, water, and position in a warm, bright spot out of direct sunlight.

Growing young plants

Sometimes it may not be practical to raise plants from seed yourself, especially if you only want to grow a handful of different plants and don't have space to sow lots of seedlings, or if a plant is hard to grow from seed. Garden centres have a good selection of young plants, but nurseries have a broader range.

Potting on

If you want to grow your herb plant in a pot, replant it when you get home from the nursery in a pot one size bigger than the one you bought it in. You will need to repeat the process when your plants outgrow their new pots.

1 *Make sure* your new pot has a drainage hole. Place a handful of gravel at the bottom, half-fill with potting compost, and remove the plant from its pot.

2 *Remove the plant* from its old pot. Set the plant into its new pot and fill with potting soil, firming in gently as you go. Water the plant well.

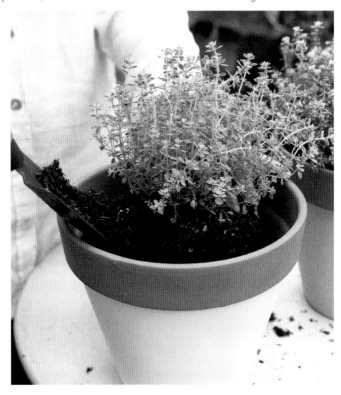

Planting into the garden

Young plants bought from a nursery should be big enough to plant outdoors in the garden immediately. Plant them out as soon as you can to allow their roots to establish.

1 *Prepare the soil* by digging into the top 15–30cm (6–12in) of soil until it becomes loose. Dig a generous hole and place the plant in the hole to the same depth it was in its pot.

2 *Backfill around the plant* and firm it in with the palms of your hands. Water the plant well.

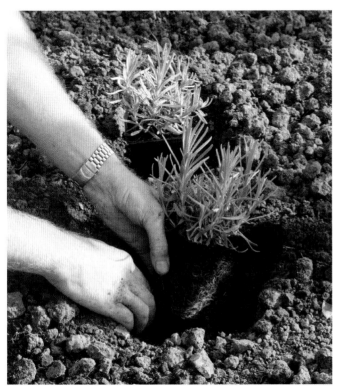

Propagation

Once your favourite herb plants are well established, you can increase their number, or grow a few insurance plants in case some do not survive a harsh winter, by using various propagation methods. See the individual entries in the A–Z section for the best technique to use for growing each plant.

Stem cuttings

Take softwood cuttings from young stems in spring, semi-ripe cuttings from ripening, stiffening stems in late summer, and hardwood ones from woody stems at the end of the growing season.

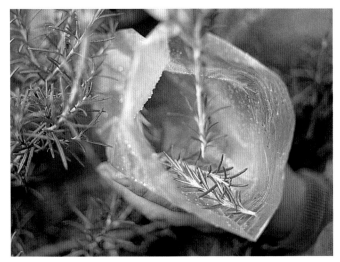

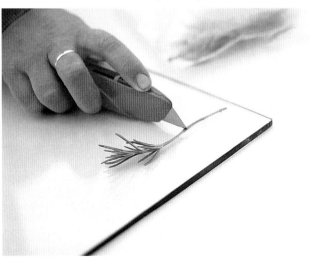

1 Select a healthy, *non-flowering stem with mature leaves, cut the stem at an angle just above the leaf attachment, and strip the lower leaves.*

2 Cut the stem *straight across 5cm (2in) below the last leaf. Plant vertically in a pot of soil. Water well. Cover with a clear plastic bag to retain moisture.*

Root cuttings

Make new plants from sections of semi-mature or mature roots of plants such as mint when they are dormant (not growing) in mid- to late winter.

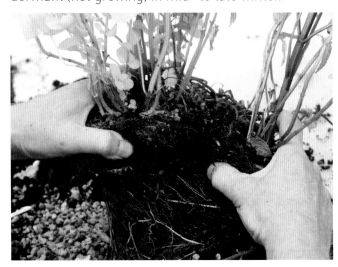

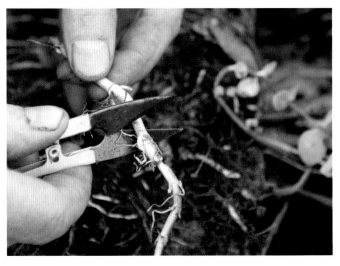

1 Lift the plant *and tease the roots apart. Cut a 5-cm (2-in) piece of root; avoid fibrous or immature roots.*

2 Trim the root *straight across at the top and diagonally at the base. Plant upright in soil. Cover with vermiculite.*

Watering and feeding

Herbs grown in pots and in the ground have different requirements. Check seed packet instructions or ask at your local garden centre or nursery about your chosen plant's specific requirements, although these general guidelines will keep all plants healthy.

Watering

Beds: You cannot always cater for the preferences of individual plants, but they will usually tolerate shared conditions as long as they have moist, well-drained soil. Work lots of compost into the soil to help it retain moisture and water it deeply when the top 5cm (2in) seems dry. The best time to water, if you are using an overhead sprinkler or a watering can, is in the morning, so that the sun has time to dry the leaves.

Pots: Herbs that are planted in pots need to be watered more often than those positioned in the ground, as their roots cannot travel as far to locate moisture. In very warm weather and on hot summer days you should water these potted plants every day, or purchase drip irrigation systems and install them in each pot with set timers to automatically water them. You can help the soil to retain more water using special granules that absorb water and release it as and when needed.

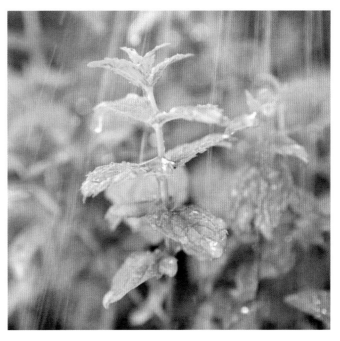

Water early Try to water your herbs in the morning to avoid mildew and rot overnight.

Feeding

Beds: Plants in open ground do not need much feeding because their roots travel to find the nutrition they require. However, you can give them a helping hand by spreading a 5-cm (2-in) layer of compost over the soil surface as a mulch over winter, then digging it into the soil in spring to restore nutrients. Herbs that are harvested frequently during the growing season benefit from the occasional fertilizer feed in midsummer too.

Pots: Potted plants also need more attention when it comes to food. Ideally, feed them with fertilizer in granules or liquid form every six weeks throughout the growing season, especially if they are harvested regularly. Start feeding in spring when new growth appears, and scrape away the top 5cm (2in) of soil in the pot and replace it with good, fresh soil. Stop feeding the plants in late summer, or you will encourage new growth when they should be slowing down before the dormant winter season.

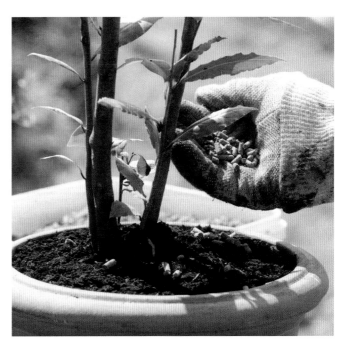

Feed well Feed potted herbs with fertilizer every six weeks during the growing season.

Weeds, pests, and diseases

Weeds compete with plants for water, sunlight, nutrients, and space – the key to defeating them is to remove them as you see them. One of the virtues of many herbs is that the aromatic volatile oils they exude are produced primarily to ward off insects; so many of the plants in your herb garden will naturally protect themselves against pests.

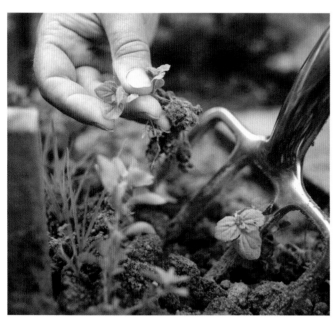

Weeding by hand This is the most effective way of removing all parts of the weeds once established.

Beating weeds

Once weeds start to appear on the surface of the soil in spring, you need to remove them by hand or with the help of a hand-fork for those that have long roots. To help prevent the weeds returning, remove them before they set seed and make sure you get as much of the root out of the soil as possible, particularly with perennial weeds. Check the soil regularly for any new shoots that may be appearing and remove them immediately.

If you want to clear a large area of weeds from the soil before planting in it, try solarizing: clear a patch of soil, water it thoroughly, then cover the area with a piece of clear plastic sheeting and bury it at the edges to prevent any air getting in and out. Over the course of the next six to eight weeks, the sun will create killing heat and steam under the plastic sheet. After that time, remove the plastic and plant your herb plants immediately.

Pests

Caterpillars: Pick off by hand, wearing a glove, and dispose of them. Encourage parasitic wasps to eat them by planting flowering herbs, or spray infested plants with 500ml (16fl oz) water blended with a peeled clove of garlic (strain the liquid before use).

Slugs and snails: Set traps of shallow bowls of beer to drown them, or pick off by hand at night when they are most active. Alternatively, use non-toxic pellets or apply copper tape to containers (right) to give them a mild electric shock as they pass over it.

Aphids: Along with scale, whitefly, mealy bugs, thrips, spittle bugs, and red spider mites, aphids weaken a plant's growth. Spritz them off plants with water from a hose or use an organic, insecticidal soap.

Vine weevils: A major pest, these grubs come out at night and chew notches out of leaf margins and devour roots. They are difficult to control biologically, but you can add nematodes to the soil to kill them.

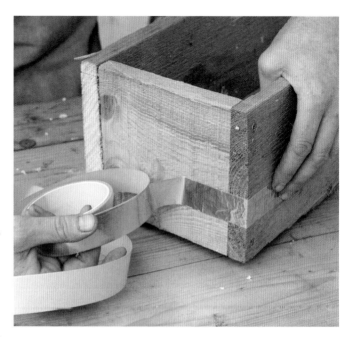

Short, sharp shock Apply copper tape just below the rim of pots or other containers to deter slugs and snails.

Avoiding diseases and bacteria

Most herbs are remarkably free of plant diseases and many can be prevented by good care and maintenance, but occasionally diseases do develop. Deal with them quickly to avoid lasting damage.

Diseases: Grow resistant varieties and apply good cultural practices and hygiene in the garden. Try not to work in the garden when it is wet as you may inadvertently spread diseases. Examine plants regularly, removing infected leaves as they fall. Dispose of any infected plant material carefully – preferably by burning it.

Bacteria: If bacteria enters a plant through a wound, spray the affected area with a simple home-made organic solution. To make the solution, purée a dozen peeled garlic cloves and then blend the garlic purée with 1.2 litres (2 pints) of water. Strain the liquid, decant it into a bottle with a spray mist nozzle attachment, and apply as necessary. If the plant does not respond within several days, clip off the infected parts and destroy them. Ensure that you sterilize your clippers or secateurs before you use them again on other plants.

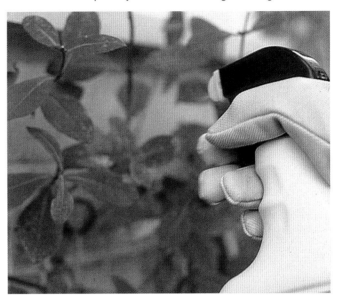

Organic spray You can easily blend your own spray and use it to treat any bacterial diseases that may affect your plants.

Fungi

Although fungi is fairly rare amongst herbs, mint is prone to rust and downy and powdery mildews can develop in warm, humid, and wet conditions. Spray with an alkaline solution to prevent fungi taking hold, and use organic controls for fungal diseases.

Viruses

Mosaic viruses cause white, yellow, or light green dots on leaves. Other viruses cause curled leaves, and ring spot viruses cause pale, yellowed ringed spots on leaves. They do not cause serious damage, but you can pull up affected plants and destroy them.

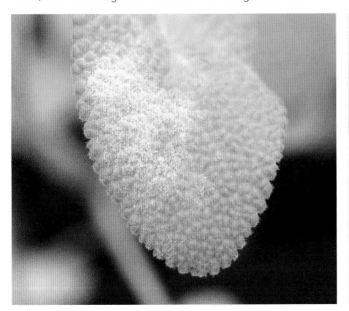

Powdery mildew A white fungus can develop on the leaves of herbs such as this sage.

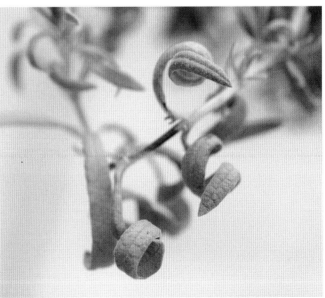

Curled leaves This can be a sign of a virus that has been transmitted by sucking insects or infected tools.

Foraging for herbs

Harvesting from the wild offers a free source of herbal remedies, and provides the satisfaction of collecting your own herbs. The active constituents of wild plants are often more concentrated, as they are likely to be growing in their preferred environment. A variety of plants can even be found growing on waste ground or in "wild zones" in urban areas.

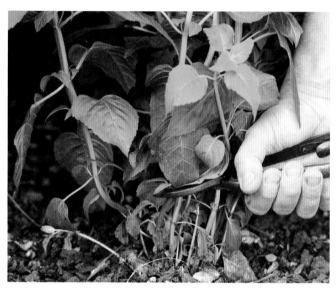

Harvesting whole plants During the growing season, do not take more than half a plant to allow it to regrow.

Sustainability

Some common plants, such as nettle or plantain, may be gathered readily from the wild. However, many rarer species are under great pressure due to over-harvesting and a decline in natural habitats. In many countries it is illegal to dig up the roots of any wild plant, and certain species may be protected.

In some countries there is a strong tradition of wild harvesting or foraging. The trade in wild plants is monitored by the CITES convention developed by the IUCN (International Union for the Conservation of Nature); any endangered species are added to their "red list" and should never be gathered.

Never pick rare plants from the wild, even if they are plentiful locally. Do not deplete a stock of plants in an area; gather only enough for immediate use. Do not harvest bark in the wild – you may damage the tree.

Safety

Proper identification of wild plants is absolutely essential. Some plants that look similar to useful herbs may be poisonous; this is especially true of plants from the Umbelliferae family, which includes angelica and gotu kola and also some toxic plants such as hemlock. Always use a field guide with clear identification charts, and if you are not absolutely certain, don't risk it.

Avoid plants growing along a main road, whether in the countryside or in the city, because of the high amounts of lead and other pollutants they may contain. Similarly, avoid plants growing at the base of trees in urban areas if they are evidently favoured spots for dogs.

It is also important to check that waste ground has not been used as a dump for toxic waste; ask locally if you are in doubt. Do not collect herb plants close to factories or any other obvious potential source of pollution. Always check that there are no signs of recent weed killer use or crop spraying.

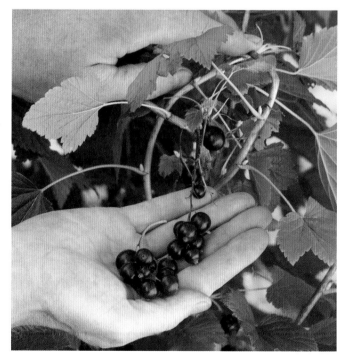

Foraging for berries Be sure to identify herbs and fruit carefully before harvesting them in the wild.

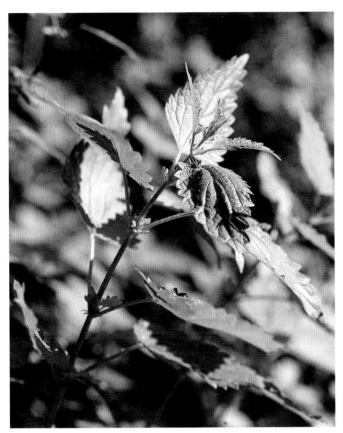

Plants in the wild Nettles are one of the plants that can be found growing in parks and on waste ground.

Where to forage

In urban areas a number of herbs known as "pioneer plants" can be found growing readily on waste ground or in wild zones, which are found in most large parks. The edges of allotments or disused railway lines can also be good places to find relatively uncontaminated plants. Avoid main roads, but if you gather young shoots in the spring and avoid the mature plant and roots, you can minimize the amount of undesired pollutants.

Most of us live in cities, and by gathering plants very close to your home you reduce the carbon footprint associated with their transportation. There is also an argument that plants tough enough to survive city conditions may be particularly appropriate and useful for city dwellers; certainly they are likely to have very concentrated levels of active constituents.

In rural areas, one of the best places to forage for herbs is the land and hedgerows around organic farms, but don't go on to a farmer's property without asking their permission first.

If you are in doubt about whether an area is suitable for foraging from a sustainability point of view, ask your local Wildlife Trust or equivalent for advice on the plants you wish to collect.

When to harvest

Herbs produce their volatile oils at night, so the best time to harvest most plants is in the early morning once the dew has evaporated. Collecting on a dry day means they will keep better and are less likely to grow mould. Pick a plant at the peak of its season and maturity to ensure it will have the highest concentration of active constituents.

Unless otherwise specified in the individual plant's page in the A–Z (pp.10–131), collect the leaves as they unfurl during the spring or early summer months; the flowers as they start to bloom; and fruits and berries just as they become ripe.

Harvest the seeds from plants such as fennel while they are still on the plant, or cut off stems with whole seedheads to dry. Smaller, dry seeds can be gathered by shaking a seedhead into a paper bag.

Most berries are ripe if they come away from the plant easily when gently tugged, or you can snip off complete trusses and separate the berries from the stems at home in your kitchen.

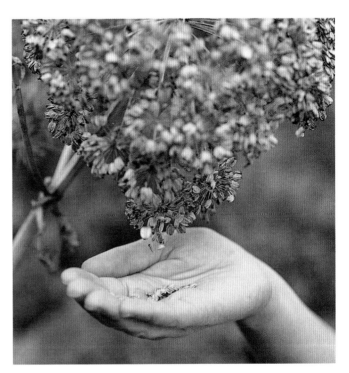

Harvesting seeds Leave seedheads on the plants and gently shake the plant over your hand to harvest the seeds.

Buying and storing herbs

Sometimes it may not be practical to raise fresh herb plants from seed yourself, so buy the plants from a reputable garden centre or nursery. Similarly, some herbs grow better in a different climate, or you may require them out of season, so buying fresh or dried versions of a herb is a better option than attempting to grow them yourself.

Pick a perfect plant

Do not buy plants with any obvious problems or diseases, such as leaves with yellow veins or mildew; all herbs should have bright, sturdy stems and foliage. Knock the plant out of its pot and check the roots, too – they should be healthy and plentiful and not fighting for space. Check each plant for any live insects, as you do not want to bring a potential problem home with you.

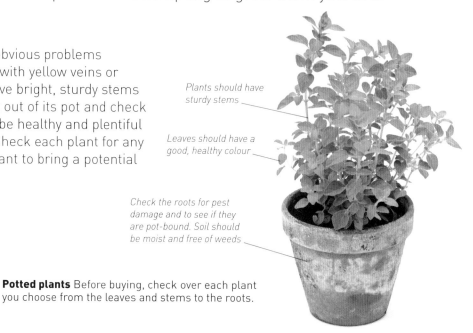

Plants should have sturdy stems

Leaves should have a good, healthy colour

Check the roots for pest damage and to see if they are pot-bound. Soil should be moist and free of weeds

Potted plants Before buying, check over each plant you choose from the leaves and stems to the roots.

Roots

Vigorous leaves and stems do not always mean that a plant is disease-free; sometimes problems lie beneath the surface of the soil. Roots are the lifeline of a plant, so it is important that they are healthy.

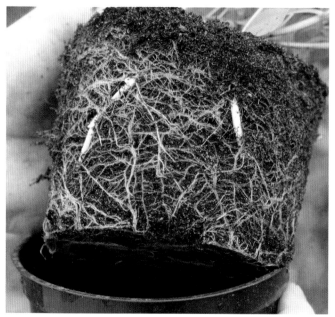

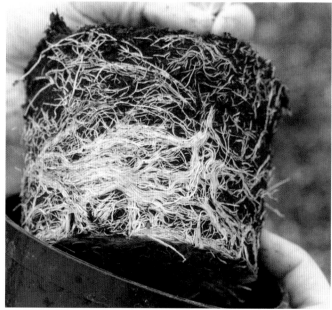

1 *A healthy specimen* *should lift easily out of its pot and its roots should be plentiful, but not overcrowded, with plenty of soil visible.*

2 *If you have a less-than-healthy plant, tease out and thin the overcrowded roots before planting it out in good soil. Remove any root weevils and grubs.*

Fresh herbs

It's worth buying fresh or cut herbs if a herb proves tricky to grow, you don't live in an ideal growing climate, the growing season for a herb is over, or you need a larger amount of a herb than you already have growing in your garden. Most supermarkets now sell a range of fresh herbs in their fresh fruit and vegetable section, or you may be able to get some herbs, such as parsley or watercress, from a farmer's market. Always buy fresh, "juicy-looking" herbs and, if possible, organically grown.

Delicate herbs such as tarragon, parsley, or mint keep well for a few days in a jug or a vase of fresh water if kept in a cool room. Many herbs, such as basil or marjoram, can be kept chilled while still on their stems, but first rinse the herbs, pat them dry with a paper towel, loosely wrap the stems in a piece of damp kitchen roll, and store in the fridge.

Most herbs keep their properties well during freezing; chop the herbs finely, coat them in a little olive oil or water, then spoon the mixture into small freezer bags or an ice-cube tray (right) and keep frozen until needed for up to six months.

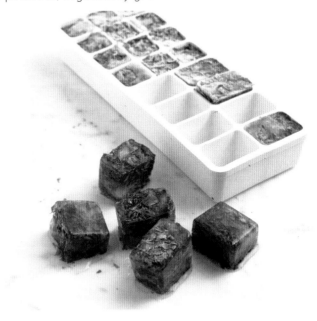

Preserving fresh herbs Cover finely chopped fresh herbs with a little water or oil in an ice-cube tray and freeze.

Dried herbs

Most herbs keep their medicinal properties well if dried carefully. It also means they can be harvested at their peak time and stored to use when out of season. Traditionally, herbs are harvested in one season – for example, spring – then grown on for a full year until they are ready to harvest again. Most herbs remain effective for six to 12 months, after which time any remaining stock should be discarded and replaced.

Always dry herbs from organically grown plants only; it is not advisable to ingest concentrated pesticides or synthetic fertilizer residues in addition to the active properties of the herb.

It is essential that you buy dried herbs only from ethical companies that actively pursue a policy of minimal environmental impact by encouraging organic cultivation and ensuring sustainable harvesting by indigenous communities. Such companies will also make sure that their herbs are fresh. Suppliers should ensure that they sell the correct species and there is no infestation present.

Store your bought dried herbs in an airtight – preferably glass – container in a dry, dark cupboard to preserve their therapeutic properties.

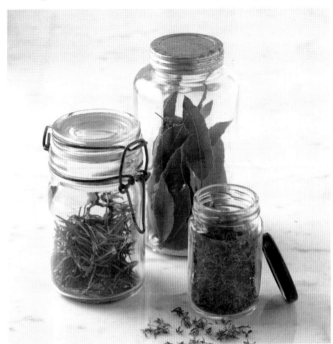

Store dried herbs in airtight jars All dried herbs should be stored out of direct light and used within six to 12 months.

HERB BASICS

Infusions

An infusion is the best way to harness the properties of the softer, green, or flowering parts of a plant. A standard therapeutic infusion is 1 heaped tsp of a single dried herb or 2 tsp of a mixture of dried herbs (for fresh herbs use double the amount) to 175ml (6fl oz) boiling water, but see individual herb entries in the A-Z (pp.10–131) for specific dosage instructions.

INGREDIENTS

1 heaped tsp dried herb, or 2 tsp chopped fresh herb
175ml (6fl oz) boiling water

METHOD

1 Place the chopped herbs in a cup or teapot, and pour the boiling water over the herbs.
2 Leave to steep for 10 minutes, preferably covered to avoid the loss of volatile oils in the steam. Strain the infusion before use.

Decoctions

To use the woodier parts of a plant, make a decoction as directed below. A standard decoction is 1 tsp dried herb or 2 tsp fresh herb to 175ml (6fl oz) water, but see individual herb entries for specific dosage instructions. Use a steel or enamelled cast iron pan if possible, as aluminium can react with anything cooked in it and could taint the decoction. This recipe makes three cups.

INGREDIENTS

15g (½oz) dried herb or mixture of herbs, or 30g (1oz) fresh herbs
750ml (1¼ pints) cold water

METHOD

1 Place the chopped herbs in a saucepan, and pour in the water.
2 Cover the pan with a lid and bring to the boil, then simmer gently for 15–20 minutes.
3 Strain the decoction and divide into 3 doses for use that day.

Macerated oils

This is the quickest, most practical method of making a macerated or infused oil, and is known as the "heat" method. Adjust the quantities below to make a larger or smaller amount of oil; there should be enough oil to completely cover the chopped herbs in the bowl.

INGREDIENTS

100g (3½oz) dried herbs or 300g (10oz) finely chopped fresh herbs
500ml (16fl oz) vegetable oil, such as organic sunflower or olive oil

METHOD

1 Place the finely chopped herbs in a heatproof bowl, and add the oil to completely cover the herbs.
2 Place the bowl over a pan of boiling water on the hob, cover the bowl, and heat gently for 2 hours. Top up the water as needed.
3 Strain the mixture and repeat by adding fresh herbs to the oil and warming again for 1 hour.
4 Strain the oil, pour into a sterilized dark glass bottle (p.370), and label with the name and date.
5 If using fresh herbs, let the oil stand for a few hours after straining to allow water from the herbs to sink to the bottom. Pour off the oil into the sterilized bottle and discard any water. Store in a cool place and use within 3 months.

Tinctures

The medicinal properties of herbs can be extracted using a mixture of water and herbs to give a preparation called a tincture. The alcohol acts as a preservative, making this an excellent way to store herbs out of season; a tincture will keep for up to 12 months.

Volume for volume, tinctures are much stronger than infusions, decoctions, or macerates, so should be used in smaller quantities. See individual herb entries in the A–Z (pp.10–131) for specific dosage instructions. Tinctures may vary in strength (eg. 1:3 or 1:5), so always follow the dosage instructions on the bottle when buying. Dosages in the A–Z are based on a 1:5 tincture unless otherwise specified. These quantities makes an approximately 1:5 tincture.

INGREDIENTS

200g (7oz)dried herb (fresh herbs will need to be dried prior to use, in order to reduce the water content of the tincture)

1 litre (1¾ pints) 37.5% proof vodka

METHOD

1 Chop the herbs finely, and place in a large sterilized sealable jar (p.370).

2 Immerse the herbs completely in the alcohol.

3 Seal the jar and store for 2 weeks away from direct sunlight, shaking occasionally.

4 Strain the mixture through a muslin cloth and then filter through an unbleached coffee filter.

5 Pour into a sterilized dark glass bottle (p.370). Label clearly with the name and date, and store in a cool, dark place.

IMPORTANT SAFETY INFORMATION

HERB SAFETY

Herbs and herbal remedies should be treated with respect. Individual herb entries in the A–Z (pp.10–131) give cautionary notes for each herb. Follow the method, dosage, and usage instructions closely.

ESSENTIAL OIL SAFETY

Essential oils contain the active ingredients of a plant in a highly concentrated form, and should be treated with respect and always diluted in vegetable base oil before use. A typical dilution for a massage oil is 2 per cent combined essential oils to 98 per cent base oil. Essential oils must be diluted before adding to a bath, e.g. 5 drops of essential oil in 15ml (1 tbsp) of vegetable oil or milk. They should never be taken internally without professional recommendation, and children under two should not be treated with essential oils. Some essential oils, such as basil and sage, should be avoided during pregnancy; consult an aromatherapist before using any essential oils at this time.

SOAP SAFETY

Soap-making requires accurate measuring and is potentially dangerous. The soap recipes in this book are not to be attempted by children. Buy 100 per cent sodium hydroxide (caustic soda) and always wear protective plastic gloves and goggles. When you first make a soap, it is extremely alkaline because of the caustic soda and has a very high pH value that drops over several weeks as the soap dries out. Test its pH value (pH testing kits are widely available) to see if it is too alkaline to use. It will eventually drop to a pH of 10–10.5, which is normal for soap but can still be an irritant to sensitive skin.

Understanding
Essential Oils

Essential oils contain the **essence of nature**. Find out what exactly is in essential oils, how these complex substances work **holistically** to heal and balance body and mind, and how to ensure you are using the purest, **very best-quality** products.

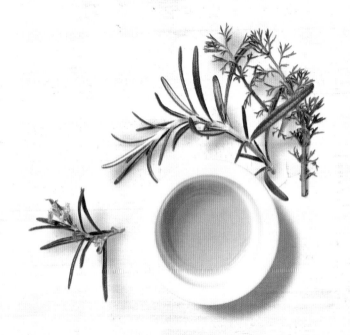

What are essential oils?

Aromatic essential oils are the **highly concentrated** essences derived from plants. Used today in **aromatherapy** and fragrances, they have a long history in **natural healing**. The oils harness a plant's **therapeutic** properties to restore **balance** to the mind, body, and spirit.

The plant's **essence**

The aromatic compounds in essential oils are thought to help plants survive, for example, by attracting pollinators and warding off fungus and bacteria. Once extracted, essential oils contain the essence of a plant in a very concentrated form, which means the essential oils often smell delightful and retain the plant's unique therapeutic benefits for our use.

Essential oils in aromatherapy

Today, there are around 150 essential oils used in aromatherapy. Each has a unique chemistry and properties that produce a distinct therapeutic, psychological, and physiological effect. As well as being anti-inflammatory, pain-relieving, decongesting, and antiseptic, oils can ease anxiety and lift the spirits. Their powerful constituents can have a profound physiological effect, restoring balance and vitality.

A single essential oil contains as many as 100 different chemical components.

Essential oil **sources**

Each plant contains essential oils. In some plants, oil is extracted from the dried seeds, peel or resin, while in others it is found in the leaves, roots, bark or flowers.

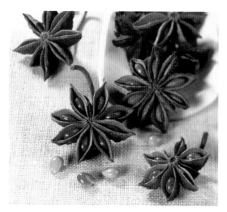

Both dried and fresh seeds can be pressed to extract the essential oils.

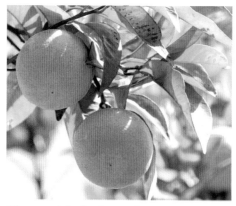

The essential oils of citrus fruits are concentrated mostly in the rinds.

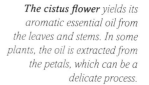

The cistus flower yields its aromatic essential oil from the leaves and stems. In some plants, the oil is extracted from the petals, which can be a delicate process.

What's in **an oil?**

A single essential oil can contain as many as 100 chemical components, which work together to give the oil its unique properties and aroma. Each component plays a role, but some are more dominant and determine how an oil will act on the body and mind.

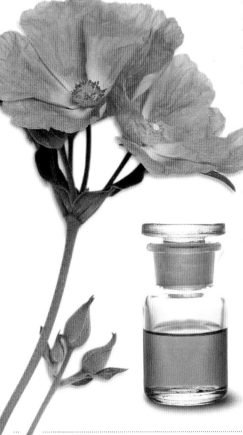

The chemistry of oils Oils are made up of major, minor, and trace components. Menthol is an example of a major component, making up around 40 per cent of peppermint oil. These major components work with the more numerous minor and trace components and all contribute to an oil's aroma and therapeutic value.

Breaking oils down Each oil's component parts split into two further categories: oxygenated compounds and terpenes. Oxygenated compounds tend to be stronger smelling and longer lasting than terpenes. They include alcohols, which are antibacterial and found in oils such as ginger and juniper; esters, which can be antiseptic, found in oils such as basil and clove; and ketones, which regenerate cells, found in oils such as rose, camphor, and vetiver. Terpenes, found in oils such as myrrh, have a range of properties, but spoil quickly when exposed to air.

The amber-hued essential oil derived from the cistus plant is rich in oxygenated compounds.

The history of essential oils

Traditionally, *highly concentrated oils from a variety of natural sources have been used to calm or stimulate the emotions and enhance wellbeing.*

The use of scented oils *in incense and candles has played a part in religious rituals throughout the ages, with many cultures believing the aromas could ward off evil or inspire us to new heights. The Egyptians used scented oils in burial rituals and as a symbol of status. The Greeks believed aromas connected them to the gods, while the Romans used scented oils for seduction.*

The modern use *of essential oils as a therapy began in the 1930s when the French chemist René-Maurice Gattefossé coined the term aromatherapy after finding that lavender oil helped heal his burned hand without scarring. In World War II, Dr Jean Valnet, a French army surgeon, used oils on wounded soldiers, while Austrian beauty therapist and biochemist Marguerite Maury prescribed oils and is credited with the idea of using essential oils in massage.*

Whether lifting the spirits *or healing wounds, aromatherapy is a safe and effective traditional practice with real relevance to our lives today.*

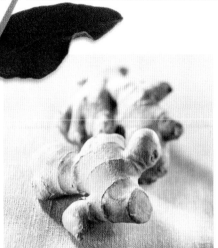

Plants such as ginger and plai produce a highly concentrated essential oil from the roots.

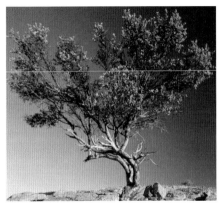

The resin from trees such as myrrh can be extracted and distilled into therapeutic oils.

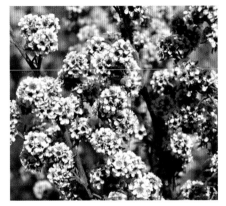

Some plants, such as fragonia, hold essential oil in the branches, as well as the leaves.

How essential oils work

Our sense of smell is more **sensitive** and immediate than any of our other senses, which is why aromas can be so evocative. Chemicals in a scent can trigger **physiological** responses and affect our mental state. These combined effects enable aromatic oils to work holistically on **mind**, **body**, and **spirit**, bringing **balance**, healing, and an often profound sense of wellbeing.

Mind

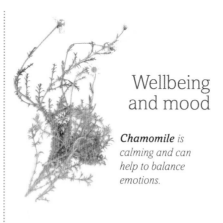

Wellbeing and mood

Chamomile is calming and can help to balance emotions.

Concentration and focus

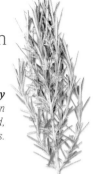

Rosemary essential oil can clear the mind, enhancing focus.

On the **mind**

Essential oils can be used to help promote a state of mind. For example, stimulating oils can be used to enhance focus, while oils that are calming enable us to relax and help to combat the effects of stress.

Enhance wellbeing and mood

Essential oils have many components that affect the nervous system, helping to lift mood and enhance wellbeing. For example, studies show that the compound linalool in lavender and clary sage reduces anxiety, while limonene, found in many citrus oils, can ease anxiety and lift depression. Chamomile and bergamot essential oils contain the compounds alpha- and beta-pinene, which also work as antidepressants, helping to lift the spirits and increase feelings of wellbeing.

When we feel anxious or depressed, it's not just our minds that are affected, our bodies can also suffer. For example, we tend to hold tension in our muscles when we are anxious. Many oils have both mood-enhancing properties and physiological effects so they treat

Relaxation

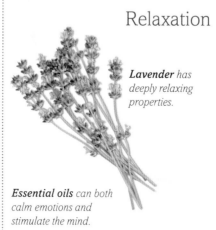

Lavender has deeply relaxing properties.

Essential oils can both calm emotions and stimulate the mind.

Balance and energy

Geranium is uplifting and balances emotions.

both the mental and physical symptoms of stress and anxiety.

An aromatherapy massage adds the inherently relaxing benefits of touch to an oil's therapeutic effects, which can be profoundly calming and uplifting. Even without the benefit of touch, simply smelling a pleasant aroma, such as a mandarin or vanilla bean, can reduce stress-induced muscle tension.

Promote relaxation The relaxing effects of oils are well documented. How they help us relax is a complicated process thought to involve several parts of the brain. One theory is that linalool, found in oils such as lavender, regulates the neurohormone GABA (gamma-aminobutyric acid). This in turn regulates levels of adrenaline, noradrenaline, and dopamine.

Rose has an uplifting and calming aroma.

Improve concentration and focus

Some oils clear and refresh the mind. For example, inhaling rosemary essential oil has been shown to improve memory by up to 75 per cent. The oil contains the compound eucalyptol, which acts in a similar way to dementia drugs by increasing a neurotransmitter called acetylcholine that helps regulate brain activity.

Balance energy

Many essential oils can either relax or stimulate as needed and are called "adaptogens". These balance body systems in a process known as homeostasis, gently calming or stimulating. Adaptogens help the body to process stress by recharging the adrenal glands, which can be over-stimulated or exhausted from stress. Lavender, rose, and geranium are examples of adaptogens.

How oils work holistically

The concept of holistic healing involves treating the entire person so that the body, mind, and spirit are in harmony. This approach is very different to the conventional one that uses targeted drugs to tackle or suppress symptoms, but doesn't always address the root cause of a symptom.

Essential oils act on the mind and body to achieve deeper healing. For example, when relaxed, the body may be better at letting go of toxins and maintaining a healthy circulation. Inhaling black pepper oil gives physical and mental support to smokers trying to quit as the oil is decongesting and also helps to reduce cravings.

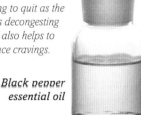

Black pepper essential oil

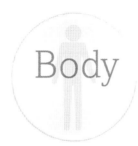

Body

On the **body**

Essential oils are natural healers, harnessing the medicinal properties that are traditionally associated with plants. For example, oils can be anti-inflammatory, antiseptic, and antifungal, and many essential oils are anti-microbial, helping to kill a whole variety of harmful micro-organisms to protect us against disease.

Work as antiseptics

Many essential oils have been shown to destroy the bacteria, viruses, and fungi that cause infection. One of the best known antiseptic essential oils, tea tree, is thought to be as effective as conventional treatments for athlete's foot, and recent research suggests that wounds infected with the *Staphylococcus aureus* bacterium heal faster when treated with tea tree oil than they do with conventional methods of treatment.

Chemical components, such as thymol found in thyme essential oil, menthol in peppermint, and eugenol in clove essential oil, to name but a few, have been shown to be powerfully antiseptic. Studies have demonstrated that inhaling these antiseptic essential oils can be as effective as applying them directly to the skin, and essential oil inhalation therapy has been used to treat the symptoms of bronchitis and acute sinusitis for many years.

In a world where many strains of bacteria are becoming resistant to conventional antibiotics, essential oils are beginning to be seen as a viable alternative.

Relieve pain and reduce inflammation

Essential oils are often used for their mild anaesthetic properties that can relieve localized pain. Oils such as thyme, rose, eucalyptus, clove, bergamot, and fennel have been shown to work on the body in a similar way to non-steroidal anti-inflammatory drugs (NSAIDs) such as ibuprofen, by inhibiting the enzymes in the body that cause inflammation, swelling, and pain. This analgesic effect makes these essential oils especially useful for soothing muscle and joint pains and for providing localized pain relief, for example from tension headaches and from sprains and strains.

Pain is often accompanied by inflammation. Many essential oils have anti-inflammatory properties. One notable example is frankincense. Several varieties of frankincense essential oil have been shown to inhibit the production of inflammatory proteins called cytokines and to prevent white blood cells, known as leukocytes, leaking into tissues, both of which cause inflammation.

Have a cleansing action

When functioning properly, our lungs, liver, digestive system, kidneys, and skin all help to remove waste products and toxins from the body. Negative factors such as stress, anxiety, poor diet, and lack of sleep can all interfere with this process. Essential oils often have detoxifying properties that help to cleanse the body and support a healthy excretory system.

For example, a chemical called D-limonene, found in citrus fruits such as oranges, lemons, mandarins, limes, and grapefruits, supports the healthy functioning of the liver, as well as helping

Star anise has strong antiseptic properties.

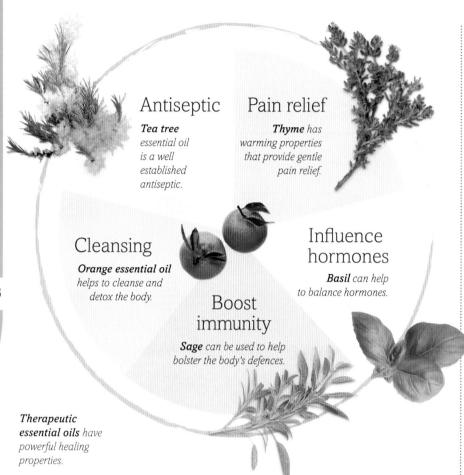

Antiseptic

Tea tree *essential oil is a well established antiseptic.*

Pain relief

Thyme *has warming properties that provide gentle pain relief.*

Cleansing

Orange essential oil *helps to cleanse and detox the body.*

Influence hormones

Basil *can help to balance hormones.*

Boost immunity

Sage *can be used to help bolster the body's defences.*

Therapeutic **essential oils** *have powerful healing properties.*

Influence hormones The endocrine system secretes hormones to regulate the body's processes. Essential oils can influence the action of hormones and smooth out imbalances. For example, relaxing rosemary has been shown to reduce levels of the stress hormone cortisol, and inhaling calming rose essential oil can help to decrease elevated levels of adrenaline. Several essential oils are thought to help regulate women's hormones during different stages of reproductive life. Lavandin essential oil is believed to help control hormone-induced mood fluctuations, and clary sage, fennel, basil, sage, cypress, and geranium have a similar balancing effect.

The concept of synergy

Blending oils *can enhance their effects. For example, mixing an anti-viral oil with one that is anti-inflammatory provides more effective relief from coughs and colds. This is sometimes called synergy, but the concept of synergy goes deeper than blending.*

Often, the therapeutic benefit of an essential oil is attributed to one or two of its major components. But increasingly evidence shows that the benefits of oils come from the interaction of major and minor components. For example, thymol, a major component of thyme, is highly antibacterial. However, studies show that the whole essential oil has a greater antibacterial effect than the isolated component. There's still much to understand about how oils work synergistically, but it is clear that while science is geared towards using single compounds, whole oils have benefits that can't be replicated in the lab.

to regulate appetite and lower cholesterol. And juniper, grapefruit, rosemary, fennel, and cypress oils have a mild diuretic effect that helps to support the work of the kidneys by encouraging the elimination of excess water. Combining these oils with a gentle massage and body brush encourages the healthy circulation of blood and lymphatic fluid, and in turn the removal of waste.

Help boost immunity

Essential oils promote wellness by enhancing and strengthening our immune response to disease. Some essential oils actually stimulate the production of disease-fighting white blood cells, such as phagocytes, T-cells, and B-cells, which are vital to the body's defences and immunity. In particular, eucalyptus and niaouli essential oils have been shown to encourage the process known as phagocytosis, where larger white blood cells called phagocytes engulf and then destroy, or deactivate, bacteria and viruses.

The compound linalool, which is found in high levels in essential oils such as lavender, sage, bay laurel, and eucalyptus has also been shown to increase the efficiency of the body's white blood cells.

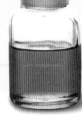

The components *in a single oil work together to greater effect.*

Essential oils work on the root cause as well as the symptom.

Spirit

On the **spirit**

Essential oils have been used for thousands of years to enhance spiritual practice. From their use in traditional ceremonies to supporting personal spiritual practices such as meditation, essential oils help to support spiritual attainment.

Promote spiritual pursuit

Essentials oils have been used for millennia to support prayer. Historically, oils such as frankincense, myrrh, cinnamon, cedarwood, and rose have been used in religious ceremonies. A well-chosen fragrance can calm breathing, settle and focus the mind, and create a sense of intent.

Enhance mindful practices

Aromas that calm the mind or help to lift the spirits, found in oils such as lavender, elemi, and bergamot, can be used to enhance focus during practices such as meditation, yoga, and breathing techniques.

Energy and chi In some traditional practices, essential oils are used to clear blockages in the "chakras", believed to be the energy centres in the body that relate to specific glands and organs. Chakras are said to be connected by meridians, which are described as channels through which vital energy, or "chi", flows.

Blockages in these areas are thought to lead to poor health in the related part of the body. The illustration, right, shows the position of the seven chakras. Specific essential oils are associated with different chakras, or centres, and are recommended to help bring balance and healing to these areas.

- **The crown chakra** at the top of the head governs the pineal gland and our "inner self". Oils such as frankincense, rose, jasmine, lavender, and elemi correspond with this area.
- **The brow chakra**, located just above and between the eyes, is connected to the pituitary gland and rules memory and mind. Oils such as myrrh, sandalwood, and jasmine can be used to treat blockages here.
- **The throat chakra** covers the area of the throat and the thyroid gland and relates to communication. Try lavender, chamomile, clary sage, cajuput, peppermint, geranium, and rosemary to treat this area.
- **The heart chakra**, located around the heart and upper body, affects wellbeing. Useful oils include rose, bergamot, lemon balm, chamomile, neroli, sandalwood, and palmarosa.
- **The solar plexus chakra** includes organs in the upper abdomen and is connected to self-esteem. Try ginger, helichrysum, manuka, coriander, lavender, marjoram, and orange.
- **The sacral chakra**, located in the lower abdomen, is linked to the reproductive system and responds to essential oils such as sandalwood, jasmine, rose, ylang ylang, orange, and geranium.
- **The base chakra**, at the base of the spine, connects to our ability to feel grounded. Oils that help healing here include myrrh, cedarwood, patchouli, petitgrain, benzoin, carrot, and vetiver.

In some practices, oils are used to clear blockages in the "chakras", or energy centres, in the body

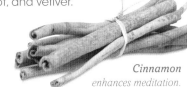

Cinnamon enhances meditation.

Chakras

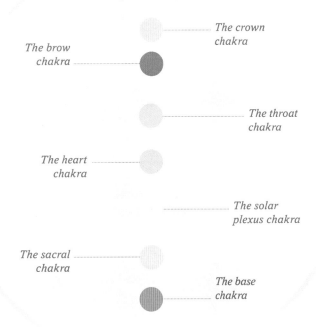

The crown chakra

The brow chakra

The throat chakra

The heart chakra

The solar plexus chakra

The sacral chakra

The base chakra

How essential oils are extracted

A plant's essential oils are contained in tiny sacs on the surface of a leaf or flower, and sometimes within bark, seeds, and roots. When you scratch a piece of lemon peel and get a spray with an **intense lemon fragrance**, you are breaking open the sacs on the peel's surface and **releasing** the lemon oil. And when you rub the leaves of a herb between your fingers to produce a smell, you are **breaking the vessels** to release the oil. Producing essential oils involves one of several methods to burst open the sacs and collect the oil.

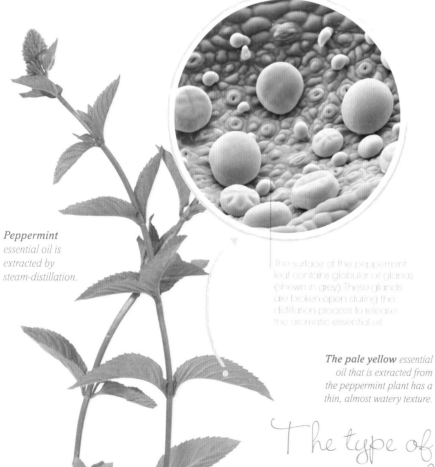

Peppermint essential oil is extracted by steam-distillation.

The surface of the peppermint leaf contains globular oil glands (shown in grey). These glands are broken open during the distillation process to release the aromatic essential oil.

The pale yellow essential oil that is extracted from the peppermint plant has a thin, almost watery texture.

Methods of **extraction**

The method used to produce an essential oil depends on the type of plant material that the oil is being extracted from. Most essential oils are produced by a process of steam-distillation, but the oil in some flowers and plants is extremely delicate and would be destroyed by the heat used in this method, so these plants require a special method of oil production known as absolute extraction.

There are four main methods of production: **steam-distillation**, the most widely used; **expression**, a simple method that is used to extract oil from rinds; **absolute extraction**, used for producing an oil from very delicate flowers; and **CO_2 extraction**, a new, evolving method.

The type of plant material determines which method of extraction is used to produce the essential oil.

Steam-distillation The most popular method for extracting essential oils is steam-distillation, a process used for herbs, roots, bark, and resins. This ancient method of extraction can be dated back around 5,000 years with the discovery of earthenware stills. Today, most stills are made of stainless steel or copper.

Firstly, the plant material is placed in a large container. Either steam is passed through the container, or water is added and heated to produce steam. As the plant material heats up, it gradually softens and pressure builds up on the surface of the plant, breaking open the tiny sacs that contain the plant's essential oil. The volatile oil rises up with the steam. The steam is then condensed, usually with cold water held in a coiling pipe, and collected in a vessel. Here, the oil and the water separate, with the oil rising and gathering on top of the water, ready to be tapped off and bottled.

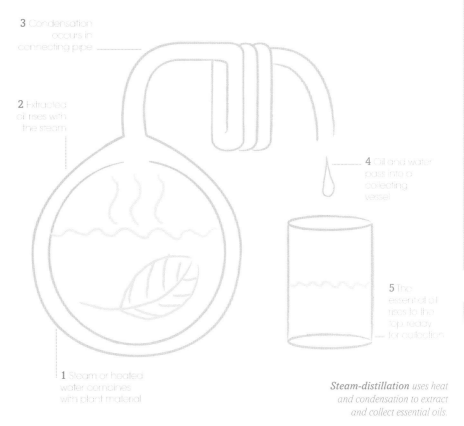

3 Condensation occurs in connecting pipe

2 Extracted oil rises with the steam

4 Oil and water pass into a collecting vessel

5 The essential oil rises to the top, ready for collection

1 Steam or heated water combines with plant material

Steam-distillation uses heat and condensation to extract and collect essential oils.

Expression The simplest way to extract an essential oil is to press the plant material and then collect the oil.

This method is used when the essential oils are found in the outer rind of a fruit and are easily released, as is the case with citrus peel. Citrus fruits, such as grapefruit, orange, lemon, and lime are mechanically pressed to extract their liquid, and then the watery juice is separated from the essential oil.

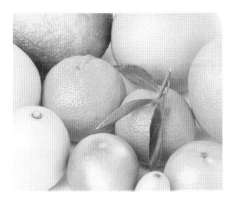

The outer rind of citrus fruits contains oil glands that can be pressed to extract the oil.

Absolute extraction The fragrance of extremely delicate flowers, such as jasmine or mimosa, is damaged by the heat involved in distillation, so these plants require a different method of extraction without steam or water. The result is a highly concentrated oil known as an absolute.

In Grasse, the perfumery capital of France, flower oils were traditionally hand-extracted using a time-consuming process known as

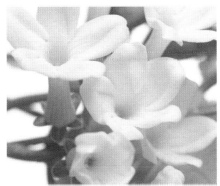

The oil from the delicate jasmine flower is obtained by solvent extraction.

enfleurage. Framed glass plates were covered with lard, and the flowers placed on top. After a few days, the lard absorbed the fragrant oil from the flower, which was then extracted by alcohol to produce the absolute.

Modern methods involve blending flowers with a solvent. The solvent is then removed to leave the absolute oil.

CO$_2$ extraction A new method of extraction called "supercritical carbon dioxide (CO$_2$) extraction" uses gas rather than heat. This involves putting CO$_2$ under pressure to convert it from a gas into a liquid that can be used as a solvent. The solvent diffuses through the plant material and extracts its aromatic constituents.

This method tends to produce additional constituents, and so more research is needed before it becomes widely used. However, it does produce an aroma closer to that of the actual plants than that acheived by other methods and so may grow in popularity.

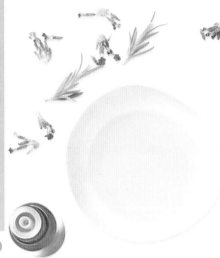

Choosing essential oils

It is not always easy, especially as a novice, to know whether or not you are buying a **pure**, **natural**, good-quality, **sustainable** essential oil. Being aware of what to look for can help you make a worthwhile purchase. The following guidelines set out key factors to consider when purchasing oils, helping you to assess **quality** and **provenance** and to choose the best oils for you.

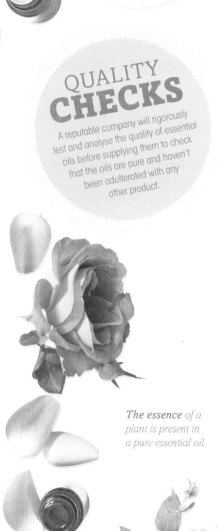

QUALITY CHECKS

A reputable company will rigorously test and analyse the quality of essential oils before supplying them to check that the oils are pure and haven't been adulterated with any other product.

Natural versus **synthetic**

A pure essential oil can be made up of a hundred or more individual chemical constituents, some of which are major constituents, others minor, which all work together "synergistically". This means that when combined they create an overall effect that is greater than their individual parts (p.176). Synthetic fragrances, or isolated compounds, such as menthol, are far cheaper than pure essential oils, and although these may have a pleasant odour, they have none of the therapeutic benefits that make essential oils so special and unique. To be sure that you are choosing a pure essential oil, try to avoid products that contain added ingredients and bulking agents, as these additions increase the volume but reduce the quality of the oil.

The essence of a plant is present in a pure essential oil.

Recognizing **quality**

Spend time researching companies and try to identify reputable ones that are likely to go to the most trouble to ensure their oils are of a high quality.

Company credentials Some companies have developed their own terminology to demonstrate that their oils are superior. For example, an oil may be described as being of "therapeutic" or "aromatherapy" grade, but ultimately these are marketing terms and not meaningful. It can be more helpful, though not a guarantee of quality, to check if a company is a member of a reputable association, such as the Aromatherapy Trade Council (ATC) in the United Kingdom or the National Association of Holistic Aromatherapy (NAHA) in the United States. Another way to check a company's credentials is to find out if it runs aromatherapy courses and/or has links with qualified aromatherapy practitioners, which indicates that the company has a deserved reputation.

All in the name If an essential oil is authentic, the botanical name should appear on the label, and compounds called chemotypes (substances that link oils to a specific plant variety), may

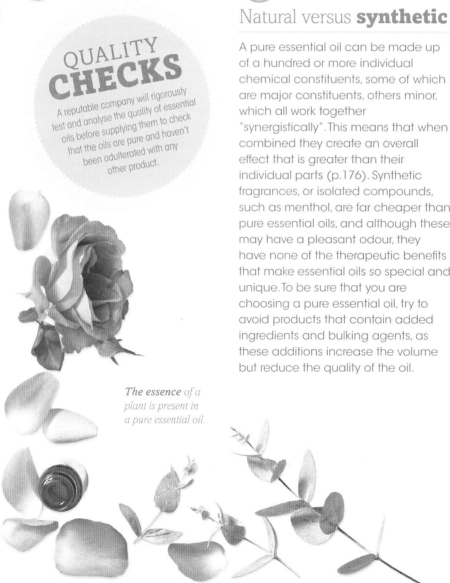

Ensure that you are buying a pure, natural, good-quality, sustainably produced essential oil.

also be listed. For example, thyme will list its botanical name *Thymus vulgaris*, and the label might also mention linalool or thymol, to indicate that the oil is from one botanical species. The label, or a company website, may also cite a country of origin, which indicates that it is a true plant oil.

Checking **sustainability**

Certain oils, such as sandalwood and rosewood, are now available only in limited amounts, or are unavailable, due to concerns about sustainability. Check the sustainability policy of a company before you buy an oil.

Endangered plants Some plants have been harvested almost to extinction. For example, spikenard (*Nardostachys jatamansi*) has a critically endangered status and so this oil should be avoided unless the supplier can guarantee that it is cultivated. You can check a plant's status at www.iucnredlist.org/search.

Supporting fair trade Fairtrade often ensures sustainability. Harvesting plants for oils can be an important source of income for some communities. With a conservation plan in place, plants are more likely to be protected as an important resource. Frankincense oil from Kenya, for example, is available as a FairWild source, a standard that protects the harvesting of wild species and ensures fair trading. When choosing oils, look

for Fairtrade or Fair for Life logos that suggest sustainability and help to ensure the benefits of producing an oil are felt by the people growing and harvesting the plants.

Choosing **organic**

Organic essential oils and base oils have a higher therapeutic value because they contain the highest levels of antioxidants and are less likely to have potentially toxic residues from pesticides and chemical fertilizers. Organic production also benefits farmers, their families, and communities, is kinder to the soil, and generally provides a more positive outlook for future crops, wildlife, and water sources. Check company literature to see if they support organic farming practices.

What's on the label?

Reading a label closely can help you to make an on the spot assessment of an essential oil. A label that has the following information suggests a high-quality oil:

The oils's botanical name and the part of the plant used.

The country of origin.

The distillation or packing date and/or expiration date.

The batch number and, if applicable, a chemotype (such as thymol).

Assessing **cost**

All essential oils require a large amount of plant matter to make just a small amount of oil. The price of an oil is connected to its yield from the plant matter, which can vary greatly, from less than 0.1 per cent to 25 per cent. For example, around 1,000kg (2,200lb) of hand-picked orange blossom produces just 1kg (2¼lb) of neroil oil – hence the high cost of exquisite neroli. In contrast, 1 tonne of cloves produces up to 200kg (440lb) clove oil, making this a less expensive oil.

Any company that sells all of their oils for the same price, or has prices that seem too good to be true, should be avoided. The good news is that because essential oils are so highly concentrated, just a small amount goes a long way, and only a few drops are used at a time. To ensure freshness, buy a small amount regularly, rather than large amounts that might go off before you use them.

Europe

Europe is a major source of essential oils. The range of climates means that a variety of plants can be grown, from citrus fruits in the hot and sunny climes of Spain and Italy to more frost-tolerant plants in northern European countries.

Bosnia	Bay laurel
	Helichrysum
Bulgaria	Parsley
	Rose
	Valerian
France	Angelica
	Caraway
	Carrot
	Cedarwood
	Clary sage
	Cypress
	Fenugreek
	Juniper
	Lavender
	Lemon balm
	Mullein
	Oregano
	Pine
	Sage
	Tarragon
	Thyme
	Tuberose
	Violet
Germany	Chamomile (blue)
Hungary	Coriander
	Dill
	Fennel
	Roman Chamomile
	Savoury
	Yarrow
Italy	Bergamot
	Helichrysum
	Lemon
	Orange
Sweden	Birch
Spain	Cistus
	Eucal. globulus
	Lemon verbena
	Marjoram
	Rosemary
	Sage
United Kingdom	Lavender
	Peppermint
	Roman Chamomile
	Yarrow

Where do oils come from?

Essential oils are extracted from a wide range of plants worldwide. Where plants grow depends on factors such as their **tolerance to frost** and if there's sufficient **rainfall** or irrigation. Many oils **thrive** in Mediterranean areas and in subtropical and tropical climates.

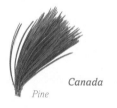

Canada
Pine

NORTH AMERICA

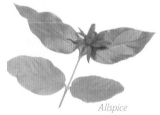

Allspice

West Indies

Americas

The humid, tropical climate in South America provides fertile growing conditions for citrus fruits, while pine forests grow abundantly in the cooler conditions in Canada.

Canada	Pine
Brazil	Eucal. citriodora
	Mandarin
	Orange
	Rosewood
Paraguay	Petitgrain
Peru	Lemon verbena
West Indies	Allspice
	Grapefruit
	Peppermint

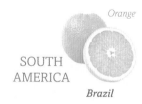

Orange

SOUTH AMERICA

Brazil

Peru

Paraguay

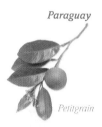

Petitgrain

Africa

The variations in climate across Africa produce a diverse range of plants, from exotic ylang ylang in the sub-tropical southeast, to myrtle and cedarwood in the north.

Comores	Ylang ylang
Congo	Geranium
Ethiopia	Myrrh
Eygpt	Basil
	Jasmine
Kenya	Tea tree
Madagascar	Clove
	Niaouli
	Palmarosa
	Ravintsara
	Vanilla
	Vetiver
Morocco	Cedarwood
	Mimosa
	Mugwort
	Neroli
	Myrtle
Réunion	Geranium
Somalia	Frankincense
	Myrrh
South Africa	Buchu
	Euc. Radiata
	Lemongrass
Uganda	Palmarosa
Zimbabwe	Eucal. smithii
	Tagetes

How crops are **grown**

Traditionally, most essential oils were harvested from the wild, and this is still the case for some abundant species such as juniper. However, as aromatherapy grows in popularity, with markets expanding in countries such as the United States, there is increased pressure on plants grown in the wild, and it can be a struggle to keep up with demand. To ensure a continuous supply of oils, many plants are specially cultivated, with suppliers creating the soil conditions and irrigation needed to grow crops.

Asia

Essential oils from Asia are *mainly from the south of the continent, where tropical conditions provide ideal growing conditions for spices such as cardamom and nutmeg.*

China	Camphor
India	Cardamom
	Cumin
	Patchouli
	Sandalwood
Indonesia	Benzoin
	Citronella
	Galangal
	Nutmeg
Iran	Rose
Nepal	Wintergreen
Oman	Frankincense
Philippines	Elemi
Sri Lanka	Black pepper
	Cardamom
	Cinnamon
	Citronella
	Ginger
	Lime
Thailand	Plai
Turkey	Rose
Vietnam	Cajuput
	Litsea
	Star anise

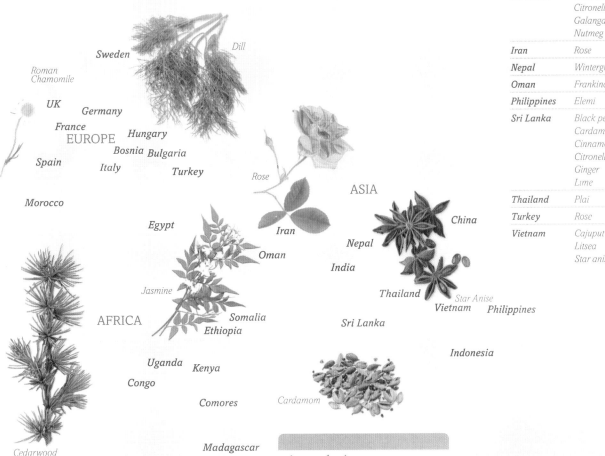

Roman Chamomile

Sweden

Dill

UK

Germany

France

EUROPE

Hungary

Spain

Bosnia Bulgaria

Italy

Turkey

Morocco

Rose

Egypt

Iran

ASIA

China

Oman

Nepal

India

Jasmine

AFRICA

Somalia

Ethiopia

Thailand

Sri Lanka

Star Anise

Vietnam Philippines

Uganda Kenya

Congo

Comores

Cardamom

Indonesia

Cedarwood

Madagascar

Zimbubwe

Réunion

South Africa

Australasia

Much of Australasia is *semi-arid, suitable for drought-resistant plants such as tea tree.*

Australia	Eucal. Globulus
	Fragonia
	Tea tree
New Zealand	Manuka

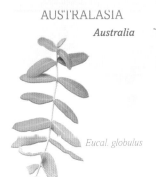

AUSTRALASIA

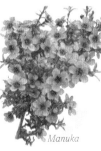

Australia

Manuka

New Zealand

Eucal. globulus

How essential oils enter the body

The quickest way to absorb essential oils is by **inhaling** their aroma, which has a direct effect on the brain. Oils can also be absorbed via the skin during a **massage**, in a **bath**, or in a cream. Both routes allow oils to enter the bloodstream, where their healing properties take effect.

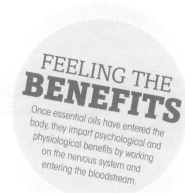

FEELING THE BENEFITS

Once essential oils have entered the body, they impart psychological and physiological benefits by working on the nervous system and entering the bloodstream.

Inhaling essential oils

Humans are believed to have the ability to distinguish between more than 10,000 different aromas. Of all the senses, smell has the most direct connection to the mind and effect on our emotions. In fact, our ability to perceive odour is so connected to our sense of wellbeing that those who have lost their sense of smell can be more prone to problems such as depression and anxiety. The entire concept of aromatherapy is rooted in how aromas directly interact with our brains and body chemistry.

Processing aromas This involves complex pathways in the brain. When we inhale a scent, we take in aromatic molecules that bind to "receptor" cells in the nasal passage. Here they send messages to the olfactory "bulb" in the forebrain and these are interpreted as a smell. Molecules are also inhaled into the lungs where they enter the blood.

The effects on the body Studies show that inhaling a scent has an immediate effect on the brain's activity. Scents breach the blood–brain barrier (the brain's protective membrane), accessing centres in the brain linked to conscious thought, and also reaching the limbic system – the brain's emotional switchboard, where memory and emotions reside, and impulses such as "fight or flight", nurturing, hunger, and arousal are controlled. The limbic system is also linked to hormones.

How the body inhales an aroma

When you inhale the aroma of an essential oil, it is processed rapidly by the brain so that you quickly receive the therapeutic benefits of the oil.

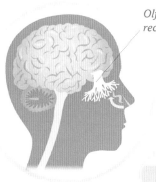

Olfactory receptor cells

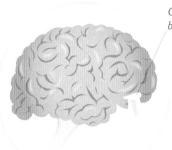

Olfactory bulb

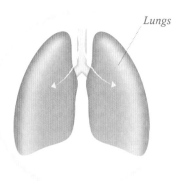

Lungs

1 Aromatic molecules travel up the nasal passage, where they bind to olfactory receptor cells in the nose. The cells send impulses to the olfactory bulb at the base of the forebrain.

2 The forebrain interprets the electrical impulses as a smell and rapidly processes and responds to the essential oil's unique aroma and properties.

Molecules are also inhaled directly from the nasal passages into the lungs, and from these enter the bloodstream, contributing to the healing effect of essential oils.

Essential oils impart their therapeutic effects on the body by being inhaled or absorbed into the skin.

Absorption into the skin

Diluted essential oils can be absorbed into the bloodstream via the skin. Many factors influence how much oil is absorbed, including skin type, the room's and the oil's temperature, and whether the base that the essential oil is mixed with is easily absorbed.

Therapeutic touch When essential oils are combined with massage, this enhances the healing effects of the oils as massage in itself can induce a state of deep relaxation. When you are stressed, physically or emotionally, your body is flooded with hormones that keep you awake and aware. In this "fight or flight" state, other processes, such as immunity, cellular repair, and the assimilation of nutrients from food, are shut down. The relaxing effect of a massage helps the body systems to start working effectively again.

During an aromatherapy massage you also inhale the aroma of the essential oil. Studies using either a plain base oil or an essential oil blend in a massage have shown that those receiving the essential oil blend usually experience greater therapeutic benefits. For example, a footbath with lavender essential oil is more relaxing and healing than a footbath with just warm water. Likewise, a massage with essential oils chosen for their specific healing properties has been shown to be more effective at healing and relieving pain from a range of causes, including post-surgical pain, cancer pain, and backache, than a massage with plain vegetable oil.

Diluting essential oils

Concentrated essences *Essential oils are highly concentrated plant essences, so as a general rule they should always be used diluted in a base oil, lotion, ointment or balm, or bath oil. In addition, while diluted oils can be used as mouthwashes and gargles, they should never be swallowed without the advice of a medically trained practitioner.*

Even when diluted, most leave-on essential oil skin preparations should avoid delicate areas of the body, such as the eyes and mucous membranes. If you have sensitive skin, or suffer from allergies, it is always good to perform a patch test of your chosen oil first. Never apply essential oils neat on babies or children. See pages 194–95 for safety guidelines.

Exceptions to the rule *Some essential oils, such as rose absolute, ylang ylang, jasmine, chamomile, tea tree, and lavender, are an exception to this rule and can be applied neat, as a scent. Likewise, tea tree can be used neat as emergency first aid for cuts, stings, and bites. Follow the guidelines in the A–Z section of this book.*

How the body **absorbs oils**

Oils can be absorbed into the bloodstream via application to the skin. During massage, you also gain therapeutic benefits from inhaling the aroma of oils.

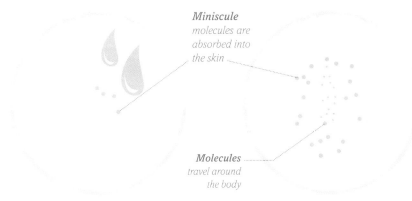

Miniscule molecules are absorbed into the skin

Molecules travel around the body

1 Tiny essential oil molecules are absorbed through the pores of the skin where they enter the bloodstream and start to take effect.

2 Once in the bloodstream, the oils travel around the body via the circulatory system. The therapeutic effects of the oils act on the body systems and promote healing.

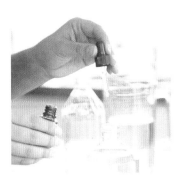

Always dilute *essential oils with a base oil before using, unless the oil's usage guidelines state otherwise.*

Applying essential oils

There are many ways to enjoy the benefits of essential oils. Languishing in a luxurious **aromatherapy** bath or enjoying an **oil-infused massage** are two popular methods. You can also disperse oils in the air, dab an oil balm on a **pulse point**, or sprinkle a few drops of oil on a tissue and **inhale** the scent deeply. Here are the main ways to enjoy your essential oils.

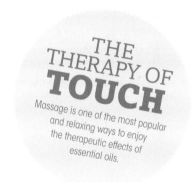

THE THERAPY OF **TOUCH**

Massage is one of the most popular and relaxing ways to enjoy the therapeutic effects of essential oils.

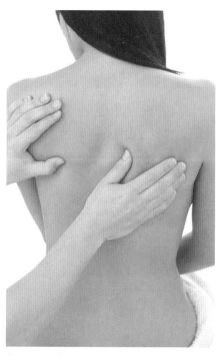

An aromatherapy massage helps to relieve tension in the body while delivering the benefits of your chosen blend of oils.

Massage

An essential oil massage has the added benefit of soothing touch. A massage from a trained aromatherapist is a wonderful treat, but you can just as easily enjoy a massage from a partner, or practise self-massage, which is a great way to nurture yourself and can become part of a daily skin- and health-care routine.

As essential oils are concentrated, they need diluting in a base, or carrier, oil (pp.294–309). For normal skin, try a light base, such as almond, grapeseed, apricot, coconut, sunflower, or canola. For dry skin, use heavier enriching oils, such as avocado, olive, wheatgerm, argan, and jojoba. Medicinal bases, such as neem, calendula, or St John's wort, provide therapeutic properties.

Mixing massage blends For a body massage, use a 2.5 per cent (for sensitive or damaged skin) to 5 per cent (for normal skin) dilution; for a facial massage use a 1 per cent dilution (see the dilutions chart on page 37). To make enough for a full-body massage, pour about 2 tablespoons base oil onto a saucer and add about 4–6 drops of your chosen essential oil, or oil blend.

Pulse point massage Pulse points are areas where blood vessels are close to the surface. Applying essential oils at these points speeds the oil's absorption.

When **to use**

Massage is ideal for addressing problems over a large surface area, for example, achy muscles and joints, digestive problems, and fluid retention. You can also home in on an area, for example, massaging the abdomen to relieve period pains or digestive upsets.

A therapeutic massage with essential oils is effective at creating a sense of calm and deep relaxation, and a feeling of being cared for.

To ease headaches, massage an essential oil balm onto the temples. You can also try massaging a balm into the pulse points on the wrist or neck to help you relax and unwind.

Mix essential oils with the base oil that best suits your needs.

Inhalation

Inhaling an essential oil, or a blend of oils, is a quick and easy way to enjoy the oils' benefits, and forms the basis of aromatherapy, as an essential oil's aroma is inhaled whichever method of application you use.

Tissue inhalation The simplest way to inhale an essential oil is to sprinkle 2–3 drops of the oil onto a tissue and then inhale deeply. You can place the tissue in a plastic bag and carry it around with you to use as and when you wish. Similarly, you can sprinkle a few drops of a soothing essential oil onto your pillowcase (or a tissue to avoid staining) at night to help you relax and induce restful sleep.

Making a steam inhalation
Make a therapeutic steam inhalation by adding about 4–8 drops of your chosen oil, or oils, to a bowl of just-boiled water. Lean over the bowl and place a towel over your head to contain the vapours, then, with eyes closed, breathe deeply for 10 minutes, or until there is no more steam. Alternatively, you can buy a special inhaler cup.
　　For epilepsy or asthma sufferers, or with young children, use caution. Instead of leaning over a bowl and covering the head with a towel, simply place the bowl of hot water nearby and capture the wafts of steam.

When **to use**

Respiratory conditions, such as hay fever, colds, congested sinuses or a chesty cough, particularly benefit from inhalations. Steam inhalations also refresh and cleanse the skin.

Try an inhalation as a quick remedy to calm or invigorate the mind or lift the spirits.

A steam inhalation scented with essential oils can help to clear congestion and soothe the mind.

Baths

Whether you are enjoying a leisurely warm bath or a quick shallow hand, foot or sitz bath (see below), adding essential oils to water is a hugely pleasurable and popular way to use them. The warmth of the water relaxes and soothes muscles, encouraging relaxation, and at the same time opens pores to help the essential oils penetrate the skin and enter the body more rapidly.

Adding oils to a bath Even though the essential oils will be diluted in the bath water, you still need to blend the oils in a base, or carrier, oil before adding them to the bath. This helps the oils to disperse in the water and also moisturizes the skin. For an average-sized bath, mix 4–6 drops of your chosen essential oil, or oils, with 1 tablespoon of a light base oil, such as sunflower, which contains waxes that act like an emulsifier, helping to disperse the oils evenly. You can also buy neutral, water-dispersing base oils, or mix the essential oils with 1 tablespoon of full-fat milk – the fats in the milk work in a similar way to the base oil, helping to disperse the oils evenly. Aim to relax in the bath for at least 15 minutes. To get the full benefits of the oils, add them once the bath has been run as they can quickly evaporate in the heat.

Hand and foot baths Hand and foot baths are a great way to target smaller areas of the body quickly. A foot bath can treat a specific condition such as athletes' foot, or soothe tired, sore feet. If your ankles are swollen, try following a hot foot bath with a cool one to improve circulation. You can also use hot and cold baths for sore, swollen hands. Fill a bowl or basin (one large enough to take both your feet, or hands) with hot water, and add 4–6 of drops of your chosen oil to a base oil or milk, as for a normal bath. Soak the hands or feet for 10 minutes.

Sitz baths A sitz (shallow) bath is an excellent way to treat conditions such as thrush, haemorrhoids, and urinary infections, or to heal stitches after childbirth. Adding tea tree oil to a sitz bath is a classic treatment for thrush. To make the bath, half-fill the bath with warm water. Use the same method of dilution as for a large bath, and sit in the water for 10 minutes.

When **to use**

Aromatherapy baths are deeply relaxing and reviving. Make sure you give yourself plenty of time to lie back and enjoy the therapeutic soak.

A sitz bath can bring immediate relief to conditions such as thrush or haemorrhoids, while a hand or foot bath is best for aching, swollen, or tired hands and feet or athlete's foot.

Soothing chamomile is perfect for baths.

Infuse your bath with your favourite blend of essential oils, then lie back and relax.

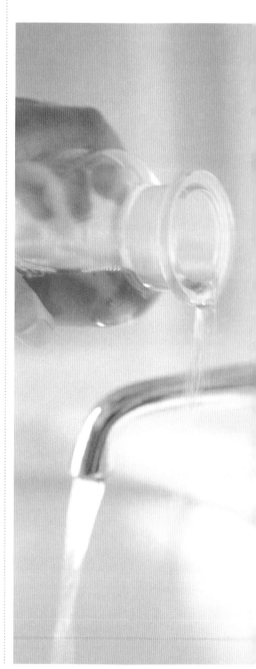

Adding calming oils to warm water soothes body and mind.

Compresses

A compress infused with therapeutic essential oils is a simple and effective way to treat local complaints such as bruises, burns and scalds, headaches, and varicose veins.

Hot or cold? Using hot or cold water can be down to preference, but some conditions do require cooling while others respond to heat.

A hot compress is ideal for complaints such as skin infections, including abscesses and boils, and muscular or joint problems, including strains, backache, rheumatism, and arthritis. For example, a hot compress with ginger, cypress, juniper, pine, and lavender essential oils is wonderfully warming and relieving for aching muscles and joints.

A cold water compress is ideal for sprains and sports injuries, especially if the area already feels hot and inflamed, and for headaches. Using essential oils such as lavender, neroli, peppermint, and eucalyptus helps to enhance the cooling process.

Making a compress Add 3–4 drops of essential oil to a shallow bowl of hot or cold water. Disperse well. Soak a flannel, wring this out well, and apply to the relevant part of the body. For a hot compress,

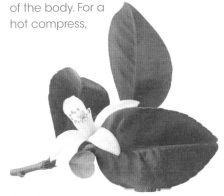

Neroli has calming properties that work well in a compress.

once the flannel is positioned, you can cover it with a towel or piece of cling film to insulate it if you wish. This also stops the water dripping onto clothes. Leave the flannel on the skin until it reaches body temperature, then repeat the whole process three times.

If you are using essential oils that can irritate the skin in a compress, it's important to always pre-dilute the essential oils in a base, or carrier, oil, such as almond or sunflower, before adding the oils to the water.

When **to use**

Try a hot compress to relieve aching and tired muscles after an exercise workout or strenuous physical activity.

A cold compress works especially well for soothing eye strain brought on by looking at computer screens for long periods of time.

Showers and saunas

Essential oils make a wonderful addition to saunas and steamy showers. Experiment with different blend combinations and aromas to suit your needs at different times. For example, if you wish to have an energizing shower to kick-start the day, choose stimulating and invigorating oils such as basil and rosemary. Or to help lift the spirits and create a sense of positivity, try uplifting oils such as bergamot, lemon, and rose.

Using oils in the shower

For a steamy aromatherapy shower, put 5–8 drops of an essential oil, or oil blend, on a warm, damp flannel, then place the flannel in the area you are having a shower, but don't use the

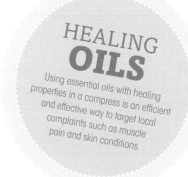

flannel to wash yourself. If possible, hang the flannel at face level to enjoy the aroma fully. Make sure the shower is hot enough to produce steam. You can also add the essential oil drops to 2 tablespoons unscented shower gel.

Using oils in a sauna Add 20–40 drops of an essential oil, or oil blend, to the pitcher of water that is used to splash the coals during a sauna. Cypress, eucalyptus, and pine essential oils all work well in a sauna.

When **to use**

Adding essential oils to a sauna or shower is a great way to clear sinuses, relieve tension headaches, and to soothe irritating hay fever and allergy symptoms.

Using oils in a shower or sauna also invigorates the mind and helps you to feel calm and relaxed.

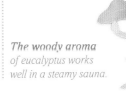

The woody aroma of eucalyptus works well in a steamy sauna.

Diffusion

This increasingly popular way to use essential oils disperses tiny molecules of the oil into the air in a fine vapour or mist. Traditionally, oil burners have been used to diffuse oils. Today, there are several types of diffuser including ultrasonic ones, vaporizers that use a small fan or warm water, electronic aromastones, and reed diffusers. Room sprays can also be used to disperse oils.

Using a diffuser, vaporizer, or oil burner To use an oil burner, pour a little warm water on the hotplate before adding the oil drops to stop the oil from burning too quickly. To use electronic diffusers or vaporizers, add the oils and use according to the manufacturer's instructions.

Making a room spray A room spray is a type of diffusion that releases a more concentrated amount of oil into the air very quickly. To make a room spray, combine 20–30 drops of essential oils with 2 tablespoons each of mineral water and vodka, and transfer the solution to a sterilized atomizer bottle.

Most essential oils can be used to fragrance a room, but citrus oils are particularly refreshing. Essential oils that have antiseptic properties, such as cedarwood, eucalyptus, lavender, and tea tree, are ideal for fumigating rooms, while lemon, lemongrass, and citronella can be used in a spray to repel insects.

When **to use**

Diffusers can deodorize or fumigate a room, or simply create a special atmosphere.

Sitting near to a burner or vaporizer is an effective way to inhale the vapours of the oils and to benefit from their therapeutic properties.

Use a room spray to change the mood in a room, either to create a feeling of calm, invigorate, or perhaps to add a little romance.

Room sprays are also useful for disinfecting and deodorizing an area such as a sick room and for repelling insects.

Cedarwood oil can be added to a diffuser to clear stale air.

Personal scents

While some oils, such as lavender, rose otto, chamomile, jasmine, vanilla, and ylang ylang, can be worn on their own as a scent, most need diluting in a base – perfumes are usually a mixture of fragranced oils in an alcohol base. You can use a single oil or several oils in a blend to create a scent that may have different "notes". When you smell a perfume, the top notes are typically the first thing you smell, followed by mid- and then base notes (p.344).

Creating a scent Don't be afraid to experiment with blends to find your favourite scent – see page 344 for essential oil blending guidelines. Essentially, try to limit your blends to no more than 4–7 oils, and try a blend for a day or so to let it settle so that you can get a better idea of its true aroma.

When **to use**

Adding essential oils to a base solution is a great way to create your own personal fragrance. You can tailor the scent to suit your unique style and preferences and to create daytime and evening perfumes.

Mouthwashes and gargles

Although essential oils should not be swallowed, you can dilute them in water or a base of aloe vera juice to make an effective mouthwash or gargle that can be used to support good oral health and hygiene.

Home-made mouthwashes are cost effective and can be tailored to your needs. They also avoid a range of synthetic ingredients that are often found in commercial mouthwashes.

Making a mouthwash To make a basic mouthwash or gargle solution, dilute 4–5 drops of essential oil (clove, fennel, ginger, lemon, mint, rosemary, and sage are all good antiseptic choices) into a tablespoon of base oil. Further dilute this blend into a tumblerful of hot water and use as needed. Do not swallow the mixture.

When **to use**

Mouthwashes and gargles are ideal for mouth ulcers, gum disease, throat infections, and to help combat bad breath.

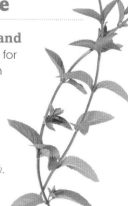

Peppermint has a fresh, menthol aroma.

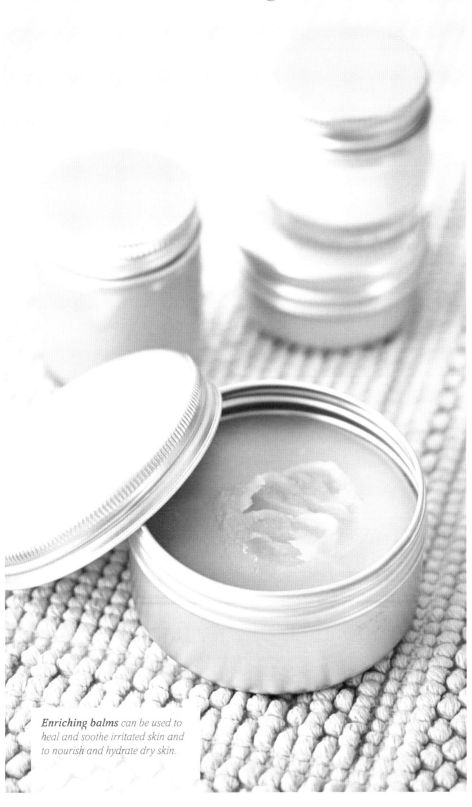

Dab a small amount of cream on irritated or itchy skin.

Enriching balms *can be used to heal and soothe irritated skin and to nourish and hydrate dry skin.*

Ointments, balms, and creams

Using oils in ointments, balms, and cream bases is an effective way to promote skin healing and to nourish skin. Ointments tend to be oil-based, while balms and creams contain extra ingredients for a creamier texture. Treat localized areas, applying a balm or ointment where needed, to encourage healing or to combat skin dryness.

When **to use**

Use for skin conditions such as eczema, psoriasis, bruising, and varicose veins, and apply to wounds to encourage healing.

Essential oils in a cream can form part of a daily skincare regime.

Use ointments with tea tree and manuka as first-aid remedies.

Hair care

Combining essential oil blends with herbal infusions, or creating conditioning hair oils by mixing essential oils with nourishing bases such as coconut oil, are great ways to enjoy a hair-care regime using natural products. Essential oil hair products can help to restore shine and lustre to hair while avoiding the many added ingredients in commercial products.

When **to use**

Use nourishing essential oil hair treatments to revive dry and dull-looking hair.

Storing essential oils

Essential oils are **volatile** substances, which means they evaporate and deteriorate more quickly when exposed to light, air, and heat. Sunlight is especially harmful to the oils as it can cause chemical reactions that degrade them. To get the complete **therapeutic** benefits from your essential oils, store them correctly so that they remain as **fresh** as possible.

Looking after
your essential oils

Following the guidelines below will help you to maximize the life span of your essential oils and enjoy their benefits to the full.

• **Avoid storing your essential oils** in plastic containers. Plastic is not recommended as it is not totally inert, which means that over time the essential oils will interact with the plastic and may become contaminated by potentially toxic ingredients that leak out of the plastic.

• **Store your essential oils** and essential oil blends in sterilized glass (or stainless steel) bottles with lids that seal tightly. Bottles with dark-coloured glass are best as ultraviolet rays of light can taint oils by reacting with chemicals in the oil. Amber, dark blue, or deep violet glass bottles offer the best protection for your essential oils, keeping them as fresh as possible.

• **Store bottles in a cupboard** out of direct light and away from heat. Some oils, such as citrus ones, should be stored in the fridge (see opposite).

• **Make a note on the bottle** of the date it was opened, or label made-up blends that you've bottled with the names of the oils that were used and the date the blend was made.

• **Essential oil bottles** should have a dropper insert, which makes them harder to spill (p.194), and easier to measure out. This is also a good safety device if a child gets hold of a bottle.

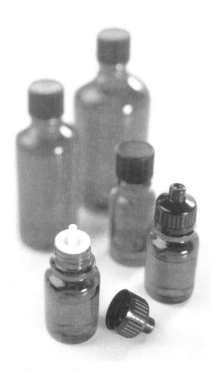

*Small, **dark-coloured bottles** help to protect oils from the damaging effects of light and air.*

Disposing of essential oils safely

If you have essential oils that are past their best or that you no longer need, contact your local authority waste disposal department, or check their web page, for advice on how to dispose of them, and follow their recommendations.

If there is no specific advice, dispose of essential oils at your local household waste recycling centre in the same way as you would do for unused paints and solvents.

• **Keep oils away from children.** Though safe if properly diluted, essential oils are highly concentrated and can irritate the skin or the eyes if they are rubbed in, and can be toxic if taken internally (see page 194 for what to do if an oil is ingested).

• **Essential oils, like alcohol,** are flammable, so should never be left near sources of ignition, such as fires, cookers, candles, or naked flames.

Follow the storage advice to ensure oils stay as fresh as possible so that you enjoy their full benefits.

Shelf life of **essential oils**

The following chart is a useful guide to how long you should keep your essential oils before they are past their best. These guidelines are based on an oil being relatively fresh when you buy it from your supplier (check the batch number or use-by date), being opened and therefore exposed to air, and on their being stored under ideal conditions (see opposite). As such tiny amounts of essential oils are used at any one time, the oils usually come in small bottles that can be replaced as needed.

If you are in any doubt about how fresh an essential oil is, avoid using it on the skin (some oils that are non-irritant when fresh may irritate the skin when oxidized) or for therapeutic use. Instead, use the oil around the house, in a diffuser perhaps, or added to a household cleanser.

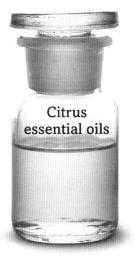 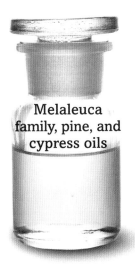 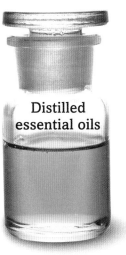 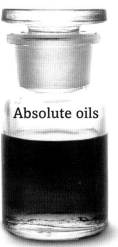

Citrus essential oils

Melaleuca family, pine, and cypress oils

Distilled essential oils

Absolute oils

9–12 months

Citrus oils such as grapefruit have the shortest shelf life. This is because they have a lot of the highly volatile components terpenes, which are prone to oxidization. Store in the fridge.

12–18 months

The melaleuca family (tea tree, niaouli) and pine and cypress essential oils have a fairly short shelf life due to relatively volatile components in their chemical composition.

2–3 years

Most of the essential oils that are steam-distilled have a shelf life of 2–3 years. Some resinous oils, such as sandalwood or myrrh, may last for longer than this.

3–5 years

Absolutes, such as rose absolute and jasmine, have the greatest longevity of all the oils and can last for up to five years.

Shelf life of **base oils**

Base oils generally have a shorter shelf life than essential oils. Unlike essential oils, they become rancid when they go off. Your nose should tell you that something is wrong, and at this point the oil is unsuitable for use on the skin.

Store base oils in dark glass bottles too, away from light and heat.

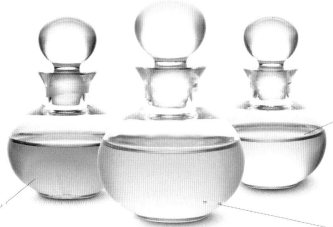

12–18 months

Most base oils have a shelf life of 12–18 months once opened.

2–3 years

Coconut and jojoba oils last the longest and should keep well for 2–3 years.

10–12 months

Borage, grapeseed, and evening primrose oils tend to oxidize at 10–12 months.

Using essential oils safely

As essential oils are **highly concentrated,** they need to be used sensibly and **diluted** properly. Follow advice on what to do if oils are spilt or misused, using oils on infants, and oils to avoid in pregnancy, when breastfeeding, and for some conditions.

TAKING CARE WITH OILS

Essential oils are perfectly safe if used sensibly. Before using an oil, carefully check the safety advice and make sure you follow the recommendations for dilution.

Spillage and **accidents**

Many essential oils irritate the skin if applied neat, without being diluted in a base, or carrier, oil, or other lotion. If you spill an essential oil, it can strip away varnish on furniture and stain fabrics such as carpets and bedding. Here are some tips for dealing with essential oil spillages and accidents and for cleaning diffusers and burners:

Accidentally ingesting oils Drink milk to dilute the oil and get medical advice quickly (see the box, below, for general information on ingesting essential oils).

Spilling oil on skin Quickly pour on a vegetable oil to dilute the essential oil: use sunflower, olive oil, or any other cooking or base oil. Once you've diluted the oil, gently wash the area with soapy water. If you don't have vegetable oil to hand, rinse the area with plenty of cold water.

Ingesting essential oils

Never take an essential oil internally without the supervision of a suitably qualified medical practitioner. Some essential oils that are totally non-toxic when applied to the skin are highly toxic when taken internally, and there can be a risk of irritation to the throat or stomach, or even liver or nervous system damage.

Splashing oil in the eyes Rinse the eye with milk or, if you don't have milk, flush the area with plenty of cool water, then seek urgent medical advice.

Spills on furniture Wearing gloves, mop up spills immediately with kitchen paper, then wash the area with soapy water. If a surface is damaged, you may need to repair or re-varnish. Place bottles on saucers or tubs, not directly on furniture.

Spills on soft furnishings and bedding Apply a stain remover for oil stains and then wash with detergent.

To clean an essential oil burner or diffuser Wipe with a cloth soaked in white spirit or white vinegar, then use a cloth dipped in soapy water to get rid of the vinegary smell. Rinse out the cloth; give the diffuser or burner a final wipe to remove any soapy residues.

Medical **conditions**

Essential oils are generally safe to use with medical conditions, but there are some cases where caution is needed. There have been concerns that oils should be avoided with **hypertension,** but there is no evidence for this.
• **If you have asthma**, avoid directly inhaling vapours in a steam inhalation (use a diffuser instead) and use essential oils extremely well diluted.
• **If you have epilepsy**, avoid hyssop and wormwood oils.
• **For atopic children** (with a tendency

to allergic reactions, or a family history of allergic responses), or those with hypersensitive skin, use no more than 1 per cent essential oils in a blend and do a patch test first (see opposite).
• **For all other contraindications**, check the safe usage for each oil in the A–Z section of the book (pp.196–293).

Safe usage terms

In the A–Z entries of the book, individual safe usage advice is given for each oil. All the recommendations are based on the essential oil being properly diluted in a suitable base oil when used on the skin (see the table, opposite). Note that though many oils are safe for most people to use and are considered non-toxic and non-irritant in general, an individual reaction or allergy to an oil is possible. If you react to an oil, or oil blend, stop using it immediately. The following terms are used in the guidance for safe usage throughout the A–Z section:

Non-toxic An oil does not represent a hazard when used as directed and an adverse reaction is unlikely.

Non-irritant Is unlikely to cause irritation or an adverse skin reaction.

Sensitizing Repeated use may cause irritation or an adverse reaction in some individuals.

Photo-toxic May cause the skin to be more susceptible to damage on exposure to the sun's UV rays.

Pregnancy and **breastfeeding**

There are a few essential oils that should be avoided in pregnancy and when breastfeeding. They may be too stimulating in the early weeks of pregnancy, as is the case with sage, or an oil may have a level of toxicity, as is the case with basil. The skin can be hypersensitive in pregnancy, so oils such as cinnamon bark oil should be avoided. Check the A–Z entries for advice on each oil.

Essential oils for pregnancy

The following essential oils are safe to use in pregnancy and when breastfeeding. Check the botanical name on the label as different varieties of a plant may not be safe in pregnancy. Also check the safe usage advice for each oil in the A–Z entries on pages 196–293.

- *Anthemis nobilis* – **Roman chamomile**
- *Boswellia carterii / sacra* – **Frankincense**
- *Cananga odorata* – **Ylang ylang**
- *Cedrus atlantica* – **Cedarwood**
- *Citrus aurantifolia* – **Lime**
- *Citrus aurantium, Citrus aurantium amara* – **Neroli / Petitgrain**
- *Citrus aurantium bergamia* – **Bergamot (bergaptene-free)**
- *Citrus limonum* – **Lemon**
- *Citrus paradisi* – **Grapefruit**
- *Citrus reticulata* – **Mandarin**
- *Citrus sinensis* – **Orange**
- *Coriandrum sativum* – **Coriander**
- *Cupressus sempervirens* – **Cypress**
- *Cymbopogon martinii* – **Palmarosa**
- *Elettaria cardamomum* – **Cardamom**

Refreshing thyme is soothing in pregnancy.

- *Eucalyptus globulus / radiata* – **Eucalyptus**
- *Helichrysum italicum* – **Helichrysum (Immortelle)**
- *Lavandula angustifolia* – **Lavender**
- *Matricaria recutita* – **Chamomile (blue)**
- *Melaleuca quinquenervia* – **Niaouli**
- *Origanum marjorana* – **Marjoram**
- *Pelargonium graveolens* – **Geranium**
- *Piper nigrum* – **Black pepper**
- *Pogostemon cablin* – **Patchouli**
- *Rosa centifolia* – **Rose absolute**
- *Thymus vulgaris CT linalool* – **Thyme**
- *Vetiveria zizanoides* – **Vetiver**
- *Zingiber officinale* – **Ginger**

Babies and **children**

Be cautious about using oils on young infants as their skin is sensitive and very permeable and babies can struggle to deal with adverse effects. Diffusers can be the best way to use oils with infants.

Guidelines for babies and children

Premature babies and infants up to 3 months old Essential oils aren't recommended on the skin. Use simple base oils such as olive and grapeseed.

3–6 months old Use only lavender or Roman chamomile. Dilute at 0.25 per cent: 2 drops of essential oil to 2 tablespoons of base oil.

6–12 months old Use only chamomile, Roman chamomile, lavender, mandarin, neroli or rose absolute. Dilute at 0.5 per cent: 4 drops of essential oil to 2 tablespoons of base oil.

1–6 years old Use only oils listed in the A–Z as non-toxic and non-irritant. Dilute at 1 per cent: 8 drops of essential oil to 2 tablespoons of base oil.

7–15 years old Use only oils listed as non-toxic and non-irritant. Dilute at 1.5 per cent: 12 drops of essential oil to 2 tablespoons of base oil.

Use olive oil to moisturize the skin of young babies.

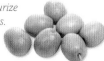

Doing a **patch test**

If you have sensitive skin or you have never used a particular essential oil, or blend of essential oils, before on your skin, do a patch test before using the oil the first time to check that you won't have an adverse reaction.

To do a patch test, make up the oil blend using the blending guidelines in the table. right. Apply a small amount to the inside of your elbow and wait for 24 hours. If no redness or irritation occurs, you can then try using the blend on a larger area of skin.

Blending essential oils and base oils

Use this table as a guide to essential oil and base oil quantities for oil blends.

	Number of drops of essential oils for base oil quantities:			
	10ml / 2tsp	15ml / 1tbsp	30ml / 2tbsp	100ml / 3½fl oz
Adults with delicate skin or for a facial blend (less than 1 per cent)	2 drops	3 drops	6 drops	20 drops
Massage blend for adults with no skin sensitivities (2.5 per cent)	5 drops	7 drops	15 drops	50 drops
Bath oil or therapeutic blend for applying to a small area of the body, for example, a joint (5 per cent)	12 drops	18 drops	40 drops	130–150 drops

A–Z of
Essential Oils

Discover the unique properties of over **80 essential oils.** Ordered alphabetically by their botanical names, each profile details a plant's origin **and properties,** the oil's appearance and aroma, and suggests some of the **best ways to use** each essential oil.

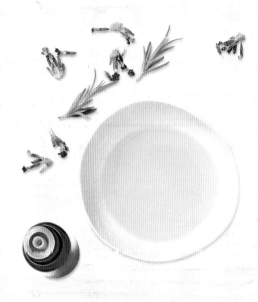

BATH OIL

FRAGRANCE

Mimosa

Acacia dealbata

Warming and **relaxing**, mimosa is a popular addition to perfumes. In skincare products, its nourishing and **soothing** properties provide a softening balm for sensitive skin, and its **calming action** helps to ease tension and lift spirits.

What is it **good for?**

Soothes skin The nourishing properties of mimosa essential oil help to soften the skin, and the oil's calming effect is useful for soothing inflamed and sensitive areas. Used as part of a daily beauty regime, mimosa oil helps to balance and tone combination skin and oily complexions.

Enhances wellbeing The deeply calming and relaxing properties of mimosa have a naturally uplifting effect on both body and mind. As well as being relaxing and soothing, the oil simultaneously energizes, and it is this ability that makes the oil a natural aphrodisiac.

Best **uses**

As a bath oil Indulge your senses and enjoy some relaxing time out by combining 4–5 drops of mimosa essential oil in 1 tablespoon base oil or full-fat milk and dispersing in a warm bath.

As a fragrance Mimosa essential oil is a good "fixative" for perfumes, helping to set the blend and make it last longer. It is often used as a "base note" in expensive scents.

Safe usage *Non-toxic and non-irritant.*

The plant

A member of *the acacia family, mimosa is native to south-eastern Australia. With its cheerful, yellow, popcorn-shaped flowers, it is now widely cultivated as an ornamental plant in warm, temperate regions around the world.*

The essential oil

Mimosa essential oil *is an "absolute", which is solvent-extracted from the tree's flowers and twigs. The thick oil is pale yellow to brown in colour with a sweet floral scent that carries slight woody undertones.*

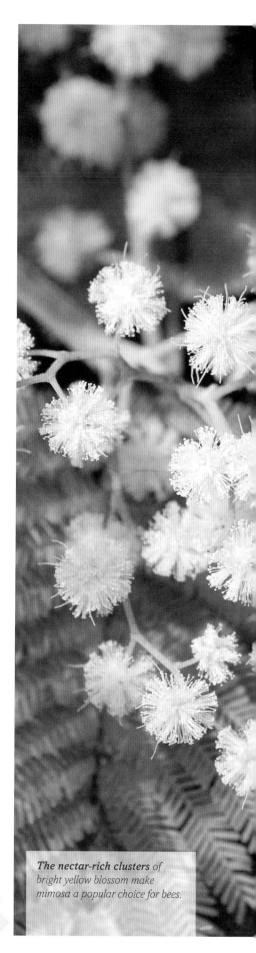
The nectar-rich clusters *of bright yellow blossom make mimosa a popular choice for bees.*

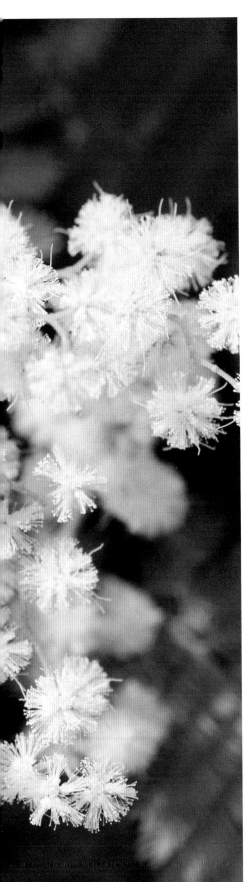

MASSAGE OIL

STEAM
INHALATION

Yarrow

Achillea millefolium

Revered by the ancient Greeks and Egyptians, yarrow is derived from the Greek *hieros*, meaning **"sacred"**. Its traditional use as a **skin healer** still holds today, and its clearing properties can relieve sinus-related headaches.

What is it **good for?**

Soothes aches and pains
Massage this natural anti-inflammatory into stiff joints to reduce pain and inflammation, or try a gentle abdominal massage to ease menstrual cramps.

Eases sinus pain
Yarrow loosens congestion, relieving sinus-related headaches and breathing problems.

Heals skin
Its antiseptic properties help treat minor cuts and wounds, and its potent healing action works on scar tissue, ulcers, slow-to-heal wounds, and itchy skin complaints such as eczema.

Balances oily skin
Add a few drops of the oil to face creams or toners to balance oily skin and help keep acne under control.

Relieves stress
With its soothing action, yarrow is an effective oil for stress-related conditions, such as hypertension or insomnia.

Best **uses**

As a massage oil
Mix 2–3 drops with St John's wort macerated oil and rub into sore, inflamed joints for pain relief.

In a steam inhalation
To relieve the symptoms of hay fever and alleviate nasal congestion, add 2–3 drops of yarrow essential oil to a bowl of hot water, place a towel over your head, and inhale the steam deeply for 2–3 minutes.

Safe usage Non-irritant in dilution. Avoid during pregnancy and breastfeeding.

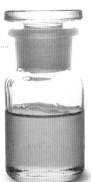

The plant

A grassland plant from the daisy family and a native of Europe and Western Asia, yarrow is now found worldwide. The oil of the Green Yarrow (Achillea nobilis) should be avoided for use in aromatherapy.

The essential oil

The herb is dried then steam-distilled to release the pale to dark blue or greeny-blue oil that has a powerful, herbaceous and slightly sweet smell, reminiscent of chamomile

DIFFUSER

OINTMENT

Buchu

Agathosma betulina

One of South Africa's best-known **medicinal** plants, buchu is a versatile essential oil that treats a wide range of ailments. Its **antiseptic, anti-inflammatory**, and detoxifying properties help to **soothe** and facilitate healing and calm digestive upsets.

What is it **good for?**

Heals skin With a potent antiseptic effect, buchu essential oil is ideal for treating skin infections.

Aids detox Buchu essential oil encourages the removal of toxins such as uric acid, which in turn relieves inflammation and sore joints. Its strong detoxifying action also helps to reduce water retention and to tackle areas of cellulite.

Eases digestive upsets Added to a massage blend, the essential oil helps to calm and soothe an irritable tummy and can also stimulate a sluggish digestion.

Acts as an insect repellent The sharp aroma of buchu oil makes this a natural insect repellent. Keep some of the oil on hand when travelling to instantly ward off pesky flies, mosquitoes, and fleas.

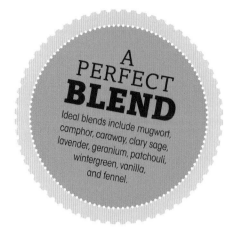

A PERFECT **BLEND**

Ideal blends include mugwort, camphor, caraway, clary sage, lavender, geranium, patchouli, wintergreen, vanilla, and fennel.

Best **uses**

In a diffuser Add 2–3 drops of buchu essential oil to an oil burner, vaporizer, or diffuser to help freshen stale air; or dilute in water and use in a spray bottle as an insect spray.

In an ointment Add 2–3 drops to 1 tablespoon ointment base to create an antiseptic skin treatment.

Safe usage Use very well diluted (less than 1 per cent). Avoid in pregnancy and when breastfeeding.

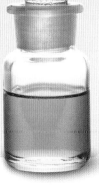

The plant

Buchu leaves are collected while the plant is flowering and fruiting, and then dried. The pungent aroma of the leaves increases as the plant dries out.

The essential oil

The golden oil is extracted from the dried leaves and flowers by steam-distillation. The oil has a sweet, medicinal aroma with hints of blackcurrant and peppermint.

STEAM INHALATION

MASSAGE OIL

COMPRESS

Fragonia™

Agonis fragrans

Relatively new to aromatherapy, Fragonia has a reputation for working at a deep level to restore **physical** and **emotional balance.** In particular, it's thought to help regulate the body clock and to boost immunity by encouraging efficient lymph circulation.

What is it **good for?**

Soothes aches and pains Reviving for tired joints and muscles, Fragonia also acts as a mild painkiller, helping to ease joint and muscle soreness and pain, mild toothache, and menstrual cramps.

Balances emotions The essential oil is an effective stress reliever. Deeply soothing, it helps to release emotional blockages.

Regulates body clock Its ability to help keep body systems in synch makes Fragonia essential oil an ideal remedy for overcoming the confusion and exhaustion caused by jetlag and coping with the demands of shift work.

Helps fight infection Its broad-acting antibacterial and antifungal properties help fight skin infections, and its antiviral action is a first-line defence against colds.

Strengthens immunity Fragonia aids lymph circulation and drainage, strengthening the immune system.

Best **uses**

In a steam inhalation Add 3–4 drops of the essential oil to hot water to create a steam inhalation to relieve respiratory and throat infections, break up catarrh, and fight infection.

In a massage oil Use in a massage blend to stimulate lymph circulation.

As a compress Add 3–4 drops to warm water and make a compress to relieve pain, congestion, cramping, and swelling and tenderness in the breasts.

Safe usage *Non-toxic and non-irritant.*

The plant

A native of Australia, *the small shrub fragonia is commonly called "coarse tea tree" by the cut-flower industry. Although the petite white flowers are fragrant, the healing essential oil is concentrated in the branchlets and leaves.*

The essential oil

Steam-distilled *from the leaves and branches, Fragonia oil is a clear to pale yellow with a similar scent to tea tree, but milder, with citrus, spicy, and floral notes.*

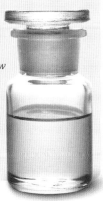

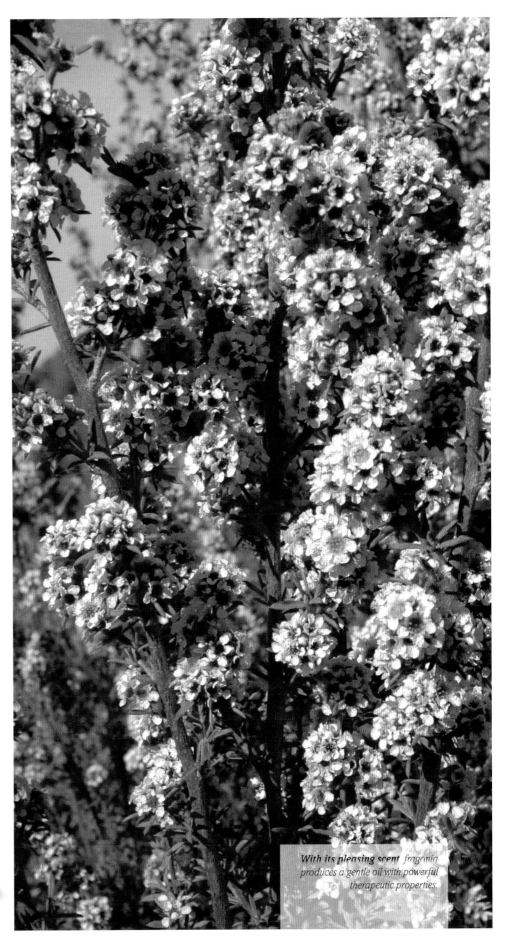

With its pleasing scent fragonia produces a gentle oil with powerful therapeutic properties.

DIFFUSER

MASSAGE OIL

SKIN CARE

Lemon verbena
Aloysia triphylla
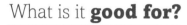

Behind the sunny, **uplifting** scent of lemon verbena lie some serious healing properties. It has a toning and **strengthening** effect on the nervous, digestive, respiratory, and immune systems. Its **antiseptic** action aids healing, while **anti-inflammatory** properties restore tired post-workout muscles.

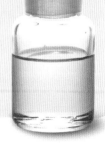

A PERFECT BLEND

Ideal blending partners include lemon, elemi, neroli, lavender, rose, bergamot, cedarwood, juniper, eucalyptus and palmarosa.

What is it **good for?**

Relieves anxiety and aids focus Lemon verbena has a wonderfully calming, sedative effect. As well as easing feelings of panic, it also aids focus, concentration, and retention when studying or reading.

Acts as an aphrodisiac The soothing effect of lemon verbena on breathing and heart rates lies behind the claim that it can be an effective aphrodisiac for both sexes.

Supports immunity As well as supporting liver function, lemon verbena helps to bring down a fever by encouraging perspiration.

Fights colds and flu With its fresh citrus scent and antiseptic action, the oil relieves cold and flu symptoms, easing irritating coughs and loosening congestion in the sinuses and lungs.

Soothes aches and pains Massaging with lemon verbena after a workout tones muscles and reduces the buildup of lactic acid. The oil also encourages the repair of weak connective tissue and speeds up the healing process of joint-related injuries. It has an anti-inflammatory effect that can help lessen the pain of arthritis and improve overall mobility.

Soothes digestion and relieves menstrual cramps A gentle massage with a lemon verbena blend eases stomach upsets and nausea. Its antispasmodic properties act on menstrual cramps, and it's thought the oil helps regulate menstrual cycles.

Best **uses**

In a diffuser Dispersed into the air, the oil helps to calm nerves, and can also be used to bolster the spirits when dealing with periods of stress, or when feeling down and depressed.

As a massage oil Lemon verbena provides skin benefits and supports health at a deeper level by lowering breathing and heart rates and boosting immunity and liver function. For a massage, blend 8–9 drops in 2 tablespoons base oil.

In a lotion Add 1–2 drops of the essential oil to 1 tablespoon lotion base to help soften and tone the skin. The oil is also useful for reducing skin puffiness and inflammation.

Safe usage Use well diluted (less than 0.5 per cent). Avoid on sensitive skin, children under 15 years old, before exposure to the sun, and during pregnancy and breastfeeding.

The plant

A native of Chile and Peru, lemon verbena now grows in many tropical areas worldwide. With its pointed pale green leaves and stems bearing tubular flowers, the plant has a strong and distinct lemon aroma.

The essential oil

The leaves and stalks are steam-distilled for the oil, which is a yellowish-green colour. It has a fresh lemony smell described as simultaneously hot and bitter. Its extremely subtle aroma has proved difficult to reproduce synthetically.

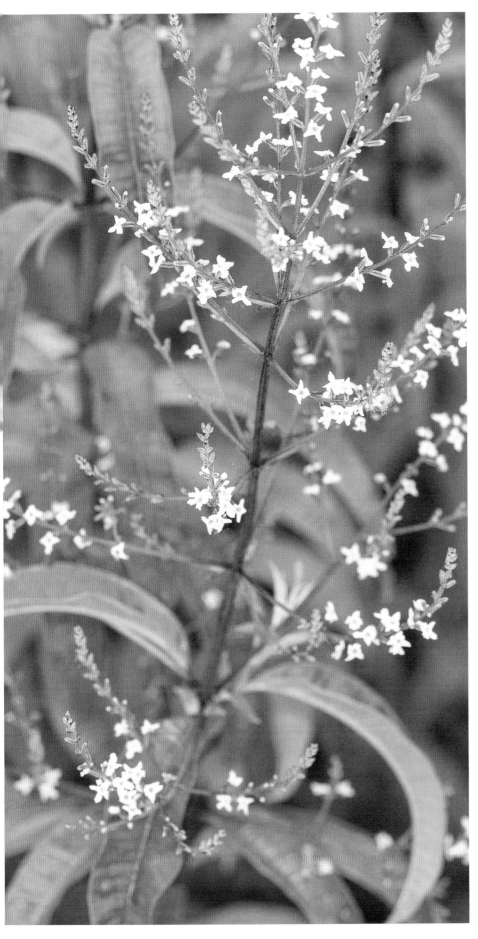

The oil's fresh, lemony aroma brings a feeling of calm and helps to enhance concentration.

This aromatic shrub flowers in the summer months, producing stems of delicate white or pale lilac flowers.

INHALATION   BATH OIL

MASSAGE OIL   BATH OIL

Galangal

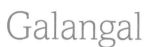
Alpinia officinarum

This previously little-known essential oil is rapidly rising in popularity thanks to its **warming**, stimulating, and **antiseptic** properties. It can relieve nausea and motion sickness, has a natural **deodorizing** quality, and also helps fight fungal infections.

What is it **good for?**

Helps fight infection The combined antibacterial and antifungal properties of galangal essential oil make it an especially useful oil for treating skin eruptions. The oil can also be used to protect wounds, keeping them clean, and helps to bring fungal infections such as athlete's foot under control.

Eases digestion and soothes tummy upsets Warming and soothing, galangal essential oil aids digestion and the assimilation of nutrients and helps to release uncomfortable trapped wind. If you suffer from travel sickness and nausea, this is a useful remedy to carry on long journeys.

Acts as a deodorant The anti-perspirant action of galangal helps reduce body odour, to keep you feeling fresh.

Energizes and lifts mood As well as lifting fatigue and jet lag, galangal has a long history as an aphrodisiac because of its warming, stimulating aroma and ability to ease anxiety.

Best **uses**

In an inhalation To relieve travel sickness, add 2–3 drops to a tissue, keep in a plastic bag, and sniff as needed.

As a bath oil Mix 3–4 drops with 1 tablespoon base oil, full-fat milk, or bath oil. Add to your bath to heal dry, cracked skin.

Safe usage Non-toxic, non-irritant in dilution. Avoid near the face or nose of children under seven years old.

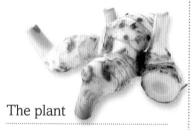

The plant

A native of Indonesia, galangal belongs to the same family as ginger and looks similar. The root (see above) is also a popular cooking ingredient and can be used like ginger.

The essential oil

The pale yellow to olive brown oil is obtained by the steam-distillation of the dried galangal root. Its aroma is reminiscent of ginger, but milder.

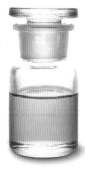

Dill

Anethum graveolens

For centuries, dill has been renowned for its impressive **healing** powers. It **stimulates** digestion, **calms** frazzled nerves, and has **antibacterial** properties that help speed the healing of wounds. It also has a mild diuretic effect that makes it a natural aid to detox.

What is it **good for?**

Supports digestion Dill has a calming, anti-inflammatory effect on the digestive tract, so has long been used as a treatment for stomach upsets and bouts of colic.

Fights infection Dill is a natural antibacterial and diuretic that can be used to relieve the symptoms of cystitis and bladder infections.

Heals skin Dill is highly effective in promoting the quick healing of cuts, grazes, and wounds, and helps to protect them from infections.

Aids restful sleep Sedating and calming on the nerves, dill essential oil helps to promote a deep sense of relaxation. This makes it a useful oil for relieving feelings of anxiety, tension, anger, and depression, and it can even ease hypertension, all of which helps to combat insomnia.

Aids detox The diuretic properties of dill essential oil aid the processes of perspiration and urination, helping to prevent a buildup of fluids and toxins.

Best **uses**

As a massage oil Add 6–8 drops of the essential oil to 2 tablespoons base oil to support a detox regime and create a state of calm.

As a bath oil Disperse 5–6 drops in 1 tablespoon base oil or full-fat milk and add to the bath. Relax in the bath and inhale the steam deeply.

Safe usage Non-toxic, non-irritant in dilution.

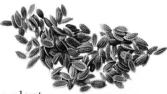

The plant

The feathery leaves *of the dill plant are commonly used to flavour food. The tiny flowers eventually give way to oil-rich seeds (see above).*

The essential oil

The pale yellow *essential oil is extracted through steam-distillation of both the dried seeds and the whole plant. The oil has an appealing grassy aroma and blends well with lime, lemon, and other citrus oils.*

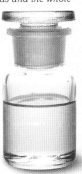

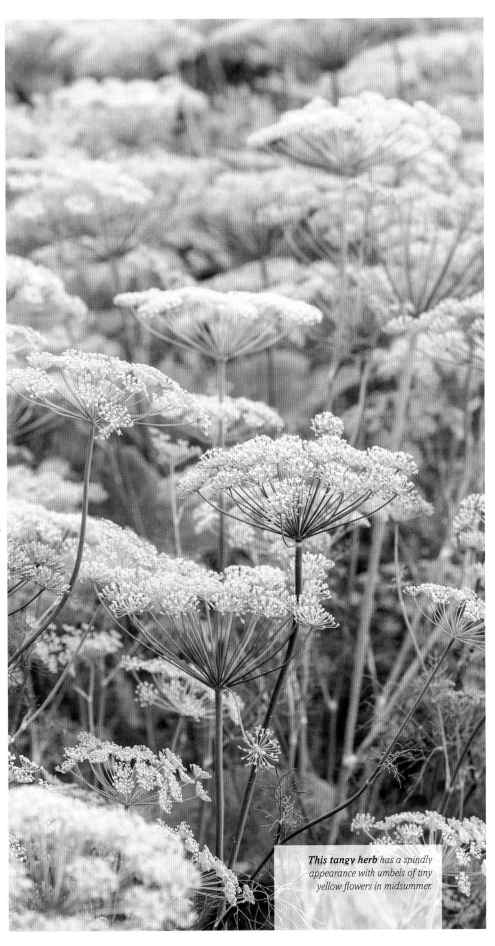

This tangy herb *has a spindly appearance with umbels of tiny yellow flowers in midsummer.*

MASSAGE OIL   COMPRESS

Angelica
Angelica archangelica

A **warming** oil, angelica is fondly referred to as the "oil of the angels" because its **uplifting** effect promotes calm, positivity, and restful sleep. It is also soothing and **clearing**, relaxing muscles and relieving congestion.

What is it **good for?**

Aids detox A mild diuretic, angelica also encourages perspiration, which promotes health by aiding the removal of toxins from the body.

Soothes aches and pains Angelica's warming properties help to boost the circulation to aching joints and muscles, and provide effective relief from menstrual cramps.

Relieves congestion Used in a chest massage oil blend or added to a steam inhalation, angelica essential oil can help to break up stubborn congestion.

Enhances wellbeing Reputed to lift flagging spirits, angelica essential oil is thought to help you "discover" your true self and can be useful during periods of upheaval or in times of transition.

Best **uses**

As a massage oil Used in a blend, angelica provides a detoxifying massage that lifts the spirits and improves wellbeing. Mix 2–4 drops in 2 tablespoons base oil.

In a compress Add 2–3 drops to warm water, dip a cloth in, squeeze out, and use to ease menstrual pain.

Safe usage Non-toxic, use well diluted (less than 1 per cent). Avoid use on skin for 12 hours prior to sun exposure.

The plant

A native of northern Europe, the dramatic umbrella-like flowerheads of the angelica plant produce a vast number of seeds. The seed oil is considered safest for aromatherapy as it contains less of the photo-toxic chemical bergapten than is found in the root oil.

The essential oil

Both the roots and seeds can be dried and then steam-distilled to produce a pungent oil with a sweet, spicy aroma. Oil from the seed is clear, while the oil from the roots is a pale yellow.

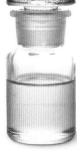

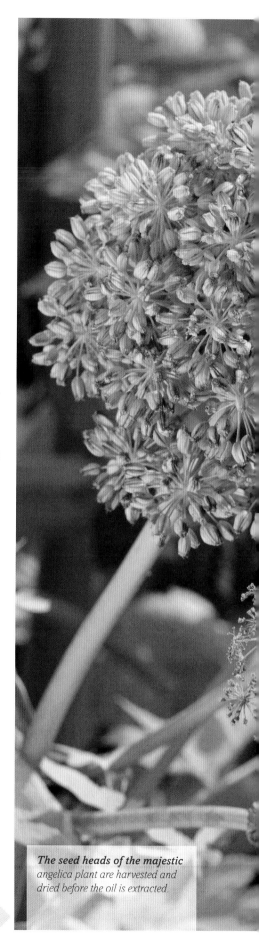

The seed heads of the majestic *angelica plant are harvested and dried before the oil is extracted.*

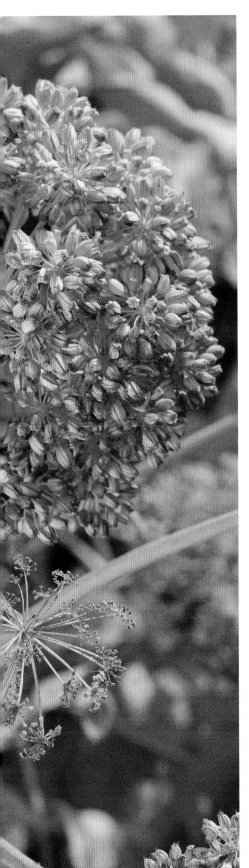

BATH OIL

DIFFUSER

Rosewood

Aniba rosaeodora

Rosewood, also called **bois de rose,** is a member of the laurel family – a relative of cinnamon and bay. A **grounding** and centring oil, it works on the mind and emotions.

A
PERFECT
BLEND

Match rosewood with geranium, patchouli, lavender, rose, bergamot, neroli, black pepper, cinnamon, and other spicy oils

What is it **good for?**

Conditions skin This oil has tissue-regenerating properties that can help slow signs of premature ageing, making this an effective treatment for dull, dry, or mature skin. Rosewood also has a healing action on wounds, making this an excellent first-aid remedy for cuts and insect bites.

Tones and calms skin Rosewood essential oil balances the levels of oil in combination or oily complexions, so helps to control pimples, acne, and blackheads.

Acts as a hair tonic As with skin, rosewood has a balancing effect on the scalp, helping to regulate excessively dry or oily hair.

Acts as a mild pain reliever The mild analgesic action of this oil means rosewood can alleviate headaches and muscle and joint pain.

Balances emotions Thought to bring emotional stability and to create a sense of calm and empowerment, rosewood essential oil also helps you to relax and is considered an aphrodisiac.

Best **uses**

As a bath oil Add 5–6 drops to 1 tablespoon base oil or full-fat milk and enjoy a restorative, steamy soak.

In a diffuser Diffuse this spicy, woody, floral aroma to calm emotions.

Safe usage *Non-toxic and non-irritant.*

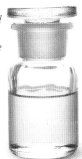

The plant

This native Brazilian tree *grows up to 40m (130ft). Now endangered, harvesting is strictly controlled. Oil from the heartwood should be avoided. A more sustainable oil from the leaves and twigs may be available.*

The essential oil

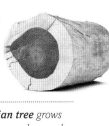

The light yellow oil *is steam-distilled from the wood chippings of the tree and has a spicy, sweet, floral aroma.*

Tarragon

Artemisia dracunculus

A popular kitchen herb, tarragon also has a long history of use as a **medicinal** herb. The oil yields a warming massage, helping to **improve circulation** to the extremities, and is mildly **analgesic**. It also offers **emotional support** in times of upheaval.

What is it **good for?**

Eases digestion In a massage blend, tarragon oil stimulates appetite and has a pronounced effect on sluggish digestion, helping food move more efficiently through the digestive tract. It also helps calm flatulence, hiccups, and nervous indigestion.

Aids detox Its mild diuretic and laxative action helps to eliminate toxins.

Eases aches and pains Tarragon contains a natural anaesthetic, eugenol, also found in clove. Like clove, it is a traditional toothache remedy. It also has a warming action that helps increase circulation to muscles, joints, and extremities, eases menstrual pains, and helps regulate periods.

Acts as a deodorant The oil's spicy scent acts on body odour, inhibiting the growth of microbes on the skin, so reducing stale, unwelcome smells.

Provides emotional support Tarragon is said to ward off feelings of despair and provide emotional support in times of change by alleviating fear and feelings of being "stuck".

Best **uses**

As a massage oil Blend 1–2 drops in 2 tablespoons base oil to ease digestive discomfort and menstrual pains.

In a foot bath Add 2–3 drops to a foot bath to boost circulation, warm the body, and inhibit foot odour.

Safe usage Use extremely well diluted (less than 0.1 per cent). Avoid during pregnancy and breastfeeding, and on children under seven years old.

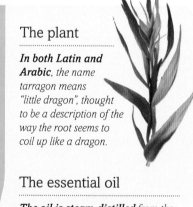

The plant

In both Latin and Arabic, the name tarragon means "little dragon", thought to be a description of the way the root seems to coil up like a dragon.

The essential oil

The oil is steam-distilled from the leaves and the flowering tops to produce a clear to pale green oil with an herbaceous aroma, somewhere between celery and aniseed.

Mugwort

Artemisia vulgaris

A **powerful** oil that should be used sparingly, mugwort can nevertheless have **profound** effects. Used in massage or simply dispersed in the air, it has a pleasant **warming** quality that stimulates circulation, clears the airways, and relaxes the mind.

What is it **good for?**

Eases aches and pains Useful for arthritis and other inflammatory joint conditions, mugwort eases stiff muscles and improves circulation.

Fights colds The oil works as a decongestant, loosening phlegm and mucus to ease bronchitis and colds.

Supports women's health With gentle massage, the oil eases cramps, relaxes abdominal tension, and encourages blood flow when periods are delayed or very light.

Provides emotional support Uplifting and relaxing, a drop on a pillow is said to bring pleasant dreams.

Best **uses**

As a diffuser Add 2–3 drops each of mugwort and lavender essential oils to a diffuser, vaporizer, or oil burner

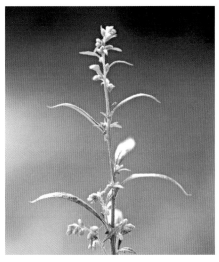

Pungent mugwort produces small clusters of white to yellow flowers in midsummer.

to produce pleasant feelings of peace and tranquillity.

As a massage oil For aching joints and muscles, massage with a warming mugwort blend for deep relief. Add 3–6 drops to 2 tablespoons base oil.

Safe usage *Use well diluted (less than 1 per cent). Avoid in pregnancy and if breastfeeding, on children under seven years old, and with epilepsy.*

The plant

A shrubby herb, mugwort is found in temperate regions, in meadows and on waysides. The name is derived from the Old English mucg wyrt, meaning "marsh plant". In Chinese medicine, the dried, compressed leaves (moxa) are burnt and briefly held close to the skin to provide warmth.

The essential oil

The oil is extracted by steam-distillation of leaves, buds, and the flowering tops of the mugwort tree to produce an amber oil with a sweet, almost floral, citrussy scent.

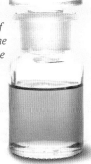

HAIR CARE   MASSAGE OIL

Birch (leaf)
Betula alba

In Scandinavia, birch leaves and twigs are bound together and used in saunas to **tone skin** and **boost circulation**. White birch oil is **stimulating** and **detoxifying**, helping the kidneys to function efficiently and promoting perspiration to hasten the removal of toxins.

What is it **good for?**

Aids detox Birch oil facilitates both perspiration and urination, which hastens the removal of toxins and impurities from the body. Added to a massage oil blend, it helps to improve a sluggish circulation.

Soothes aches and pains
A natural anti-inflammatory and analgesic, birch essential oil can help to ease sore muscles and joints after a work-out and numb pain locally. These same properties also help to ease the discomfort caused by arthritis and rheumatism.

Acts as an antiseptic The antiseptic properties of birch essential oil make it a useful remedy for skin eruptions such as cold sores. The oil is also an effective healer for irritating skin conditions, such as eczema and psoriasis, but ensure it is well diluted before using.

Tones skin and hair Birch has a balancing effect on combination skin, and can soften and tighten skin, giving mature skin a youthful appearance. Used in a hair rinse, it helps promote shine and tackles stubborn dandruff.

Best **uses**

In a hair rinse Add 4–5 drops to a final rinse to combat dandruff.

As a massage oil Mix 6–10 drops with 2 tablespoons base oil for a full-body massage to help improve circulation and remove toxins.

Safe usage *Use well diluted (less than 2 per cent). Avoid in pregnancy and if breastfeeding; on children under 15 years old; if on anticoagulants or sensitive to salicylates.*

The plant

European white birch or silver birch is native to the northern hemisphere. The distinctive papery bark can be distilled into a highly antiseptic birch tar oil, unsuitable for aromatherapy. The young leaves produce the milder white birch oil.

The essential oil

The oil, which has a slightly spicy, woody aroma, is steam-distilled from the leaf buds and is pale yellow in colour.

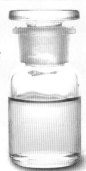

OINTMENT

SKIN CARE

DIFFUSER

MASSAGE OIL

Frankincense (Olibanum)

Boswellia carterii, B. sacra, B. frereana, et al

This is an important oil for **toning** and **invigorating** the complexion, particularly for mature or sun-damaged skin. Frankincense can be used as both an antiseptic and anti-inflammatory, and its distinct aroma helps to **soothe** and **calm** frayed nerves, making it useful for treating anxiety.

What is it **good for?**

Soothes aches and pains The potent anti-inflammatory action of frankincense has been found to ease arthritis and rheumatic pain.

Tones skin The oil helps to close pores and tone skin. Its rejuvenating qualities make it an excellent choice for mature skins, helping to minimize wrinkles and fine lines and reduce the appearance of blemishes and long-term sun damage.

Acts as an antiseptic Diluted, frankincense oil can be used topically to heal wounds and skin ulcers.

Fights colds Frankincense essential oil helps to soothe the mucous membranes, calming and deepening breathing, and easing coughs, bronchitis, and laryngitis.

Relieves anxiety This calming oil lifts the spirits, increases energy and focus, and aids meditation, ideal when feeling stressed, tired, or overwhelmed.

Best **uses**

In an ointment The powerful anti-inflammatory properties of frankincense make it an effective ointment to use on sore joints, helping to reduce pain and increase movement.

As a toner Make a facial toner by adding 2 tablespoons aloe vera juice to 6 tablespoons water and 4 drops of frankincense.

In a diffuser Add 3–4 drops to a diffuser, vaporizer, or oil burner.

In a massage oil Add a few drops of the oil to a base oil for a soothing and toning massage.

Safe usage Non-toxic, non-irritant in dilution.

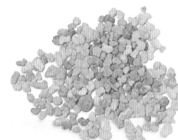

The plant

Frankincense trees grow wild in north-east Africa and Oman. They produce an aromatic sap that, when dried, is called the "pearl of the desert", and is traditionally burned as incense.

The essential oil

The rich fragrant oil is steam-distilled from the tree resin (above). It produces a pale yellow or greenish oil with a sweet, spicy, resinous odour.

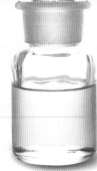

Frankincense promotes feelings of positivity, enhancing wellbeing.

SKIN CARE

HAIR CARE

FRAGRANCE

MASSAGE OIL

BATH OIL

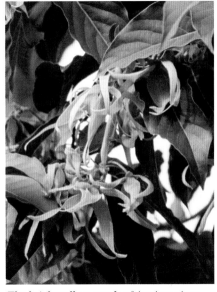

The bright yellow petals of the ylang ylang yield an exceptionally floral essential oil.

Ylang ylang
Cananga odorata

With its **exotic**, highly floral aroma, ylang ylang is **uplifting** and **arousing**, and at the same time eases feelings of anxiety. A key constituent of the traditional hair preparation, macassar oil, its **balancing** properties make it suitable for all skin types.

What is it **good for?**

Improves complexion Ylang ylang has a balancing action on the secretion of sebum, helping to regulate its production, making it an ideal skin cleanser for both oily and dry skin types. It is a particularly effective tonic for acne-prone complexions.

Tones skin With its stimulating effect, ylang ylang helps to improve the structure and appearance of tired or sagging skin, restoring a youthful glow.

Nourishes hair The essential oil has a long history as a treatment for dry hair. It nourishes and stimulates the scalp, and conditions dry, brittle hair. It is even reputed to promote hair growth.

Aids relaxation Stimulating and calming, ylang ylang essential oil is well placed for increasing feelings of wellbeing. Its calming properties have demonstrable effects, helping to lower blood pressure and breathing rates, in turn reducing feelings of anxiety.

Acts as an aphrodisiac The arousing aroma of ylang ylang and its renowned relaxing effect make this oil a popular aphrodisiac, as it helps to release inhibitions and ease tension, while arousing the olfactory senses. Traditionally, petals were scattered on the beds of newlyweds to help shed inhibitions and dispel anxiety.

Treats depression The sedating and calming properties of ylang ylang make it a useful support in the treatment of depression and tension.

Best **uses**

As a skin toner Add 1–2 drops of the oil to 2 teaspoons witch hazel and 3 tablespoons water. Dab on skin with a cotton ball.

As a hair tonic For a dry scalp, add 1–2 drops to 1 teaspoon olive oil and massage into the scalp before bed. Brush through with a natural-bristle brush, and wash out in the morning.

As a perfume The essential oil can be used neat as a simple perfume. Or you can mix 1–2 drops in a teaspoon of a base oil, such as apricot kernel, and apply it to the pulse points.

In a massage oil For a skin-toning and relaxing massage, add 1–2 drops of ylang ylang oil to a base oil blend.

As a bath oil Add 1–2 drops of the oil to 1 tablespoon base oil or full-fat milk and disperse in the bath.

Safe usage *Non-toxic and non-irritant. As it has a powerful odour, use well diluted, unless using neat as a perfume.*

The plant

A native of Asia, *ylang ylang means "flower of flowers"; the waxy petals have been used in medicines and skin creams for millenia. Now grown mainly in Madagascar and the Comoros, it is a base of high-end oriental scents and a key ingredient in Chanel No.5.*

The essential oil

The pale yellow oil *is steam- or water-distilled from the flowers to create an oil with an intensely sweet, exotic floral scent. The scent can be overpowering, so use sparingly at first to discover how strong you like it.*

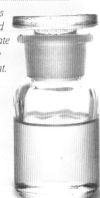

SKIN CARE

STEAM
INHALATION

MASSAGE OIL

SKIN CARE

Elemi

Canarium luzonicum

Elemi has a long history in skin care, traditionally used in **healing** skin salves in the Middle East and Europe. Today, its ability to **tone** and **firm** skin makes it a favourite ingredient in high-end beauty products. It also helps to relieve congestion in the lungs.

What is it **good for?**

Combats signs of ageing Elemi is ideal for dry or sun-damaged skin. It accelerates skin-cell renewal and supports collagen synthesis, helping to prevent sagging and the appearance of premature fine lines. In skin-care products, elemi helps to harmonize both dry and oily skin types.

Heals skin The healing properties of elemi can help to reduce scarring, and its effective antiseptic action helps prevent infection in cuts and wounds.

Eases respiratory problems With expectorant and antiviral properties, a few drops of the oil added to a steam inhalation brings relief to respiratory problems such as chest infections, catarrh, sinusitis, and bronchitis.

Lifts moods Calming and uplifting, this a good oil to choose when stressed, or suffering from nervous exhaustion.

Best **uses**

In a cream Add 2–4 drops of elemi essential oil to 2 tablespoons unscented cream or lotion base for a revitalizing skin treatment to apply before bedtime as part of an evening skincare regime.

In an inhalation Add 3–4 drops to a bowl of hot water and inhale for welcome relief from the symptoms of hay fever, as well as to ease the congestion that leads to coughs and sinus-related headaches.

Safe usage *Non-toxic, use well diluted (less than 0.5 per cent).*

The plant

A relative *of frankincense and myrrh, the elemi tree is native to the tropical forests of the Philippines and neighbouring nations. The name means "above and below" in Arabic, suggesting that it was valued both spiritually and physically.*

The essential oil

Steam-distilled *from the resin of the elemi tree, the essential oil is pale yellow and has a distinctive sharp, citrussy, pine aroma.*

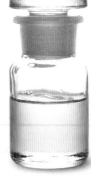

The honey-coloured resin produces the oil.

Caraway

Carum carvi

This **warming** essential oil works on both mind and body, **relieving** mental strain and emotional fatigue. It also supports the digestive and urinary systems, helps **clear** the respiratory system, and can be used to treat stubborn skin and scalp conditions.

What is it **good for?**

Soothes nerves Caraway oil is a natural tonic for frayed nerves, calming the mind and soothing mental fatigue. It also settles nervous digestion, colic, flatulence, and gastric spasms.

Helps fight infection Its expectorant action means that caraway can help to clear bronchitis, bronchial asthma, and irritating coughs. It also helps to soothe sore throats and laryngitis, supports the healthy function of the urinary system, and helps to flush out toxins.

Heals and soothes skin The tissue-regenerating qualities of caraway essential oil can be harnessed to help disperse bruises, reduce boils, and clean infected wounds. The oil is used to combat oily skin, help clear acne and flaky scalps, and relieve itching.

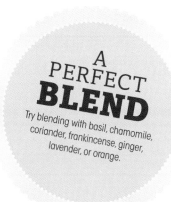

A PERFECT BLEND

Try blending with basil, chamomile, coriander, frankincense, ginger, lavender, or orange.

Best **uses**

As a massage oil Blend 3–6 drops with 2 tablespoons base oil for a soothing massage to relieve abdominal discomfort.

In a cream Add 3–6 drops to 2 tablespoons base cream and use to relieve dry, itchy skin and scalp.

Safe usage Non-toxic. Use well diluted (less than 1 per cent).

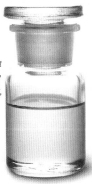

The plant

A native of south-eastern Europe, caraway now grows in the wild and is cultivated all over Europe and temperate Asia. A member of the Umbelliferae family, it is related to cumin, fennel, and dill.

The essential oil

Caraway oil is extracted by steam-distillation from the dried ripe seeds. It produces a clear to pale yellow oil that has a sweet, spicy aroma with a hint of pepper.

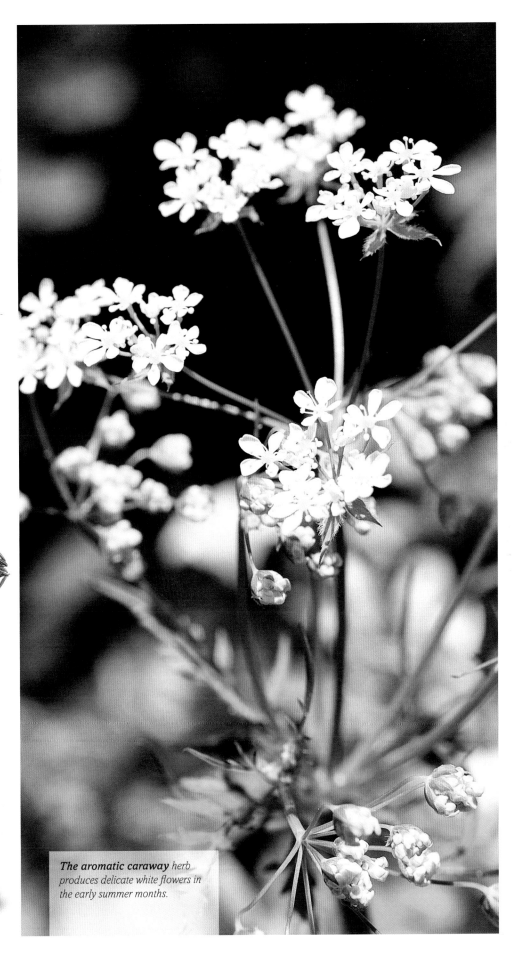

The aromatic caraway herb produces delicate white flowers in the early summer months.

HAIR CARE

FRAGRANCE

OINTMENT

MASSAGE OIL

Cedarwood

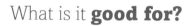
Cedrus atlantica

A long-established essential oil, cedarwood has an impressive range of benefits. Both **antiseptic** and **astringent**, it balances and tones complexions and facilitates healing in infections and skin eruptions. Its **uplifting** aroma makes it a perfect pick-me-up, helping to release tension and lift feelings of lethargy.

A PERFECT BLEND

Blends well with rose, black pepper, bergamot, jasmine, neroli, juniper, cypress, clary sage, frankincense, and mimosa.

What is it **good for?**

Soothes skin Cedarwood contains the highest level of the anti-inflammatory substances known as sesquiterpenes of any essential oil. This makes it helpful for easing itchy, irritated skin, especially in cases of acne, dandruff, or athlete's foot.

Relieves pain Cedarwood essential oil has a warming, regenerative effect, making it a useful treatment for chronic degenerative conditions, such as arthritis.

Tones and heals skin The astringent properties in this essential oil can help to balance oily or acne-prone skin and make it an effective tonic for oily hair. It also promotes healing of wounds and skin ulcers.

Supports women's health The stimulating effect of cedarwood can help regulate the menstrual cycle and is a useful antiseptic treatment for unwanted vaginal discharges.

Aids detox Cedarwood helps to stimulate the flow of lymph, reduce water retention, and aid the removal of toxins from the body.

Fights colds and coughs Used as an inhalation or in a diffuser, the oil can help break up excessive catarrh, and soothe coughs and bronchitis.

Lifts moods Grounding and calming, cedarwood can combat feelings of negativity. Its uplifting qualities treat nervous tension, anxiety, depression, and tiredness, as well as aid focus. For men, it is considered an aphrodisiac.

Best **uses**

As a hair tonic Add 10–20 drops to a bottle of unscented shampoo or conditioner to combat dandruff.

As a room fragrance Use 3–4 drops in a diffuser, vaporizer, or oil burner to cleanse the air and lift anxiety, depression, and feelings of exhaustion.

In an ointment Add 12–16 drops to 2 tablespoons base oil or an ointment base and apply several times a day to provide fast relief and healing for itchy, irritated skin conditions.

As a massage oil Add 12–18 drops cedarwood essential oil to 2 tablespoons base oil for an uplifting and skin-soothing massage.

Safe usage Non-toxic, non-irritant in dilution.

The plant

The sacred Cedars of Lebanon *in the Atlas Mountains are large imposing trees that can live for up to 2,000 years. As a symbol of protection and power, they have been so highly prized and sought after over the years that they are becoming an endangered species, so ensure the oil you buy is harvested sustainably.*

The essential oil

The tree bark *is the source of a thick, pale, yellow to amber essential oil with a sweet, mild, balsamic– woody odour that becomes gradually more woody while the oil dries out.*

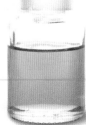

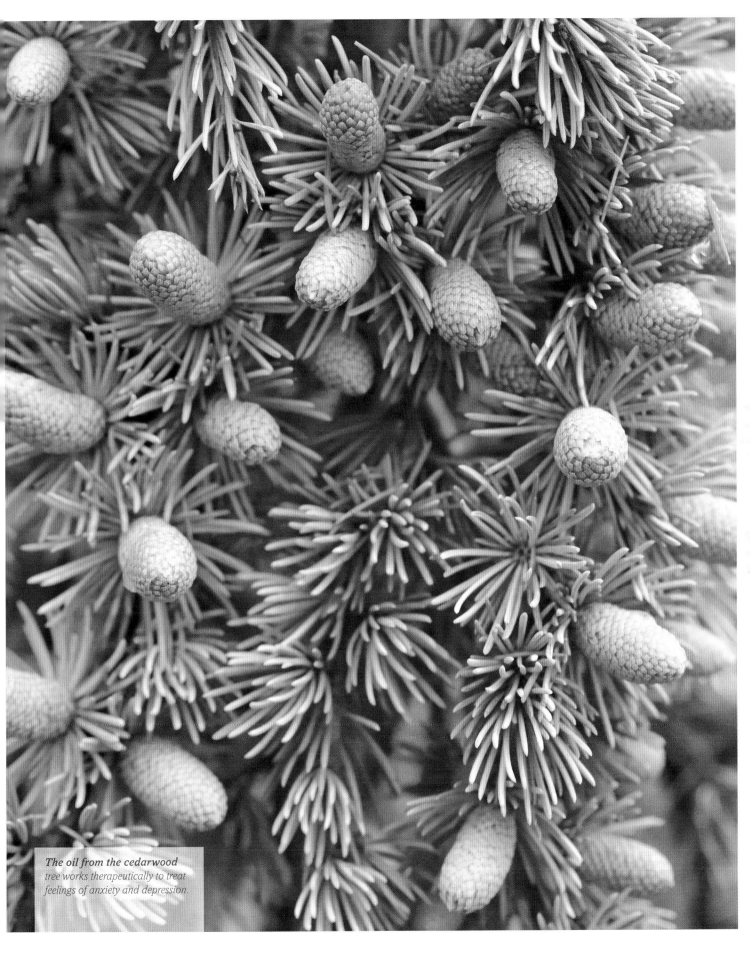

The oil from the cedarwood tree works therapeutically to treat feelings of anxiety and depression.

MASSAGE OIL   OINTMENT

FOOT BATH   DIFFUSER

Camphor

Cinnamomum camphora

With its **medicinal** aroma, camphor is a very useful oil. It has a dual action on skin, at first **cooling** then deeply **warming**, and stimulates the circulation, metabolism, and digestion. It's an effective pain reliever and also helps to clear the head and calm the mind.

What is it **good for?**

Improves circulation The stimulating effect of camphor essential oil helps to boost a sluggish circulation and digestion, and also balances the metabolic rate.

Soothes aches and pains A natural anaesthetic, camphor can provide relief from nerve pain and inflammation. It is also an effective antispasmodic and eases cramps and muscle spasms.

Fights colds and flu Camphor helps clear blocked sinuses and respiratory complaints, making breathing easier.

Best **uses**

As a massage oil If you are chilly or achy, add 2–4 drops to 2 tablespoons base oil for a warming massage that instils a sense of wellbeing.

In an ointment Add 2–4 drops to 2 tablespoons ointment base for a rub to relieve pain and sore muscles.

Safe usage *A strong oil, use well diluted and use only "white" camphor essential oil.*

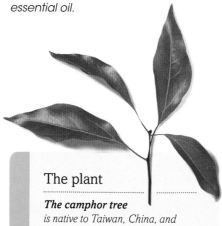

The plant

The camphor tree *is native to Taiwan, China, and Japan and grows to a great age. It must be at least 50 years old to produce the oil, which is present in all parts of the plant.*

Ho Sho, or Ho Leaf, *oil is distilled from the leaves of the camphor tree and is a much milder oil than the oil from the rest of the plant, and is soothing for the skin and mind. It is non-toxic and non-irritant in dilution.*

The essential oil

When the wood*, branches, and leaves of the camphor plant are steam-distilled, they produce a brown oil that must be distilled twice more before it becomes the clear oil, known as "white camphor" that is safe to use in aromatherapy.*

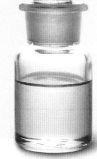

Cinnamon

Cinnamomum zeylanicum

This spicy, **warming** oil was used by the ancient Egyptians as an aromatic foot massage. It is used in very small amounts in cosmetics for its antiseptic properties, and its **energizing** and **stimulating** aroma makes it ideal for lifting flagging spirits.

What is it **good for?**

Soothes aches and pains Cinnamon is warming if you feel particularly chilly, as it helps to boost circulation to the extremities. It's especially effective for reviving and soothing sore joints aggravated by cold, damp weather.

Aids digestion Massaged over the abdomen, cinnamon oil can stimulate circulation, improve sluggish digestion, and relieve constipation. It also has an antispasmodic action that helps to calm stomach cramps and spasms.

Acts as an antiseptic Cinnamon is effective against a broad range of bacteria, viruses, and parasites, especially lice and scabies.

Balances emotions An uplifting room scent, the oil can help to counter exhaustion and depression.

BATH OIL

MASSAGE OIL

Best **uses**

As a foot bath Warm cold feet by adding 1–2 drops of cinnamon oil to a relaxing foot bath.

In a diffuser Add 1–2 drops to a diffuser to disinfect air in a sick room or to get rid of unpleasant smells.

Safe usage Use very well diluted (less than 0.5 per cent), and use only cinnamon leaf oil on the skin (not cinnamon bark).

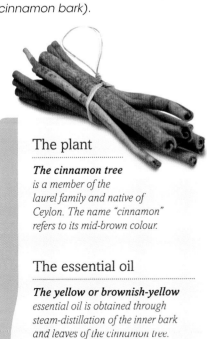

The plant

The cinnamon tree *is a member of the laurel family and native of Ceylon. The name "cinnamon" refers to its mid-brown colour.*

The essential oil

The yellow or brownish-yellow *essential oil is obtained through steam-distillation of the inner bark and leaves of the cinnamon tree. It has a warm and spicy aroma. The leaf oil is considered milder and is therefore safer for use in aromatherapy.*

Cistus

Cistus ladaniferus

Derived from the flowering plant also known as rock rose, Rose of Sharon, and labdanum, **fragrant** cistus has powerful **skin-toning** and **healing** properties. It is a useful immune stimulant, and its antiseptic properties fight infection. It also helps centre the mind.

What is it **good for?**

Aids detox Used in massage oils, blended with a favourite base oil, cistus helps to encourage effective lymphatic drainage, improves circulation, and boosts immunity.

Heals skin Known for its healing properties, cistus oil can help to speed up tissue healing in wounds. Its astringent properties also make it useful for treating bleeding gums, bruises, and mouth ulcers.

Tones skin Rich in antioxidants, cistus essential oil is beneficial for your skin and brightens tired-looking complexions. A good astringent, it can help tighten and tone mature skin.

Acts as an antiseptic Cistus oil has an effective antiviral action that is especially useful in the treatment of respiratory congestion caused by colds and flu and other infections.

Helps balance emotions The oil has a centring effect that facilitiates meditation and contemplation. Its earthy aroma stimulates the senses and strengthens emotions after loss.

Best **uses**

As a bath oil Add 4–6 drops to 1 tablespoon base oil or full-fat milk for a refreshing, toning soak.

In a massage oil Add 8–12 drops to 2 tablespoons base oil for a toning and detoxifying massage that helps eliminate a build-up of toxins.

Safe usage Non-toxic, non-irritant in dilution.

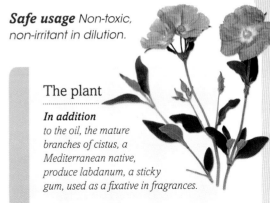

The plant

In addition *to the oil, the mature branches of cistus, a Mediterranean native, produce labdanum, a sticky gum, used as a fixative in fragrances.*

The essential oil

Steam-distilling *the leaves and twigs yields an amber oil that has a warm, earthy aroma with honey overtones.*

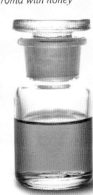

217

SKIN CARE

DIFFUSER

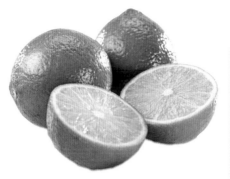

DIFFUSER

SKIN CARE

FRAGRANCE

Lime

Citrus aurantifolia

Stimulating and **refreshing**, lime can be relied on for its **cleansing** properties, and its fresh aroma calms and clears the mind. Like its relatives, grapefruit and lemon, it is a key oil for reducing water retention and puffiness. It also balances oily skin and hair.

What is it **good for?**

Aids detox Lime's strong detoxifying action helps tackle cellulite and the puffiness linked to water retention. As with grapefruit oil, inhaling lime oil has been shown to help weight loss by boosting the metabolism.

Balances oily skin and hair Lime has a toning effect that helps clear oily and acne-prone complexions. Added to a hair rinse, it conditions and removes excess oil to refresh the scalp. Treat dandruff by mixing lime juice in water and use it as a final rinse.

Has a cooling effect Lime oil "turns down the heat", helping to calm cold-related fevers. It also boosts the immune system, and eases bronchitis, coughs, sinusitis, and asthma.

Acts as an antiseptic The oil's soothing and antiseptic properties help to heal cold sores, insect bites, and cuts. Treat cuts by putting two drops of the oil in a cold compress and pressing on the affected area.

A stress reliever The refreshing and stimulating scent relieves stress, exhaustion, and anxiety, and its ability to calm promotes creativity and focus.

Best **uses**

As a lotion Added to a skin cream or lotion, lime essential oil clears and brightens dull, congested skin.

In a diffuser Add 1–3 drops to a diffuser, vaporizer, or oil burner to lift the spirits and keep the mind sharp.

Safe usage Non-toxic, use very well diluted (less than 1 per cent). Avoid use on skin 12 hours prior to sun exposure.

The plant

The lime tree, grown widely in tropical and subtropical areas, produces an acidic green fruit that is a popular food and drink flavouring.

The essential oil

Lime oil, which is cold-pressed from the rind of the fruit, has a sharp citrus scent, and is either pale yellow or light olive in colour.

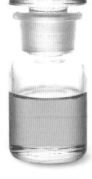

Neroli

Citrus aurantium

The blossom of the bitter, or Seville, orange tree is the source of a **calming**, refreshing, and uplifting oil that has long been considered a treatment for anxiety and depression. It is intense, yet **refreshing** and light, and a component of Eau de Cologne.

What is it **good for?**

Relieves stress Neroli has a long history as a remedy for anxiety. Its power to balance and revive makes it a first choice in cases of acute shock. It alleviates the effects of chronic stress on the adrenal, circulatory, and digestive systems.

Hydrates and tones skin Mixed in an oil-based elixir or cream, the oil balances moisture levels in the skin, helping to reduce fine lines caused by dehydration. Its gentle toning action makes it ideal for fine skin, helping to maintain elasticity, and for oily and acne-prone skin.

Promotes healing The oil's antiseptic and antibacterial properties speed the healing of cuts and wounds.

Improves digestion A gentle massage with a neroli blend soothes stomach cramps and diarrhoea.

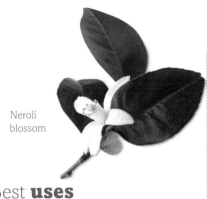

Neroli blossom

 SKIN CARE MASSAGE OIL

Best **uses**

In a diffuser If you have anxiety, add 3–4 drops of calming neroli to a diffuser, vaporizer, or oil burner.

As a skin toner Make a simple toning facial spritz by combining 2 teaspoons aloe vera juice with 6 tablespoons water and 4 drops of neroli in a spray bottle.

As a perfume Neroli has sufficient complexity to be worn neat as a scent in its own right, a trail il shares with rose and jasmine.

Safe usage Non-toxic and non-irritant.

The plant

This species of orange tree is native to China, but has been cultivated for hundreds of years in the countries bordering the Mediterranean. It takes at least 450kg (1000lb) of orange blossom flowers to make just 450g (1lb) of neroli oil.

The essential oil

With delicate blossoms, the best quality oil is water- rather than steam-distilled. The pale yellow oil darkens with age, and its sweet floral smell is powerful yet refreshing.

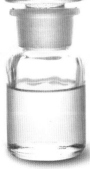

Petitgrain

Citrus aurantium amara

Another **beneficial** oil from the bitter orange tree – the other being neroli from the flowers. One of its most valuable properties is its **balancing** and toning effect on oily skin and hair. The relaxing aroma of petitgrain helps calm body and mind.

What is it **good for?**

Tones skin and hair Added to lotions and toners, petitgrain balances greasy skin by inhibiting the over-production of oil, helping to brighten and lift a dull complexion. Added to a rinse, it helps manage greasy hair.

Acts as an antiseptic Petitgrain oil helps to calm acne outbreaks and other skin eruptions. Its antiseptic action keeps wounds clean while they go through the healing process.

Acts as a deodorant Its astringent properties help to regulate perspiration, and its antibacterial action helps to control unwelcome body odour.

Calms body and mind Petitgrain's woody aroma has a relaxing sedative effect on body and mind. It counters nervous exhaustion and stress-related conditions, especially anger and panic, and helps to calm a rapid heartbeat.

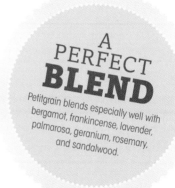

A PERFECT **BLEND**

Petitgrain blends especially well with bergamot, frankincense, lavender, palmarosa, geranium, rosemary, and sandalwood.

Best **uses**

As an acne treatment To control oily skin and to help clear up existing pimples and acne outbreaks, add 2–4 drops to a skin toner or lotion.

Massage oil A gentle massage with a petitgrain oil blend restores calm and balance when you are feeling angry or anxious. Add 12–18 drops to 2 tablespoons base oil.

Safe usage Non-toxic, non-irritant in dilution.

The plant

In the past, the oil was extracted from the cherry-sized unripe oranges, hence the name "petitgrain", meaning "little grains".

The essential oil

Petitgrain oil is extracted from the green twigs and leaves to produce a pale yellow to amber oil whose floral aroma has woody and green undertones.

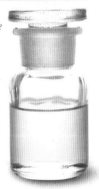

MASSAGE OIL

COMPRESS

Bergamot
Citrus aurantium bergamia

An aromatherapy favourite, this oil has a balancing effect on body and mind. Soothing and **cooling,** bergamot is ideal for dry or itchy skin conditions, and its fruity aroma helps to **elevate** a low mood, enhancing wellbeing.

What is it **good for?**

Soothes skin Bergamot essential oil is useful for balancing combination and oily skin and improving skin tone. Its strong soothing effects help to calm dry, itchy skin, and its natural healing properties can reduce the appearance of scars over time.

Enhances wellbeing The sweet aroma of bergamot acts as an antidepressant by balancing mood and easing anxiety. It is a popular ingredient in colognes.

Cools fevers Bergamot has a cooling action that can help to bring down fevers.

Acts as an antiseptic The oil has antibacterial and antiviral properties. Dab, diluted, on cold sores (it is active against the herpes virus) and pimples.

Best **uses**

As a massage oil To promote feelings of relaxation and help ensure a restful sleep, make a refreshing blend by mixing 2–4 drops with 2 tablespoons base oil and use to massage your feet before bedtime.

In a compress Add 2–3 drops to cool water and add to a compress, then apply directly to the skin to help relieve heat stroke or a fever.

Safe usage *Non-toxic, non-irritant in dilution. Ensure you buy bergaptene-free (also called Bergamot FCF), otherwise it is photo-toxic.*

The plant

Named after *the Italian city of Bergamo, these oranges are very sour, but with a deeply scented rind. The familiar aroma is used, among other things, as an ingredient in Earl Grey tea and Eau de Cologne.*

The essential oil

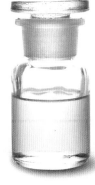

The rind *of the bergamot fruit is cold-pressed to produce either a light yellow or pale green oil which carries an extremely rich, sweet, fruity smell.*

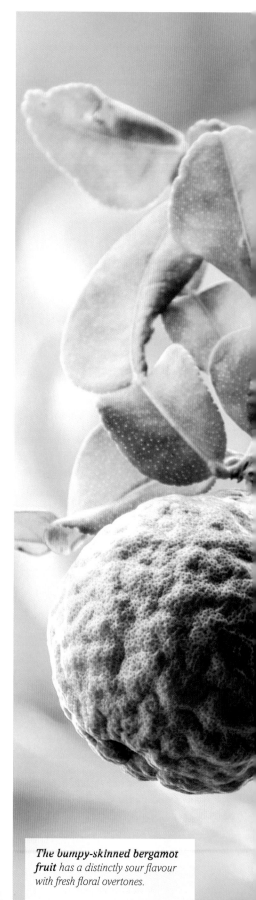

The bumpy-skinned bergamot fruit *has a distinctly sour flavour with fresh floral overtones.*

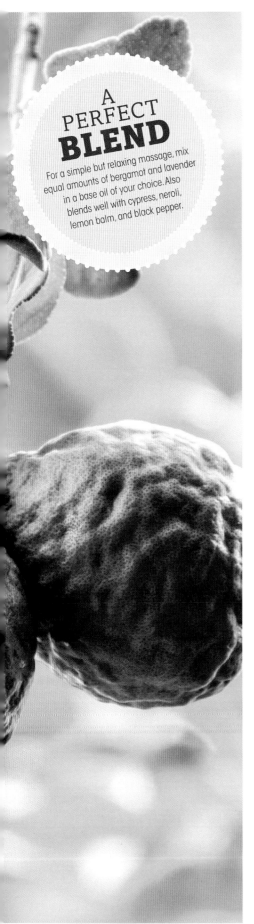

A PERFECT BLEND

For a simple but relaxing massage, mix equal amounts of bergamot and lavender in a base oil of your choice. Also blends well with cypress, neroli, lemon balm, and black pepper.

MASSAGE OIL

COMPRESS

Lemon

Citrus limonum

Fresh and **invigorating**, lemon stimulates the senses and clears the mind. **Detoxifying** and **toning**, the oil lends itself naturally to massage blends and skin products, and its citrus aroma and antiseptic properties make it a natural deodorizer.

What is it **good for?**

Tones skin Lemon boosts circulation, helping to reduce varicose veins and prevent chilblains. It cleanses oil-prone skin and hair, and tones, helping to ward off wrinkles and "spider" veins.

Acts as an antiseptic Lemon acts as an antiseptic, stimulating the defences against bacteria and viruses and killing germs. Use in a compress for boils and skin eruptions, or apply neat to warts and verrucas.

Aids detox A lemon oil massage supports the liver, aids lymphatic cleansing, and reduces cellulite and fluid retention.

Eases digestion It stimulates the digestive system, helping to combat obesity and loss of appetite.

Lifts moods A cheerful, deodorizing scent, lemon is great for busy days when you need mental focus and positivity.

Best **uses**

As a massage oil Add 8–12 drops to 2 tablespoons base oil for a detoxifying body massage.

In a compress Dilute 5–6 drops of lemon oil in almond oil or calendula tincture, and add to water to use as a compress to sooth skin eruptions.

Safe usage *Non-toxic, use well diluted (less than 2 per cent). Avoid using for 12 hours prior to sun exposure.*

The plant

The lemon tree *is native to India, but arrived in Europe with the Crusaders in the 12th century. As well as being a natural remedy, the rind is used in baking and cooking, and the essential oil, expressed from the rind of the fruit, has a long history of use in perfumery.*

The essential oil

The clear oil *with its fresh, citrus smell, is pressed from the peel of the lemon fruit.*

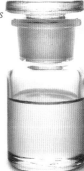

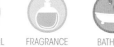

Grapefruit
Citrus paradisi

Grapefruit has an **energizing** and stimulating effect on body and mind. It makes an **uplifting** room spray, and in a massage blend boosts circulation, aids detox, and reduces water retention. Gently antiseptic and astringent, it is useful for controlling oily skin and hair.

What is it **good for?**

Aids detox The oil aids lymphatic drainage, helps boost metabolism, and assists weight loss. Massaged into skin, its diuretic and cleansing properties combat cellulite and water retention, and it stimulates, boosting circulation.

Tones skin and scalp The oil's gently antiseptic and astringent effects make it ideal for oily complexions, open pores, and acne, as well as oily hair. It helps to tone and tighten skin.

Combats tiredness With its fresh, zesty scent, grapefruit oil can help lift emotions and is revitalizing if you are suffering from mental exhaustion or are recovering from a late night.

Soothes aches and pains Add a few drops of the oil to a favourite base oil and use as a massage blend to help provide relief from muscle and joint pain, and tension headaches.

Acts as an air freshener Its uplifting, zesty aroma can help eliminate unpleasant odours in kitchens and bathrooms.

Best **uses**

As a massage oil Add 6–8 drops to 2 tablespoons base oil to cleanse skin.

In a room spray Clear stale air by adding 8–10 drops to water in a spray bottle. Shake well before use.

In a bath oil Add 5–6 drops to 1 tablespoon base oil or full-fat milk and disperse in a bath.

Safe usage Non-toxic, non-irritant in dilution (less than 3 per cent). Avoid using 12 hours prior to sun exposure.

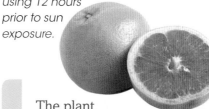

The plant

Unlike other citrus fruits, grapefruit originates from the Caribbean, and not Southeast Asia. Its name comes from the grape-like cluster in which the fruits grow.

The essential oil

The oil, which is cold-pressed from the peel of the fruit, can be yellow, pale green, or pale orange, with a zesty, sweet, citrussy smell.

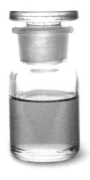

Mandarin
Citrus reticulata, Citrus nobilis

Mandarin (also known as tangerine) has **antiseptic** and anti-fungal properties, similar to other citrus fruits. It has a tonic effect on the digestive system, nourishes the skin, and its sweet, **cheerful** aroma is almost instantly **uplifting**.

What is it **good for?**

Tones skin Mandarin essential oil nurtures skin. It can help reduce the appearance of stretch marks and tone areas of flabbiness.

Aids detox In a massage oil, mandarin encourages lymphatic drainage and helps improve circulation. Its diuretic action helps combat water retention and cellulite.

Heals skin This stimulating oil helps regenerate skin cells. Its antiseptic and gently astringent properties make it useful for combating oily skin and outbreaks of acne.

Aids digestion Mandarin has a tonic effect on the digestive system. It helps food move along the digestive tract and eases indigestion and constipation, especially if these are stress-related. If you feel nauseous, it can calm your stomach.

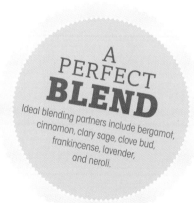
Enhances wellbeing A gentle, relaxing yet uplifting oil, mandarin is especially good for calming restless children, and is safe to use in pregnancy.

Best **uses**

In a diffuser Add 3–4 drops to a diffuser to freshen air or calm nerves.

In a massage oil Add 2–3 drops to a base oil for a soothing massage.

Safe usage Non-toxic, non-irritatant in dilution.

The plant

A native of China and the Far East, the mandarin tree was introduced to Europe in the nineteenth century. From Europe, the tree was shipped to the United States, where it was renamed tangerine.

The essential oil

An orange or amber colour with a tangy sweet, floral aroma, the oil is cold-pressed from the rind of the fruit.

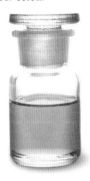

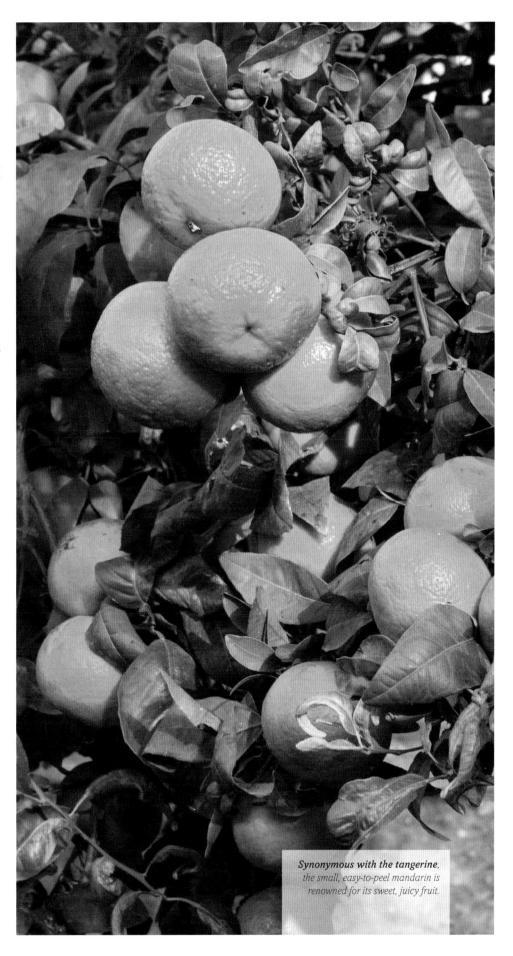

Synonymous with the tangerine, the small, easy-to-peel mandarin is renowned for its sweet, juicy fruit.

BATH OIL

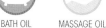
MASSAGE OIL

DIFFUSER

Orange
Citrus sinensis

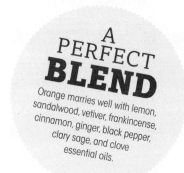

A
PERFECT
BLEND

Orange marries well with lemon, sandalwood, vetiver, frankincense, cinnamon, ginger, black pepper, clary sage, and clove essential oils.

Sometimes called sweet orange, this **versatile** oil is widely used for its **uplifting** and **detoxifying** effects. It is also **calming**, it may help ease tense muscles, and its **rejuvenating** properties help skin maintain a youthful appearance. Cheering and familiar, its aroma acts as a reviving tonic.

What is it **good for?**

Aids detox Orange essential oil has a detoxifying and cleansing effect throughout the body. Used as part of a massage blend, the oil helps to improve the circulation, stimulates the lymphatic system, and supports the action of the bladder and kidneys, facilitating the removal of toxins and waste from the body.

Tones skin Used in skincare products, orange essential oil helps to promote the production of collagen and supports the skin's natural repair process. The oil has inherent healing properties that are attributed to the aromatic compound limonene, also an effective antiseptic.

Revitalizes and brightens skin Orange essential oil has toning and slightly astringent properties that can help to clarify oily-looking skin and revitalize a dull or tired-looking complexion.

Boosts immunity Orange supports the immune system, and its cooling and refreshing properties can also help to relieve the symptoms of a feverish cold or flu virus.

Improves digestion As with other citrus oils, orange calms the digestive system, helping food to move efficiently through the gut, and in turn relieves constipation and trapped wind, and eases indigestion.

Relieves anxiety Orange essential oil has a sweet, uplifting scent that can calm nervous tension, lift feelings of depression, and promote restful sleep in cases of insomnia.

Best **uses**

As a bath oil Enjoy a relaxing bath that smoothes and tones skin by blending 6–8 drops in 1 tablespoon base oil or full-fat milk and dispersing in a warm bath.

As a massage oil To relieve nausea and indigestion if you have over-indulged and to release trapped wind, add 4–6 drops to 1 tablespoon base oil and massage the abdomen.

In a diffuser Used in a diffuser or room spray, the oil can help clear the air and mind. Its disinfectant action is useful in sick rooms, while its calming aroma can aid restful sleep for both adults and children.

Safe usage Non-toxic, non-irritant in dilution.

The plant

Like most citrus trees, the sweet orange tree originated in China. Today, however, most of the commercial production of orange essential oil takes place in Brazil, the USA, and Cyprus.

The essential oil

Orange oil is cold-pressed from the rind of the fruit. A fine oil, it is a pale orange-greenish colour with the same sweet, fresh, and fruity smell you get when you peel an orange.

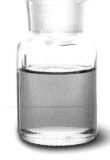

Sweet-smelling citrus oil is reviving and uplifting, enhancing feelings of wellbeing.

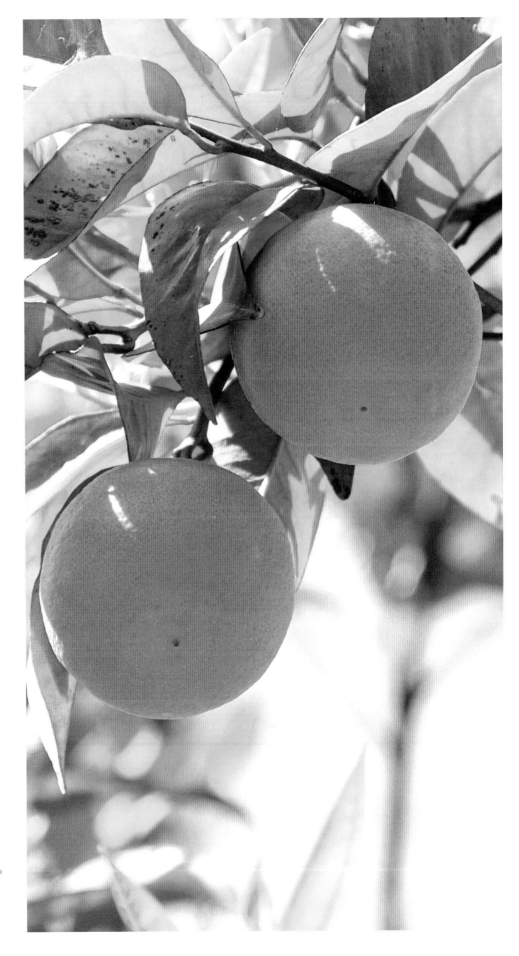

The sweet orange tree grows
*abundantly in warm, temperate
climates around the world.*

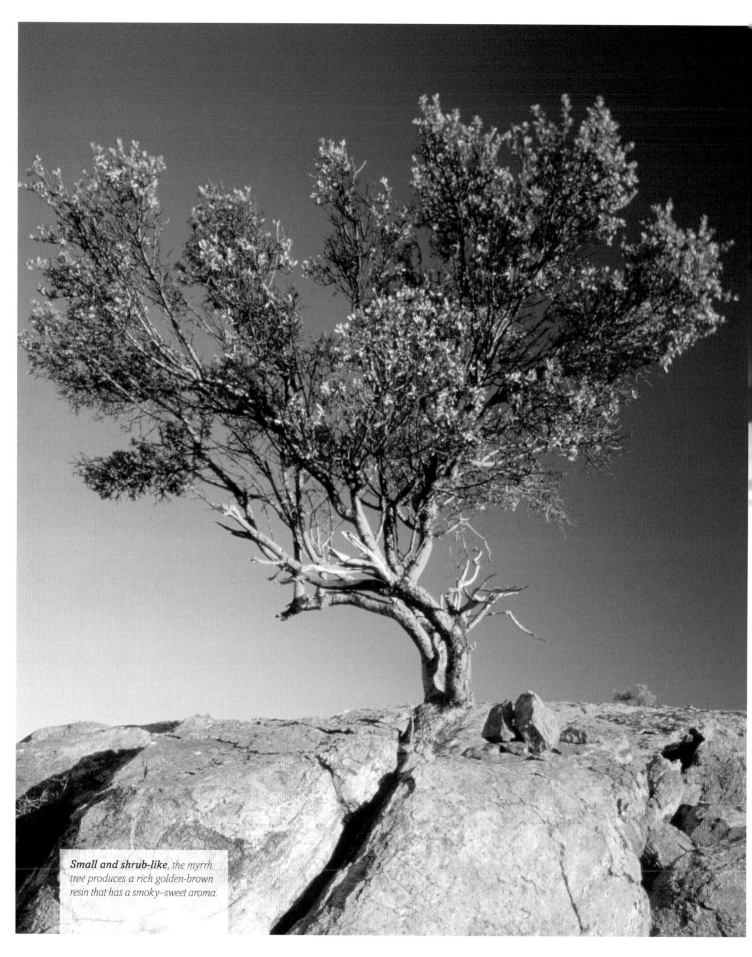

Small and shrub-like, the myrrh tree produces a rich golden-brown resin that has a smoky–sweet aroma.

SKIN CARE   MOUTHWASH

Myrrh

Commiphora myrrha, C. molmol

The **antiseptic** properties of myrrh make it a popular remedy for healing cuts and wounds. As a well-established **anti-ageing** treatment, it is added to skincare products to help prevent the premature appearance of fine lines. A grounding and centring oil, it both stimulates and **fortifies** the emotions.

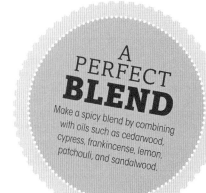

A PERFECT BLEND

Make a spicy blend by combining with oils such as cedarwood, cypress, frankincense, lemon, patchouli, and sandalwood.

What is it **good for?**

Heals skin Myrrh has an established history treating various types of skin eruptions, such as acne, athlete's foot, weeping eczema, and cold sores. Its healing properties make it useful for cuts, burns, and wounds. A non-irritating oil, myrrh can be applied neat to skin.

Tones skin Its ability to preserve skin tone helps delay wrinkles and other signs of ageing. It is also ideal for healing chapped and broken skin.

Cares for teeth and gums As part of a mouthwash, the antiseptic properties of myrrh help tackle infection and inflammation, soothing ulcers, sore throats, bleeding gums, bad breath, and oral thrush.

For coughs and colds Myrrh makes an excellent expectorant, particularly when coughs and colds produce thick, white mucus. Try using myrrh in a steam inhalation to ease chronic lung conditions, coughs, colds, and bronchitis.

Enhances wellbeing The aromatherapeutic properties of myrrh are purported to help strengthen confidence in overcoming difficulties and to enhance focus and provide a strong sense of purpose.

Best **uses**

As a skin toner Add 2–4 drops of myrrh essential oil to 2 tablespoons facial lotion or toner to improve skin tone and quality, especially for mature and sun-damaged skin.

In a mouthwash Add 1–2 drops of the oil to water for a mouthwash to fight gum disease and bad breath.

Safe usage Non-irritant in dilution. Only use extremely well diluted (less than 0.2 per cent) in pregnancy and when breastfeeding.

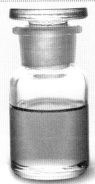

The plant

The myrrh tree *belongs to a family of small spiky shrubs and bushes native to the Middle East, North Africa, and northern India. The resin is gathered by making incisions in the tree that allow it to flow freely.*

The essential oil

Dried lumps of resin *are steam-distilled to produce the essential oil, which is pale orange to amber in colour.*

Strengthening and healing, myrrh has a rejuvenating effect on skin.

MASSAGE OIL

MOUTHWASH

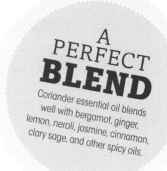

A
PERFECT
BLEND

Coriander essential oil blends
well with bergamot, ginger,
lemon, neroli, jasmine, cinnamon,
clary sage, and other spicy oils.

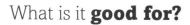

A-Z OF ESSENTIAL OILS

228

Coriander

Coriandrum sativum

This highly **aromatic** oil has a long history in traditional medicine, especially in Ayurvedic and Chinese medicines. Its **antiseptic** action helps clear pimples and fungal infections, and when used in a mouthwash, the oil freshens breath. Its light, **herby aroma** energizes and is a natural tonic for flagging spirits.

What is it **good for?**

Relieves pain Coriander has a warming effect that helps stimulate circulation and relieve stiffness and pain in muscles and joints. The oil's analgesic properties help relieve general headaches and localized neuralgia pain, and can ease menstrual cramps.

Acts as an antiseptic Coriander essential oil is useful for dealing with occasional spots, pimples, and fungal infections. The oil's strong antiseptic and deodorizing effect also makes it especially helpful for dealing with the bacteria that cause smelly feet, bad breath, and gum disease.

Enhances wellbeing Used as a room spray, coriander's soothing herbal aroma has an energizing effect that helps lift apathy and feelings of nervous exhaustion.

Best **uses**

As a massage oil Add 6–12 drops to 2 tablespoons base oil for a warming and deodorizing massage.

In a mouthwash Mix 1–2 drops of the essential oil in a teaspoon of glycerine or calendula tincture and add to water before using as a gargle or mouthwash to treat gum infections.

Safe usage Non-toxic and non-irritant.

The plant

Both the leaves and seeds of the coriander plant produce useful oils. When the oil is distilled from the leaves it is known as cilantro essential oil. The leaves are also a popular culinary ingredient.

The essential oil

Steam-distillation of the crushed ripe seeds produces a clear to pale yellow oil with a sweet, spicy, slightly fruity, warm herbaceous scent that is warming, uplifting, and calming.

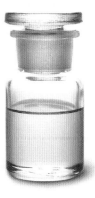

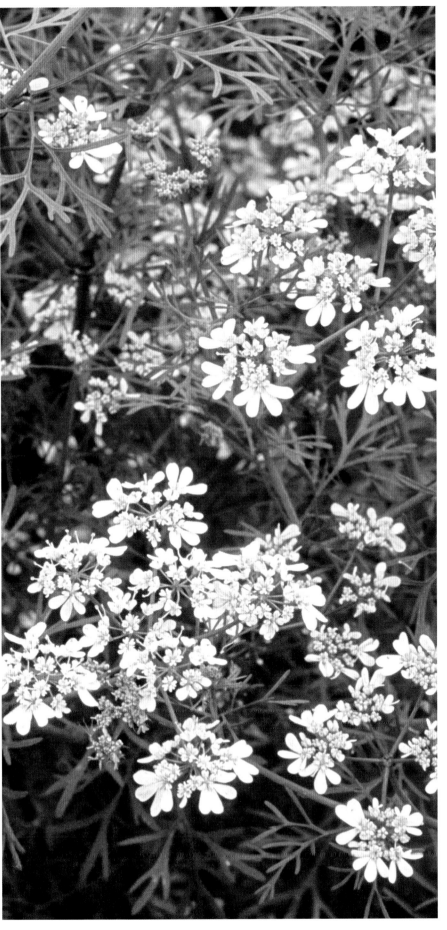

Warming coriander makes a gently stimulating and soothing oil, perfect for lifting the spirits.

The seeds produced from the flowering coriander plant are used to make the aromatic essential oil.

MASSAGE OIL

COMPRESS

Cumin

Cuminum cyminum

The use of cumin can be traced back to the Ancient Egyptians and Assyrians. This **warming** essential oil helps to **relax** muscles and relieve aching joints. It stimulates circulation and helps **calm** the nerves and **lift** the spirits. It is also a useful antiseptic that can support healing.

What is it **good for?**

Aids detox The detoxifying action of cumin makes this a useful massage oil for fighting stubborn cellulite. Cumin also supports liver function, aiding the removal of toxins.

Boosts circulation Cumin has a tonifying effect on the body. It helps to boost the general circulation and can also be useful for helping to control high blood pressure.

Eases pain and digestive discomfort Cumin helps to fortify the digestive tract, relieving nausea, bloating, and constipation. It brings relief to mild headaches.

Heals skin Added to skin preparations, cumin essential oil has an antiseptic action that helps to heal dry or cracked skin, reduce bruising, and control acne, eczema, and psoriasis. It also revitalizes mature and tired-looking skin.

Fights fatigue The stimulating aroma provides a welcome lift if you feel lethargic, weak, or unable to focus.

Best **uses**

As a massage oil Add 2–4 drops to 2 tablespoons base oil for a massage to relieve joint and muscle pain.

In a compress Add 2–3 drops to some glycerine or almond oil, add to cool water, and use as a compress to relieve itchy skin and bruises.

Safe usage *Dilute very well (less than 0.5 per cent). Avoid using for 12 hours prior to sun exposure.*

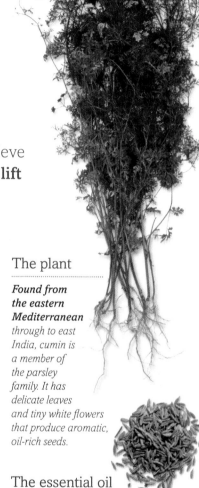

The plant

Found from the eastern Mediterranean *through to east India, cumin is a member of the parsley family. It has delicate leaves and tiny white flowers that produce aromatic, oil-rich seeds.*

The essential oil

The crushed seeds *of the cumin plant are steam-distilled to produce a pale yellow oil that darkens with age. The oil has a pungent spicy–woody aroma that is musky and sensual as well as stimulating.*

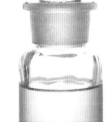

This relaxing oil is ideal for easing and soothing muscular pains.

COMPRESS

MASSAGE OIL

FRAGRANCE

Cypress

Cupressus sempervirens

With a well-deserved reputation as a **warming** and **uplifting** oil, cypress also soothes and relaxes, making it a useful remedy for relieving muscular aches and pains. It helps to **stimulate** circulation and its strong **toning** action works on skin and veins. The fresh, woody aroma creates a feeling of **positivity**.

A PERFECT BLEND

Clary sage, bergamot, lemon, lavender, ginger, juniper, pine, and geranium essential oils are all natural blending partners for cypress

What is it **good for?**

Improves circulation Cypress oil has a powerful toning action on the veins and helps to regulate blood flow. This makes it especially useful for treating spider veins, varicose veins, and troublesome haemorrhoids.

Tones skin The oil's balancing properties make it ideal for evening out oily and puffy complexions and also for toning areas of loose skin, for example, after weight loss.

Aids detox Strongly astringent, cypress oil is useful in combating water retention and cellulite. It also supports healthy circulation and helps flush out toxins.

Acts as a deodorant Its astringent quality makes the oil an effective antiperspirant and deodorizer. Added to a foot bath, the oil helps control perspiration and foot odour.

Supports women's health The soothing action of cypress helps ease menstrual discomfort and cramping.

Soothes aches and pains Diluted in a base oil and massaged over

affected areas, cypress can relieve rheumatism and osteoarthritis, as well as general muscle and joint pain. It can help control spasms, relieve menstrual cramps, and may be used for injury rehabilitation.

Heals wounds A popular ingredient in antiseptic lotions and creams, cypress essential oil has antiseptic properties that help heal wounds. Its astringent properties can slow bleeding, such as nosebleeds.

Calms nerves Refreshing and mentally toning, cypress oil helps to ease stress-induced nervous strain and tension and to lift weariness.

Best **uses**

As a compress To stem nosebleeds, apply 4–5 drops to a cold compress. Keeping your head level, gently press your nostrils together with the compress.

As a massage oil Dilute 16–20 drops in 2 tablespoons base oil for a warming massage to relieve rheumatism, arthritis, menstrual cramps, and varicose veins.

As a cologne The masculine notes suit men's colognes and aftershaves.

Many women also enjoy using this essential oil as an alternative to heavy floral scents.

Safe usage *Non-toxic, non-irritant in dilution.*

The plant

This coniferous evergreen tree *can grow up to to 35m (115ft) tall and live for more than 1000 years. A native of the Mediterranean regions, cypress has long been an important ingredient in incense for ritual uses as well as being a source of the therapeutic healing oil.*

The essential oil

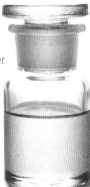

The clear to very pale yellow *oil has a woody, nutty aroma with a hint of spice. It is produced by steam-distilling the fresh leaves and cones.*

SKIN CARE

DIFFUSER

FIRST AID

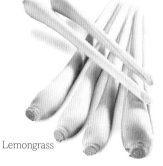
Lemongrass

Lemongrass

Cymbopogon citratus, C. flexuosus

This essential oil works on body and mind to **refresh** and **stimulate**. It has antiseptic and astringent effects that work on oily or acne-prone skin. Lemongrass is **deodorizing**, **antibacterial**, and makes an effective **insect repellent**.

What is it **good for?**

Acts as an antiseptic Its astringent and antiseptic effects cleanse skin: a few drops in a facial steam work on open or blocked pores. Its antiseptic properties and fresh scent also help control sweating and the bacteria that cause body odour, and it relieves acne, eczema, and athlete's foot.

Acts as an insect repellent Lemongrass is one of the key active ingredients in natural insect repellents.

Aids digestion Lemongrass is a natural appetite stimulant. It is also a good remedy for gastric infections.

Eases aches and pains Diluted in a blend, a lemongrass massage strengthens muscle tone and slack tissues, ideal for a pre-sport massage or to treat aching muscles or muscle strain. It can also soothe headaches.

Enhances wellbeing Lemongrass calms and fortifies nerves and eases depression and stress.

Best **uses**

As a toner Add 4–8 drops to 2 tablespoons witch hazel or a light lotion to refresh and tone skin.

In a diffuser Disperse into a room to raise spirits and lift exhaustion.

As an insect repellent Dilute 10–12 drops in a small spray bottle of witch hazel. Or mix 4–8 drops with 2 tablespoons lotion to dab on skin.

Safe usage Use only very well diluted (less than 0.5 per cent). Avoid use on hypersensitive skin and on children less than seven years old.

The plant

Lemongrass is a native of India. *Its oil is used in cosmetics and scents. There are two main types: West Indian (Cymbopogon citratus) and East Indian (Cymbopogon flexuosus), both with similar properties. After distilling the oil, the grass is used as cattle feed.*

The essential oil

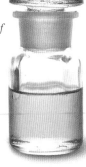

The essential oil *is produced by steam-distillation of the chopped grass. The liquid is pale yellow to amber in colour, and has a fresh, herbaceous, lemony aroma.*

BATH OIL

MASSAGE OIL

DIFFUSER

Palmarosa

Cymbopogon martinii

Palmarosa comes from a wild grass native to India. The pleasant floral aroma has hints of rose. Its **balancing** action makes it a popular skincare product: it **hydrates** dry skin, **rejuvenates** tired or mature skin, and helps controls sebum secretions in oily skin.

What is it **good for?**

Nourishes and tones skin Palmarosa hydrates and balances. By stimulating cell regeneration and controlling sebum, it helps keep skin supple and elastic and improves the appearance of scar tissue and stretch marks. A natural toner, the oil helps to reduce the appearance of wrinkles and fine lines and to brighten tired complexions. In a facial steam, it can unclog pores and tone sagging skin.

Aids recuperation A gentle tonic, the oil helps to hasten recovery after illness. It aids digestion and boosts poor appetite. Diluted and massaged over the abdomen, it may also relieve symptoms of diarrhoea.

Acts as an antiseptic Its antiseptic properties are specifically active against the bacteria that cause acne. It can also treat athlete's foot, dermatitis, and minor skin infections.

Enhances wellbeing A palmarosa massage helps relieve stress, anxiety, and tension, and is a mild aphrodisiac, countering strong negative emotions that interfere with sexual fulfilment.

Best **uses**

As a bath oil Mix 4–6 drops with 1 tablespoon base oil or full-fat milk for a fortifying bath when you are tired, recuperating, or have a digestive upset.

As a massage oil Add 16–24 drops to 2 tablespoons base oil to tone skin.

In a diffuser Diffuse to freshen air, fight fatigue, and focus the mind.

Safe usage Non-toxic, non-irritant in dilution (less than 5 per cent).

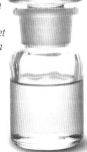

The plant

Also called Indian or Turkish geranium, palmarosa grass is a relative of lemongrass, but has a floral, rather than citrus, scent. Native to India, it is now cultivated in Indonesia, East Africa, the Comoro Islands, and Brazil.

The essential oil

The thin, pale yellow essential oil can be steam- or water-distilled from the fresh or dried grass. It has a sweet floral aroma with a subtle hint of rose.

DIFFUSER

SKIN CARE

Citronella

Cymbopogon nardus

Best known as an **insect repellent** used in a variety of candles, potpourri, and lotions, citronella has other important uses. As a room scent it helps to **clear** and **refresh** the mind, and its antiseptic properties make it effective in deodorants.

What is it **good for?**

Tones skin The toning properties of citronella help balance skin that is prone to oiliness.

Acts as an insect repellent This popular insect repellent is a very useful holiday companion. Carry a citronella-infused tissue to help keep annoying bugs at bay.

Freshens and clears air The antiseptic properties of citronella help to clear the air of viruses, which is especially useful during the cold and flu season or to clear the air in a sickroom. Its antiseptic effect also makes it a useful ingredient in deodorants.

Enhances focus Citronella essential oil can lift the emotions when you feel downcast and also helps you to keep a clear head and maintain focus.

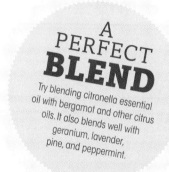

A PERFECT **BLEND**

Try blending citronella essential oil with bergamot and other citrus oils. It also blends well with geranium, lavender, pine, and peppermint.

Best **uses**

In a diffuser Add 2–3 drops to a diffuser or to water for a room spray to make an effective insect repellent.

In a lotion For a foot lotion to combat odours, add 3–6 drops to 2 tablespoons unscented lotion base.

Safe usage Non-irritant in dilution (less than 15 per cent). Avoid using on hypersensitive skin.

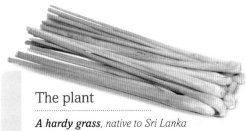

The plant

A hardy grass, native to Sri Lanka and Java, citronella is distinguishable from its cousin, lemongrass, by its reddish-coloured stems.

The essential oil

Citronella oil is steam-distilled from the finely chopped fresh, dried, or part-dried grass. It is a pale to dark yellow oil with a sweet, lemony scent.

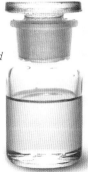

DIFFUSER

SKIN CARE

Carrot seed

Daucus carota

This unusual oil has a **rejuvenating** effect on many body systems. A **grounding** oil, it can relieve feelings of stress and lift exhaustion. It also has a mild diuretic action that helps to eliminate toxins, and its **healing properties** can be harnessed to **revitalize** problem complexions and nourish dry and mature skin.

What is it **good for?**

Aids detox The mild diuretic effects of carrot essential oil help to reduce excess fluid retention. This detoxifying oil also supports the efficient functioning of the liver, and strengthens the digestive system.

Relieves stress The earthy aroma of carrot essential oil is grounding and calming, helping to relieve feelings of stress, and give the body stamina to fight feelings of exhaustion and general lethargy.

Soothes aching muscles As part of a massage oil blend or diluted in the bath, carrot seed oil is deeply warming, helping to ease aches and pains and boost the circulation.

Repairs skin Highly valued in cosmetics, carrot essential oil is added to face and body creams to nourish, tighten, revitalize, tone, and rejuvenate tired-looking skin. Its calming properties also make it suitable for itchy and irritated skin.

Best **uses**

In a diffuser Add 3–4 drops of carrot seed oil to a diffuser, vaporizer, or oil burner to impart a very subtle, grounding aroma to the air.

In a cream Add 6–8 drops of carrot seed essential oil to 2 tablespoons cream or lotion base and use to help soften dry skin, and also to encourage healthy cell growth and skin rejuvenation.

Safe usage Use in dilutions of less than 2 per cent. Avoid using during pregnancy or while breastfeeding.

The plant

Wild carrot, also known as "Queen Anne's lace" is a European native that has hairy leaves and delicate white lacy flowers with purple centres that spread out in a distinctive umbrella shape. Though wild carrot bears little resemblance to the commercial root vegetable, it does share the same aroma.

The essential oil

Steam-distilling the dried seeds of the wild carrot plant produces a yellow–brown oil that has a fairly viscous texture. The oil has an understated, mildly sweet, dry, and distinctly earthy aroma with some noticeable herbaceous undertones.

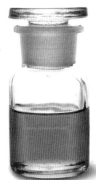

With its subtle aroma, this oil holds potent healing properties.

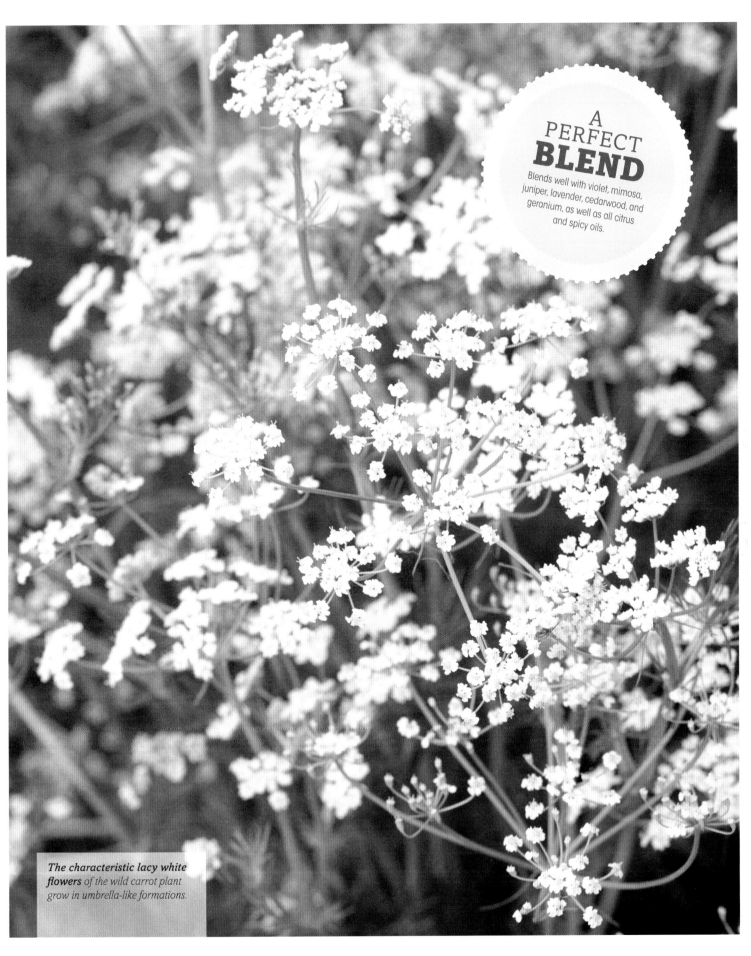

A
PERFECT
BLEND

Blends well with violet, mimosa, juniper, lavender, cedarwood, and geranium, as well as all citrus and spicy oils.

The characteristic lacy white flowers of the wild carrot plant grow in umbrella-like formations.

MASSAGE OIL

MOUTHWASH

Cardamom
Elettaria cardamomum

A natural **diuretic** and digestive stimulant, cardamom **boosts** the metabolism and helps the body to metabolize fat efficiently. It is also an effective **antiseptic**, making it a popular component of natural mouthwashes and deodorants.

What is it **good for?**

Acts as a deodorant Cardamom essential oil is a good addition to deodorants, helping to eliminate the bacteria that cause body odour.

Cares for teeth and gums Its antiseptic properties are useful for treating bad breath and for helping heal sore, bleeding gums.

Aids detox Diluted with a base oil, cardamom makes a stimulating massage blend, helping to boost circulation. Its mild diuretic action also helps facilitate the removal of toxins.

Soothes digestive upsets Cardamom has a calming action ideal for an upset stomach and nausea. It also relieves heartburn.

Combats tiredness The oil relieves stress and is refreshing, helping combat fatigue. A reputed aphrodisiac, especially if you are overtired.

Best **uses**

As a massage oil Add 6–8 drops to 2 tablespoons base oil for a refreshing, detoxifying full-body massage.

In a mouthwash Mix 1–2 drops in a teaspoon of glycerine or calendula tincture; add to water for a mouthwash.

Safe Usage *Non-toxic and non-irritant. Avoid using in children under seven years old.*

The plant

A native of India, cardamom seeds and pods have been used for centuries as a culinary spice and a healing remedy. Cardamom is also used in traditional Chinese medicine.

The essential oil

The essential oil is extracted by steam-distillation from the seeds and produces a colourless to pale yellow oil that has a sweet–spicy aroma with woody notes.

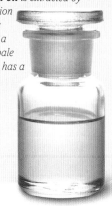

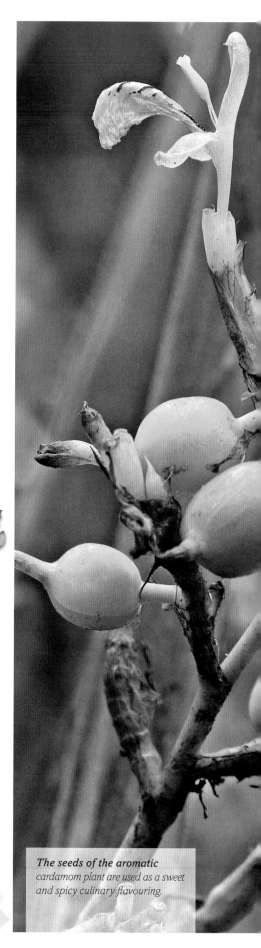

The seeds of the aromatic cardamom plant are used as a sweet and spicy culinary flavouring.

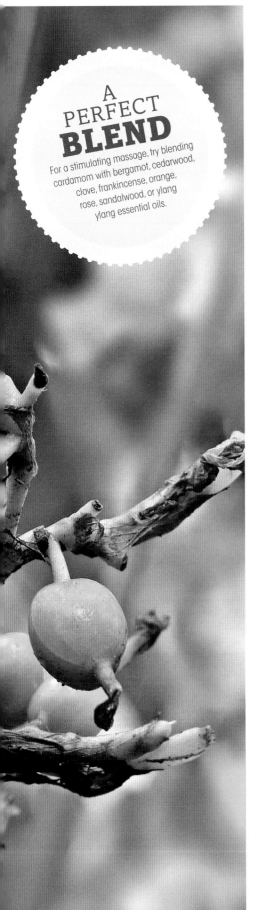

MASSAGE OIL

STEAM
INHALATION

DIFFUSER

A PERFECT BLEND

For a stimulating massage, try blending cardamom with bergamot, cedarwood, clove, frankincense, orange, rose, sandalwood, or ylang ylang essential oils.

Eucalyptus

Eucalyptus globulus

This **warming** and **antiseptic** oil is great for relieving aches and pains as well as healing mouth ulcers and insect bites and stings. The oil **tones** and balances the skin, and its sharp aroma helps **increase concentration** and lift feelings of depression.

What is it **good for?**

Acts as an antiseptic Dab onto skin to heal bacterial and fungal infections and wounds and soothe bites. In a bath, it can relieve cystitis. The oil makes a good sick-room spray.

Tones skin A facial steam with a few drops of the oil helps to cleanse and tone oily or acne-prone skin.

Eases aches and pains Add the oil to a base oil or an ointment to warm and loosen tight muscles and joints.

Improves focus Eucalyptus refreshes the mind, banishing headaches and improving concentration.

Best **uses**

As a massage oil Blend 2–3 drops in an ointment to rub on the chest to clear sinuses and aid sleep when congested.

In an inhalation Add 6–8 drops to hot water and use as a facial steam to unclog pores, cleanse and tone, and leave you clear-headed and refreshed.

In a diffuser Diffuse 3–4 drops to combat tiredness.

Safe usage Non-toxic externally; non-irritant in dilution (less than 20 per cent). Avoid near nose or face on children under seven years old.

The plant

The blue gum eucalyptus, a tree native to Australia, is the most widely cultivated of hundreds of species of eucalyptus.

Several other varieties are used in aromatherapy, notably the slightly gentler Eucalyptus radiata and the more cooling Eucalyptus citronella.

The essential oil

This oil is steam-distilled from the leaves of the tree. It has a clear to pale yellow hue and has a strong, camphorous, woody smell.

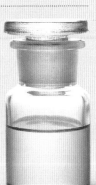

MASSAGE OIL

MOUTHWASH

Fennel (sweet)

Foeniculum vulgare

With a long history as a sacred and medicinal herb, fennel is a **cooling** and **cleansing** essential oil. Its main action is to **unblock**, where it works on both body and mind, easing constipation and other complaints and providing the courage to express held-in emotions.

What is it **good for?**

Aids detox Fennel has a diuretic effect and helps to stimulate circulation. Diluted in a base oil, it provides a good detoxifying massage that helps tackle stubborn cellulite.

Cares for teeth and gums Well diluted, fennel essential oil can be gargled in a mouthwash to help fight the bacteria that causes tooth decay and bad breath.

Soothes digestion Fennel has unblocking properties. A massage blend containing fennel helps relieve flatulence, bloating, digestive cramps, and constipation. The oil also stimulates appetite, and eases nervous indigestion brought on by a rushed meal or emotional upset.

Fights colds A mild expectorant, fennel essential oil helps loosen phlegmy coughs. Blend with a base oil for a chest rub, or add to a diffuser, vaporizer, or oil burner.

Best **uses**

As a massage oil For indigestion, blend 4–6 drops of fennel essential oil in 1 tablespoon light base oil and gently massage the abdomen in a clockwise direction.

In a mouthwash Mix 1–2 drops in a teaspoon of glycerine or calendula tincture and add to water to use as a mouthwash.

Safe usage Dilute well before use (less than 2 per cent). Avoid during pregnancy and if breastfeeding. Not suitable for children under seven years old.

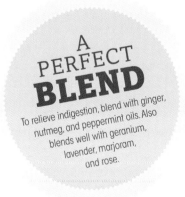

A PERFECT **BLEND**
To relieve indigestion, blend with ginger, nutmeg, and peppermint oils. Also blends well with geranium, lavender, marjoram, and rose.

The plant

The fennel plant grows up to 2m (6ft) high. Its green feathery leaves and golden yellow flowers attract insects and bees and eventually produce the oil-rich seeds.

The essential oil

The essential oil is steam-distilled from crushed fennel seeds. It is pale yellow with a sweet–spicy smell that is reminiscent of aniseed.

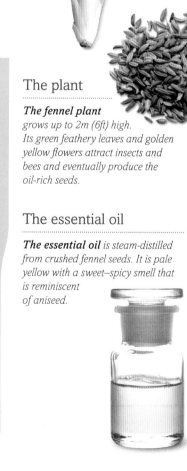

COMPRESS

DIFFUSER

OINTMENT

Wintergreen

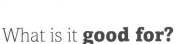
Gaultheria procumbens, G. fragrantissima

A pungent **medicinal** oil, wintergreen should be used sparingly. Its strong minty aroma can clear the head and even small amounts applied topically can provide **pain relief**.

What is it **good for?**

Relieves pain The oil is a popular ingredient in muscle ointments and rubs. It contains a natural aspirin-like analgesic that can help to relieve pain locally. Used in a compress, the oil can alleviate headaches, muscle cramps, joint pain, and tendonitis, and can also bring some relief to pain caused by chronic conditions such as arthritis and rheumatism.

Aids digestion Once absorbed through the skin, the oil can stimulate the digestive process by triggering the release of digestive juices.

Tones skin and hair Arguably too strong for use on the face, when well-diluted, wintergreen's astringent and antiseptic action can help to treat acne on the body. Its antifungal properties also help prevent dandruff and can work to clear athlete's foot.

Clears the head A few drops of wintergreen essential oil in a vaporizer or diffuser aids breathing and helps relieve stress and tension.

Best **uses**

In a compress Blend 3 drops each of wintergreen and lavender oils for an effective hot or cold compress to relieve localized aches and pains.

In a diffuser Used in a diffuser, vaporizer, or oil burner, the oil opens up the nasal and respiratory passages.

In an ointment Add 1–2 drops to an ointment base to relieve pain locally.

Safe usage Dilute well before use (less than 2 per cent). Avoid during pregnancy and if breastfeeding. Not suitable for young children. Avoid if on anticoagulant medication and if sensitive to aspirin.

The plant

A shrubby evergreen, wintergreen is native to North America. It has glossy, green, oval leaves and abundant white blooms in the summer, which turn into bright red berries during the winter, often lasting through to spring. The berries were used traditionally in herbal medicine to help relieve muscular aches and pains.

The essential oil

Steam-distilled from the chopped-up leaves, wintergreen essential oil has a sweet, fresh, and pleasant minty aroma. The oil is pale yellow or pinkish yellow in colour. Wintergreen blends well with other minty oils, such as peppermint, and also complements bergamot, basil, lavender, and lemongrass essential oils.

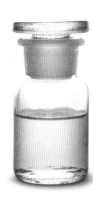

This essential oil has strong anti-bacterial and antifungal effects.

FIRST AID

COMPRESS

STEAM INHALATION

DIFFUSER

SKIN CARE

Helichrysum (Immortelle)

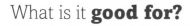
Helichrysum italicum

Also known as immortelle, or **"everlasting" oil**, this is a fantastic, **regenerative** oil that **cools** and soothes the skin. Its antiseptic and **anti-inflammatory** properties help heal scars and skin eruptions. Deeply **de-stressing,** it's perfect for relieving anxiety, nervous exhaustion, and feelings of depression.

What is it **good for?**

Enhances wellbeing The oil's therapeutic properties help treat tension, depression, exhaustion, and other stress-related conditions. Uplifting, it curbs negativity and promotes a feeling of safety, helping to heal old emotional wounds.

Relieves pain An effective anti-inflammatory, this is a good choice for joint pain, arthritic conditions, and general strains and sprains.

Heals wounds and fights infections Helichrysum can be applied in a cream to wounds to help reduce swelling, disinfect, and promote healing through tissue regeneration. It has demonstrated antibacterial properties.

Heals and protects skin The anti-inflammatory and regenerative properties of helichrysum oil make it useful for treating skin problems such as acne, dermatitis, bruises, boils, and abscesses. It can also help to fade scars, stretch marks, and blemishes. The oil's antioxidant properties protect the skin from harmful free radicals that cause premature skin ageing.

Soothes skin The oil's calming action helps soothe allergic skin breakouts and numbness and tingling in nerve-related conditions.

Boosts circulation The oil stimulates circulation. It can also help to control blood pressure and provide relief from conditions such as varicose veins.

Relieves coughs and colds The oil has an antispasmodic effect that relieves asthma and persistent coughs. It may act as a decongestant in cases of sinusitis and catarrh, especially when these are allergy- or stress-related.

Best **uses**

As first aid The oil can be applied in a cream as an effective emergency treatment for burns, grazes or cuts.

As a compress Add 6–8 drops to a cool compress and hold over skin flare-ups and bruises.

As an inhalation Add 8–10 drops to a steam inhalation to help clear blocked sinuses.

In a diffuser Add 3–4 drops to a diffuser to create a calming ambience.

As a skin toner Added to facial spritzers, toners, or lotions, helichrysum essential oil leaves skin feeling fresh and toned and helps to reduce the appearance of fine lines and skin blemishes.

Safe usage Use well diluted (less than 0.5 per cent).

The plant

A Mediterranean herb, helichrysum's small, cheerful flowers are popular with florists. Part of the sunflower family, the oil's names, "everlasting" and "immortelle", come from the reputation of the flowers for retaining their brilliant colour even when dried.

The essential oil

This watery yellow essential oil that occasionally has a tinge of red is steam-distilled from the flowers. It has a distinctive straw-like aroma with hints of fruit, tea, and honey.

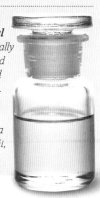

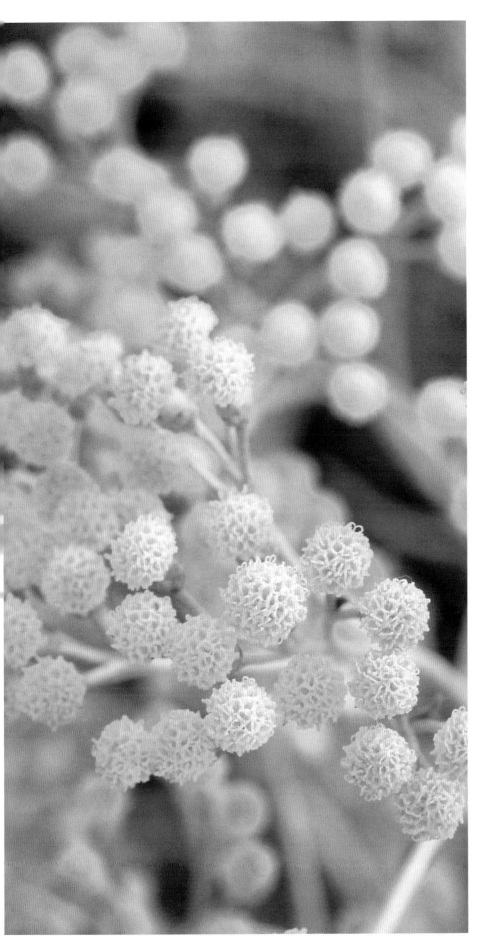

This cooling and soothing oil nourishes, rejuvenates, and heals skin.

This fragrant evergreen shrub produces clusters of bright yellow flowers in the summer months.

STEAM
INHALATION

MOUTHWASH

Star anise

Illicium verum

Star anise has been in use since ancient times in Europe, the Middle East, and Asia, favoured for both its **therapeutic benefits** and distinctive flavour. With its sharp aroma, the essential oil acts as a mild **pain reliever** and also makes an effective **antiseptic**.

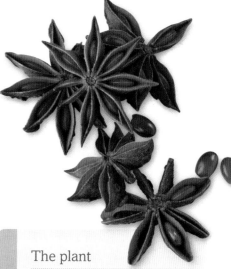

What is it **good for?**

Relieves aches and pains Star anise has pain-relieving properties that provide localized relief from muscular aches and pains, and help to ease rheumatism and arthritis.

Acts as an antiseptic The essential oil has a strong antibacterial action. It also has potent antifungal properties that can help heal skin infections such as athlete's foot, and it can be used to treat head lice and mites.

Acts as a deodorant Star anise is often added to soaps to combat body odour, and the oil makes a natural breath freshener.

Tones skin Its skin-balancing properties are useful for calming oily and combination skin.

Promotes restful sleep The oil has a sedative action that helps to calm, slowing the heart rate and aiding sleep, making it especially useful for anxiety-related sleep problems.

Best **uses**

In an inhalation Add 3–4 drops of star anise oil to a steam inhalation to provide temporary relief from bronchitis, cold, and flu symptoms.

In a mouthwash Add 1–2 drops to a teaspoon of glycerine or calendula tincture. Add to a glass of water and rinse in the mouth to fight the germs that cause bad breath. Do not swallow.

Safe usage Use well diluted (less than 1 per cent). Avoid during pregnancy and if breastfeeding. Not suitable for children under seven years old.

A PERFECT **BLEND**

Star anise blends well with vetiver, palmarosa, orange, and other citrus oils, as well as neroli, frankincense, lavender, ylang ylang, and tea tree.

The plant

An evergreen tree from China and Vietnam, star anise produces distinctive star-shaped fruits that are commonly used in Asian cooking as well as in traditional medicine.

The essential oil

The pale yellow oil has an aroma similar to black liquorice and is steam-distilled from the fresh and partly-dried fruits.

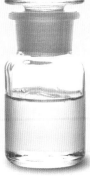

FRAGRANCE   SKIN CARE

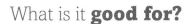

Jasmine
Jasminum officinale

The heady aroma of jasmine is highly prized by perfumers. The essential oil is one of the most **uplifting**, and its deeply **relaxing** effects account for its reputation as an aphrodisiac.

What is it **good for?**

Soothes skin Added to skin lotions, the oil can be a calming treatment for sensitive and inflamed skin that feels hot to the touch.

Tones skin Naturally toning, jasmine improves skin elasticity. Diluted in a massage blend and used regularly, it can help to fade stretch marks and scars.

Enhances wellbeing The warm, floral aroma of jasmine has a powerfully uplifting effect, helping to increase feelings of alertness, relieve tension, stress, and anxiety, and disperse feelings of negativity. It is traditionally regarded as an aphrodisiac for men and women.

Fights coughs and colds
A few drops of jasmine oil added to a steam inhalation can help to soothe irritating coughs and hoarseness and relieve laryngitis.

Best **uses**

As a perfume Jasmine oil can be applied neat as a perfume, creating a sense of relaxation and imbuing the wearer with a feeling of enjoyment.

As a toner Make a simple facial toner by adding 2–3 drops of jasmine absolute to a teaspoon of glycerine or witch hazel, then add to water. Soak a piece of cotton wool in the solution and apply to the skin.

Safe usage *Non-toxic and non-irritant.*

The plant

*A **native** of northwest India, the name "jasmine" is derived from the Persian "yasmin", which means "fragrant flower". The waxy flowers are esteemed in perfumery for their exotic, intensely floral aroma.*

The essential oil

*The **flowers** are too delicate to be steam-distilled so solvent extraction is used to create a thick orange–brown oil known as an absolute.*

 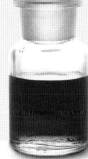

Fresh and floral, the sweet aroma of jasmine is instantly uplifting.

MASSAGE OIL

DIFFUSER

COMPRESS

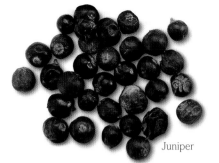

Juniper

STEAM
INHALATION

MASSAGE OIL

Juniper

Juniperus communis

A distinctive, crisp-smelling oil that stimulates and **strengthens** the nerves and **bolsters spirits**. It has a mild diuretic effect that helps relieve water retention, a **warming** action that **soothes** aching muscles and joints, and a toning and **balancing** effect on the skin.

What is it **good for?**

Tones skin and hair Juniper oil is stimulating, astringent, and detoxifying. It helps to unblock pores, and balances oily skin and skin prone to blackheads and acne. Diluted, it can be applied to eczema and psoriasis, and in a hair rinse it helps treat dandruff.

Aids detox Juniper's purifying action reduces water retention. As a diuretic, it helps to dispel toxins, making it useful for gout, rheumatism, and arthritis.

Treats urinary infections A few drops in a warm, shallow bath can ease symptoms of cystitis. Try as a massage or compress on the lower back to ease kidney stone discomfort.

Eases aches and pains Juniper essential oil soothes rheumatic and arthritic pain. Its tonic effect helps regulate the menstrual cycle and can ease cramps.

Relieves varicose veins Its gentle astringent action can help to shrink varicose veins and haemorrhoids.

Relieves anxiety Juniper eases tension and mental exhaustion. It is reputed to dispel negative emotions such as insecurity, loneliness, and guilt.

Best **uses**

As a massage oil Add 6–8 drops to 2 tablespoons base oil to enjoy the benefits of this oil in a massage.

In a room freshener Add 2–3 drops to a diffuser or spray to clear stale air.

In a compress In a cool compress the oil can soothe skin eruptions.

Safe usage Non-toxic, non-irritant in dilution.

The plant

Evergreen juniper trees produce seed cones called berries. While oil can be distilled from the needles and twigs, the sweetest oil comes from the berries.

The essential oil

Steam-distilled from the berries, the colourless or pale yellow oil has a fresh, warm, woody, herbaceous smell. If it smells like a cocktail, that's because the berries also flavour gin.

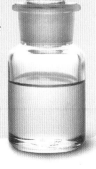

Bay laurel

Laurus nobilis

The same bay leaves that flavour cooking can, when distilled in an essential oil, produce a remedy that is **warming** and **pain-relieving** and that can lift spirits and **relax** the mind. The oil is an effective **antiseptic**, especially useful in the cold and flu season.

What is it **good for?**

Soothes aches and pains With a mild analgesic action, bay laurel can relieve sore muscles and lower back ache and ease tension headaches and migraines.

Fights cold and flu symptoms An effective expectorant and decongestant, bay laurel essential oil is an excellent choice for treating congested lungs and blocked sinuses and for disinfecting sick rooms.

Acts as a sedative Try putting a drop or two of the essential oil on your pillow or a tissue before bedtime to promote relaxation and aid a restful night's sleep.

Enhances wellbeing Bay laurel has long been associated with peace, wisdom, and inner confidence, and is thought to help you to maintain courage and focus when dealing with challenges in life.

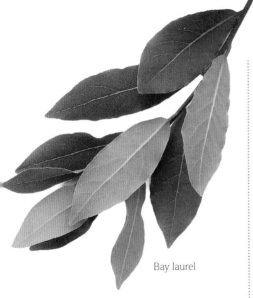

Bay laurel

Best **uses**

In an inhalation Add 3–5 drops to a steam inhalation to ease sinus congestion, breathing, and coughs.

Massage Dilute 1–2 drops of the oil in a teaspoon of base oil and massage into the temples to relieve headaches.

Safe usage *Use well diluted (less than 0.5 per cent). Not suitable for hypersensitive skin or for children under seven years old.*

The plant

The tree, *with its familiar deep green, sword-like leaves, originates from Asia Minor, but is established throughout the Mediterranean. Both the fruits and leaves are used medicinally and as food flavourings.*

The essential oil

The leaves are steam-distilled *to produce a clear oil with a spicy, floral aroma, popular in colognes and aftershaves.*

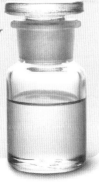

BATH OIL

MASSAGE OIL

Lavender

Lavandula angustifolia

A versatile and popular essential oil, lavender has a **calming** fragrance and is particularly renowned for its ability to relax and promote restful sleep. Its **rejuvenating** and **soothing** effects make it an effective skin treatment and a good skin healer.

What is it **good for?**

Soothes skin Lavender oil has a softening and conditioning effect on the skin. Try adding to creams, base oils, and bath preparations.

Heals skin Lavender is regenerative, making it useful for wounds and mouth ulcers. Applied neat, the oil makes an effective first-aid remedy for cuts, burns, bites, and stings. Its healing effects can ease acne, eczema, acne rosacea, and psoriasis, and reduce scarring.

Promotes restful sleep Deeply relaxing, lavender helps reduce stress levels and anxiety and is a popular remedy for promoting restful sleep.

Acts as a painkiller Mild analgesic properties make lavender a good treatment for headaches and migraine, as well as muscular and nerve pain. As an anti-spasmodic, it eases menstrual cramps.

Acts as an antiseptic It keeps wounds, ulcers, and sores clean. In a shallow bath, its antibacterial and anti-inflammatory properties make it excellent for infections such as cystitis.

Freshens the air It makes an ideal deodorizing and antiseptic room spray.

Best **uses**

As a bath oil Add 8–12 drops to 1 tablespoon base oil or full-fat milk and disperse in a relaxing bedtime bath.

As a massage oil Add 12–20 drops to 2 tablespoons base oil.

Safe usage *Non-toxic and non-irritant. Can be used neat on small areas.*

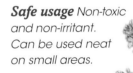

The plant

Lavandula augustifolia *is commonly used for essential oils.* ***Lavandin*** *or spike lavender is a hybrid with a medicinal aroma and antiseptic and tonic properties.*

The essential oil

Colourless *or pale yellow, lavender oil has a floral, slightly harsh, sweet aroma. Some oils have synthetic compounds. Check the label for the name Lavandula angustifolia.*

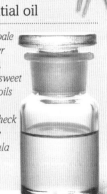

HAIR CARE

FIRST AID

Manuka

Leptospermum scoparium

Strongly **antiseptic**, manuka is ideal for use on cuts and wounds. It also contains a natural **antihistamine** that can bring welcome relief to hay fever sufferers. A sharp, **earthy aroma** clears the mind and dispels anxious or angry feelings.

What is it **good for?**

Heals skin The powerful antiseptic action of manuka speeds the healing of cuts and abrasions, as well as insect bites and stings. The oil is also strongly antifungal and can be added to ointments to treat athlete's foot, and to hair rinses to treat dandruff.

Fights colds and flu Added to a steam inhalation, manuka oil's antibacterial action makes it a good remedy for colds and coughs.

Acts as a deodorant Well diluted, manuka can control perspiration and the bacteria that cause body odour.

Soothes aches and pains An anti-inflammatory, the oil relieves joint and muscle pain and stomach cramps.

Soothes allergies Manuka contains a natural antihistamine that can calm reactions to pollen, dust, and irritants of the respiratory tract and the skin.

Enhances wellbeing If you suffer from anxiety or feelings of anger, use the oil to ground yourself, promote calm and relaxation, and help clear emotional and mental blockages.

Best **uses**

In a hair rinse Add 3–5 drops to warm water and use as a final rinse to balance excessively dry or oily hair.

As first aid Add 6–12 drops to 2 tablespoons of ointment and use to kill bacteria and speed the healing of cuts.

Safe usage Non-toxic, non-irritant in dilution.

The plant

Manuka is a shrubby tree, native to New Zealand. Its copious pink, dark-red or white flowers attract the bees, but it's the understated leaves that produce the aromatic essential oil.

The essential oil

Steam-distilled from the leaves and twigs, the yellow to light brown oil has a sharp, earthy aroma with honey-like and herbaceous undertones.

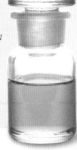

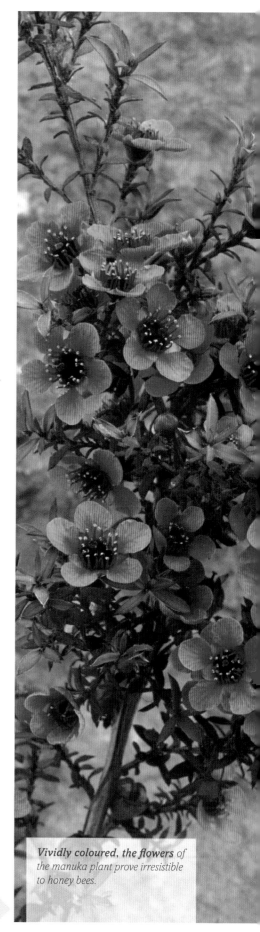

Vividly coloured, the flowers of the manuka plant prove irresistible to honey bees.

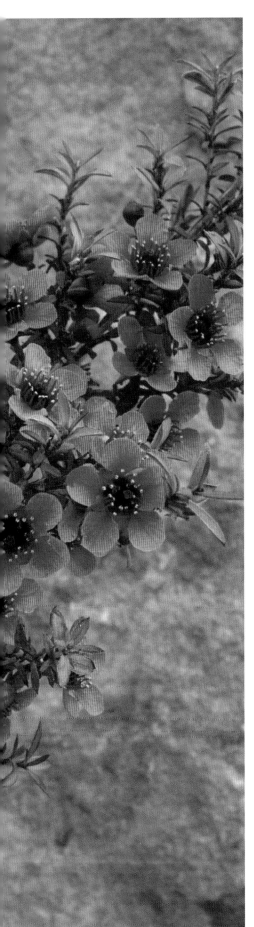

MASSAGE OIL

SKIN CARE

Litsea

Litsea cubeba

Also known as May chang, litsea is a warming, refreshing, uplifting oil that helps to calm and **soothe** frayed nerves. Its antiseptic and **skin-balancing** properties are particularly valued in skincare preparations.

What is it **good for?**

Tones skin Astringent and anti-inflammatory, litsea helps control acne and assists healing in existing breakouts, and also balances oily and combination skins.

Aids digestion The oil stimulates digestion and eases nausea. A good remedy for those with a poor appetite.

Acts as a deodorant In a body spray or footbath, the oil helps control perspiration and the bacteria that lead to body odour.

Relieves stress Litsea helps lift depression and calms the rapid heartbeat that comes with panic or stress, enabling you to think more constructively about a situation.

Soothes aches and pains The oil has a warming effect that boosts circulation and reduces inflammation in sore, tired muscles.

Best **uses**

As a massage oil A gentle massage with a litsea oil blend leaves you feeling warm, relaxed, calm, and balanced.

As a toner Add to a toner to leave skin feeling clean and refreshed.

Safe usage *Use well diluted (less than 0.5 per cent). Not suitable for children under seven years old or for hypersensitive skin.*

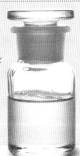

The plant

Litsea is also *called Mountain, or Chinese, pepper, because its berries resemble peppercorns. All the parts of the plant contain oil, but it is the hard berries that yield the highest quality. In spite of its lemony scent, it is a relative of cinnamon and other fragrant members of the laurel family.*

The essential oil

The fruit *are steam-distilled to produce a yellow oil with a complex and refined lemony scent.*

BATH OIL

MASSAGE OIL

COMPRESS

SKIN CARE

Chamomile (blue)

Matricaria recutita

Popular as a herbal tea, chamomile essential oil makes an effective skin treatment thanks to its **calming** and **toning** properties. It has a strong **anti-inflammatory** action that penetrates the skin's layers to **soothe** and repair, useful for skin conditions such as eczema, and for healing.

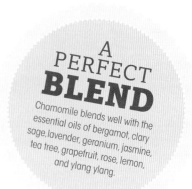

A
PERFECT
BLEND

Chamomile blends well with the essential oils of bergamot, clary sage, lavender, geranium, jasmine, tea tree, grapefruit, rose, lemon, and ylang ylang.

What is it **good for?**

Soothes skin A deeply soothing and calming oil, chamomile has anti-inflammatory properties that make it ideal for treating allergic skin conditions and sensitive skin and scalps. It helps to relieve the itchy, inflamed skin caused by rashes, cracked nipples, and conditions such as chicken pox. Its efficacy in treating eczema rivals treatments such as hydrocortisone.

Heals and cleanses skin A repairing oil, chamomile helps heal scratches and wounds, and also has been shown to promote faster tissue regeneration than corticosteroids. Its mildy astringent properties help to clean blocked pores.

Acts as a mild pain-reliever The anti-inflammatories present in chamomile, bisabolol and apigenin, work in a similar way to painkillers such as ibuprofen, providing effective mild pain relief and helping ease conditions such as arthritis.

Soothes digestion Chamomile is a natural soother and a popular remedy for calming digestive upsets. It can be used to treat a range of digestive complaints such as indigestion, peptic ulcers, and bouts of colic.

Strengthens immunity Use chamomile as a first line of defence against viruses and infection. It boosts immunity by stimulating leucocyte (white blood cell) production.

Promotes restful sleep Chamomile helps to calm irritability, nervousness, and tension headaches, helping promote relaxation and sleep.

Best **uses**

As a bath oil Mix 8–10 drops with 1 tablespoon base oil or full-fat milk and disperse in a warm bath to relax muscles and help calm anxiety.

In a massage oil Add 16–24 drops to 2 tablespoons base oil for a gentle massage to ease insomnia, back pain, stomach upsets, and period pains, to boost immunity, and to lift depression.

In a compress Add a few drops of chamomile essential oil to a wet, squeezed out cloth to make a cool compress that can help heal sores and calm allergic skin reactions.

In a skin cream Add 8–16 drops to 2 tablespoons cream for a skin cream.

Safe usage *Non-toxic, non-irritant in dilution.*

The plant

Also known as *German chamomile, the plant, which has delicate feathery leaves and simple daisy-like white flowers on single stems, is cultivated widely throughout central and northern Europe.*

Roman chamomile *(Anthemis nobilis) is a milder, sweeter oil with similar anti-inflammatory properties that is particularly suitable for infants and children.*

The essential oil

A deep ink-blue *viscous liquid, the oil is steam-distilled from the flowers. The heavy, herbaceous sweet smell has a fruity note. Roman chamomile makes a paler oil.*

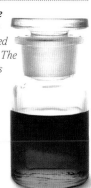

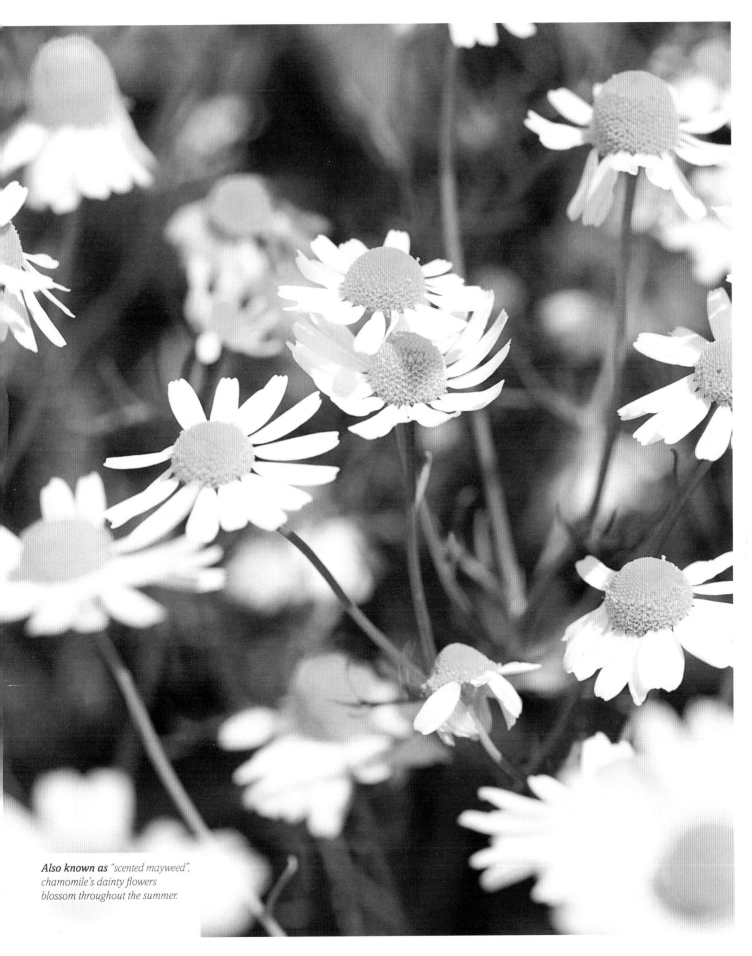

Also known as "scented mayweed", chamomile's dainty flowers blossom throughout the summer.

FIRST AID

FOOT BATH

Tea tree

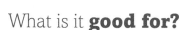

Melaleuca alternifolia

Best known for its powerful **antiseptic** properties, tea tree essential oil is a great all-rounder to keep in your first-aid kit, ready to use on wounds and sores. Studies show it is effective against a range of bacteria and fungi that can lead to infection. It also has a strong **deodorizing** action that can combat body odour.

What is it **good for?**

Boosts immunity Tea tree has immune-stimulating properties that help the body to fight off infection. A massage with a tea tree blend can aid recovery during convalescence.

Fights skin infections The oil acts as a barrier against bacteria, viruses, and fungi. It can be added to an ointment to help treat athlete's foot and ringworm, or can be dabbed on neat to cold sores, warts, and verrucas.

Heals cuts, scrapes, and bruises Tea tree promotes the formation of scar tissue to aid healing.

Helps to control acne A popular ingredient in skin remedies, the oil can be applied to pimples as an immediate treatment.

Acts as a hair tonic A tea tree scalp massage can help bring dandruff under control, and used in a rinse, tea tree can restore the balance of oils to combat greasy hair.

Mouth and gum care Use well diluted to treat bad breath, mouth ulcers, and gum infections.

Fights body odour A natural deodorizer, tea tree can be added to baths, body sprays, or creams to combat body or foot odour.

Fights cold and flu symptoms This antiseptic is effective in warding off colds and flu. Once a cold has set in, a steam inhalation with the oil eases congestion and breathing.

Eases urinary tract infections Tea tree can help to fight cystitis and other genital infections, including thrush, herpes, warts, pruritus, and trichomonas.

Best **uses**

As first aid Use tea tree essential oil in a dilution of 10 per cent (1 part tea tree to 10 parts witch hazel) to rinse and clean infected wounds and sores.

In a foot bath For tired, hot, smelly feet, or for athlete's foot, add 20 drops of tea tree oil to a small basin of warm water and soak feet for 15 minutes. Dry thoroughly.

Safe usage *Non-irritant in dilutions of less than 10 per cent. Non-toxic externally.*

A PERFECT BLEND

Try blending tea tree with clove, eucalyptus, lavender, lemon, pine, rosemary, or thyme essential oils.

The plant

A hardy tree, native to New South Wales in Australia, tea tree was an important medicine in Aboriginal tribes. Similar to the cypress in appearance, it has needle-like leaves with white flowerheads.

Two close relatives also produce essential oils: niaouli, also native to Australia, is primarily used to treat skin complaints and respiratory illnesses, and cajuput, native to Indonesia and the Philippines, is used to treat respiratory conditions.

The essential oil

Steam-distilled from the leaves of the tree, the essential oil is a clear liquid with a medicinal scent reminiscent of eucalyptus.

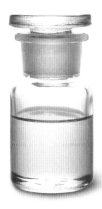

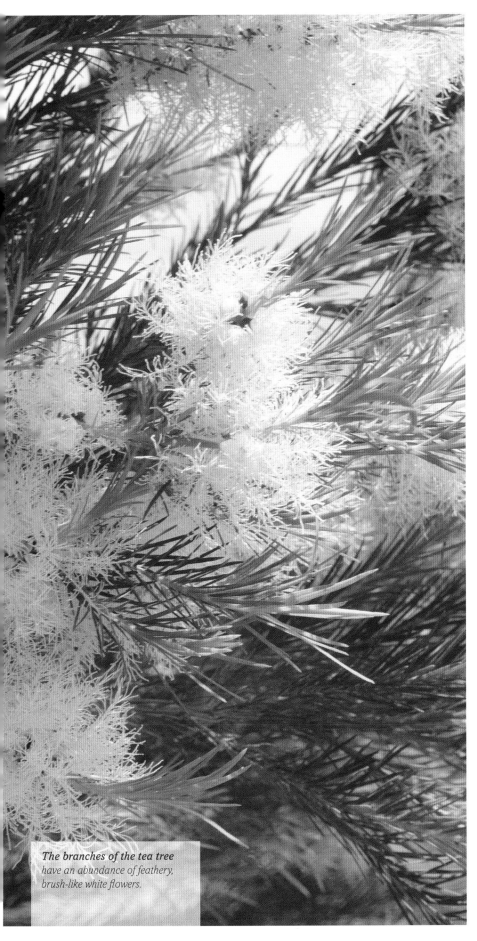

This healing essential oil, commonly used for its antiseptic effect, has a distinctive medicinal scent.

The branches of the tea tree have an abundance of feathery, brush-like white flowers.

MASSAGE OIL

DIFFUSER

252

Cajuput

Melaleuca cajuputi

A member of the tea tree family, cajuput has a **milder** and less overpowering aroma, but many of the same benefits. Its **antiseptic** properties are useful for fighting respiratory and urinary infections, and, as a natural **pain-reliever**, it can ease headaches and muscle and joint pains.

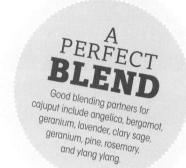

A PERFECT **BLEND**

Good blending partners for cajuput include angelica, bergamot, geranium, lavender, clary sage, geranium, pine, rosemary, and ylang ylang.

What is it **good for?**

Acts as an antiseptic Its broad antiseptic properties make cajuput useful for fighting cold and flu viruses, bacterial urinary tract infections, and fungal infections, such as athlete's foot. Diluted, the oil can also be applied to cuts and wounds to keep these clean and infection-free.

Acts as a decongestant Cajuput makes an excellent decongestant and expectorant that helps to clear blocked sinuses and congested lungs.

Acts as a pain reliever Cajuput has soothing analgesic properties that can provide local pain relief from tension headaches and muscle and joint aches and pains.

Tones skin The oil helps to brighten oily or combination skin and keeps the bacteria that cause acne at bay.

Aids detox By promoting sweating, cajuput aids the removal of toxins from the body and also provides a pleasant cooling sensation that is especially helpful for soothing fevers.

Aids focus Cajuput helps to clear the mind and to fight mental exhaustion and apathy.

Best **uses**

As a massage oil Dilute cajuput essential oil in a massage oil blend and massage into achy, painful areas.

In a diffuser Add a few drops of the oil to a diffuser, vaporizer, or oil burner to relieve sinusitis and a blocked nose and to clear germs in the air. Or add a few drops to a steam inhalation.

Safe usage Non-irritant, non-toxic externally. Avoid use near the nose of children under seven years old.

The plant

***Also called** white tea tree, cajuput is a native of Malaysia now found throughout Southeast Asia and parts of Australia. From the Malaysian "kayu-puti" (white wood), its name describes its white bark. The oil is concentrated in its pointed leaves.*

The essential oil

The clear to pale yellow *essential oil is steam-distilled from the fresh leaves and twigs. Cajuput has a penetrating, slightly sweet aroma with hints of camphor.*

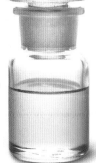

This relatively mild oil has many therapeutic benefits.

BATH OIL

FIRST AID

MASSAGE OIL

STEAM INHALATION

Niaouli

Melaleuca viridiflora, M. quinquenervia

Chiefly a **disinfectant** and astringent, niaouli helps to fight a range of infections. **Stimulating** the body and mind, it increases concentration, clears the head, and lifts the spirits. Think of niaouli as a gentler version of tea tree – suitable even for sensitive skin.

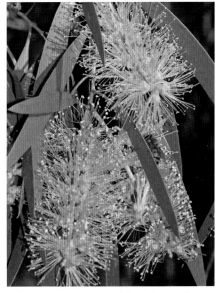

A large evergreen, niaouli has clusters of yellow flowers amid distinctive pointed leaves.

What is it **good for?**

Heals wounds Niaouli's disinfectant properties make it valuable for cleaning wounds, cuts, and applying to ulcers. Use it to help calm acne and balance oily skin.

Reduces the appearance of scars Niaouli encourages tissue regeneration, which in turn helps to minimize the appearance of scars, including the marks left by acne, pimples, or chickenpox.

Fights cold and flu symptoms A decongestant and expectorant, the oil helps to break up congestion in the lungs, bronchi, and nasal passages. Its antiviral and immune-boosting properties make it an important oil in the treatment of colds and flu.

Aids detox Niaouli stimulates the release of digestive juices as well as the circulation of blood and lymph, aiding the absorption of nutrients and encouraging the healthy excretion of waste and toxins.

Acts as a pain reliever An effective analgesic, niaouli can provide localized pain relief by numbing sensitive areas. It's useful for headaches, migraines, muscle and joint pain, and pain due to sprains.

Aids focus The sharp aroma of niaouli essential oil clears unwanted thoughts from the mind and enhances focus. This quality makes it a useful aid to meditation and helpful for concentration.

Best **uses**

As a bath oil If you feel as though you might be coming down with a cold virus, add a few drops to a bath oil blend to help fight the infection.

As first aid Dilute a few drops in a tumblerful of water and use as an antiseptic wash for cuts and other minor skin irritations.

As a massage oil Add to a base oil and use for an all-over body massage to strengthen the whole body, or use specifically, for example to help fight an infection, relieve pain, or stimulate a sluggish circulation.

In a steam inhalation Add 2–3 drops to a steam inhalation (or add to a diffuser or vaporizer) and inhale for several minutes to help you fight cold and flu symptoms, bronchitis, whooping cough, sinusitis, catarrh, and other respiratory conditions.

Safe usage Non-toxic and non-irritant.

The plant

A popular tree *for planting on streets and in parks, niaouli has fluffy spikes of flowers and a papery bark that periodically peels. It is native to New Caledonia, Papua New Guinea, and Australia and belongs to the same family as tea tree and cajuput.*

The essential oil

Niaouli oil is extracted *from the young leaves and twigs by steam-distillation. It has a mildly sweet, fresh, camphorous smell and its colour varies from clear to a pale yellowy-green hue.*

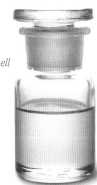

SKIN CARE

MASSAGE OIL

Lemon balm

Melissa officinalis

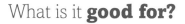

Lemon balm, also known as melissa, is often added to **skincare** products because of its calming, **anti-inflammatory** action on irritated skin. Its antiseptic effect makes it useful to have on hand for treating bee and wasp stings, and its cheerful **"feel-good"** aroma ensures it is a popular choice in aromatherapy.

254

What is it **good for?**

Soothes skin Lemon balm helps to calm inflamed skin and allergic skin conditions. It can be used, well diluted, to treat skin ulcers and eczema, especially when stress-related, and to reduce redness and irritation from insect bites and stings, and sunburn.

Tones skin With a stimulating action on the circulation, the oil brightens dull-looking complexions and has a tightening and toning effect on the skin. Lemon balm is exceptionally high in the antioxidants that help fight ageing caused by free radical damage.

Heals skin This antibacterial oil can be useful for treating acne and other skin eruptions such as cold sores.

Relieves headaches Uplifting and soothing, lemon balm can be a useful remedy for headaches and migraines, especially when a headache is associated with stress and held-in tension in the neck and shoulders.

Acts as an antiseptic Lemon balm has an antiviral action that works on the cold sore virus. If used at the first sign of a cold sore, it can limit its impact.

Aids digestion Added to a gentle abdominal massage blend, the essential oil can help relieve wind, colic, and dyspepsia, and is also useful for treating feelings of nausea.

Eases breathing Lemon balm has a mild antihistamine effect, helpful for hay fever and asthma. It also calms anxiety-induced respiratory problems.

Reduces anxiety A sedative action makes lemon balm especially useful in cases of panic. It can calm a racing heartbeat and help lower blood pressure. The oil makes a soothing massage when you feel overwhelmed.

Cools fevers A cooling action makes lemon balm useful for relieving heat exhaustion and soothing fevers.

Best **uses**

As a skin toner To hydrate skin, add 20 drops of lemon balm to 1 tablespoon witch hazel, or 1 teaspoon glycerine. Add to 3 tablespoons water and put in a spray bottle for a cooling spray.

In a massage oil Use 2–3 drops in 1 tablespoon base oil for a massage oil that counters the effects of over-indugence, such as indigestion trapped wind, and nausea.

Safe usage *Non-toxic externally. Sensitization possible. Use well diluted (less than 1 per cent).*

The plant

A native of central and southern Europe, lemon balm is a member of the mint family. Its leaves are a similar shape to mint, but when you rub them between your fingers, they release a tart sweet smell, like lemons.

The essential oil

This pale yellow oil with a pleasant lemony, fresh, sweet, and herbaceous smell can be steam-distilled from the fresh leaves and flowers. Because the plant yields very little oil, lemon balm is often adulterated with other lemon-scented essential oils. Pure lemon balm oil is very expensive.

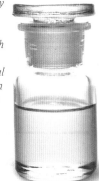

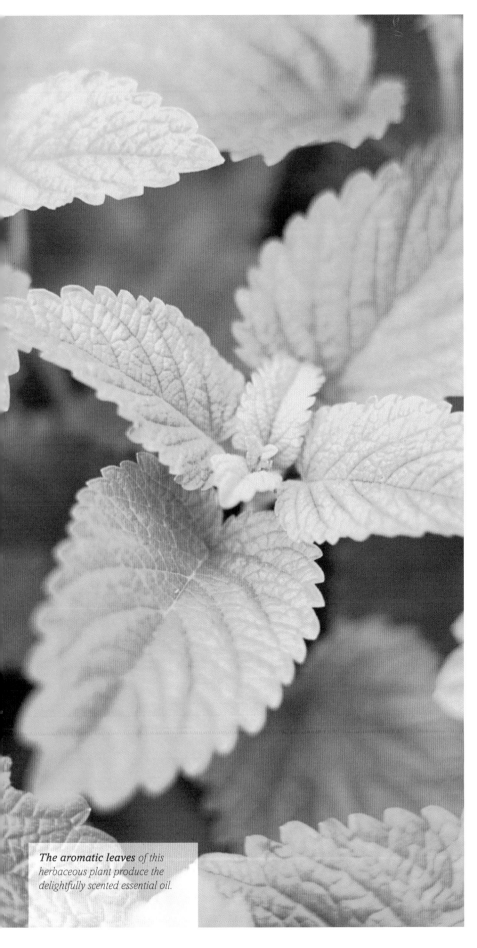

The aromatic leaves of this herbaceous plant produce the delightfully scented essential oil.

A calming oil, lemon balm is helpful for soothing insect bites or patches of irritated skin.

MASSAGE OIL

STEAM
INHALATION

Peppermint

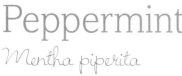

Applied to the skin, peppermint feels initially cooling and **refreshing,** then gently warming. Its **stimulating** and analgesic properties make it an effective remedy for neuralgia and muscular pains and headaches. It's also a first-class **antiseptic**, and a popular addition to all types of beauty products.

A PERFECT BLEND

Try blending peppermint essential oil with eucalyptus, lavender, lemon, pine or rosemary essential oils.

What is it **good for?**

Fights odour Peppermint is an effective body deodorant. Used in toothpaste, mouthwashes, and other dental preparations, its antiseptic and deodorizing properties can also help combat bad breath.

Soothes skin Diluted peppermint oil has cooling and toning effects on the skin and can be particularly soothing for skin that is irritated after excessive exposure to the elements. It can also be used to relieve hives and other allergic skin reactions.

Acts as an antiseptic Its antiseptic and antiviral properties make this a useful oil for treating cold sores, even for resistant strains of the herpes virus that causes them, and for products such as lip balms and hand creams.

Eases digestive upsets A tummy massage with a peppermint blend can ease indigestion and flatulence, calm nausea and travel sickness, and improve a sluggish digestion.

Fights cold symptoms The oil acts as an expectorant to help alleviate coughs and clear sinuses.

Soothes bites and stings Peppermint essential oil makes an effective insect repellent, and it can also be used to help soothe mosquito bites and other skin irritations.

Relieves headaches Peppermint oil has long been recognized as a safe and effective treatment for tension headaches.

Best **uses**

As a massage oil Add 1–2 drops of peppermint essential oil to 1 tablespoon base oil and gently massage the abdomen in a clockwise motion to help bring relief to symptoms of indigestion, constipation, and nausea.

In an inhalation Add 3–4 drops of peppermint essential oil to a steam inhalation (not suitable for children or those suffering with asthma) or to a diffuser, vaporizer, or oil burner, and use as a decongestant to help clear sinuses and congested lungs.

Safe usage *Use well diluted (less than 2 per cent). Avoid use in cardiac fibrillation and near the nose in children under seven years old.*

The plant

This popular herb *is actually a hybrid of Mentha aquatica (water mint) and Mentha spicata (spearmint). It has been used as a medicinal herb for thousands of years, particularly as an infusion for digestive disorders, though in modern times it is mostly used in the flavouring and toothpaste industries. The essential oil is extracted from the flowering herb.*

The essential oil

Peppermint essential oil *is steam-distilled from the flowering herb. The thin, almost watery oil has a fresh, sharp, strongly menthol aroma with a sweet-smelling undertone and it is a clear to pale yellow in colour.*

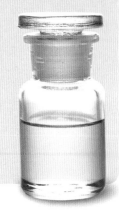

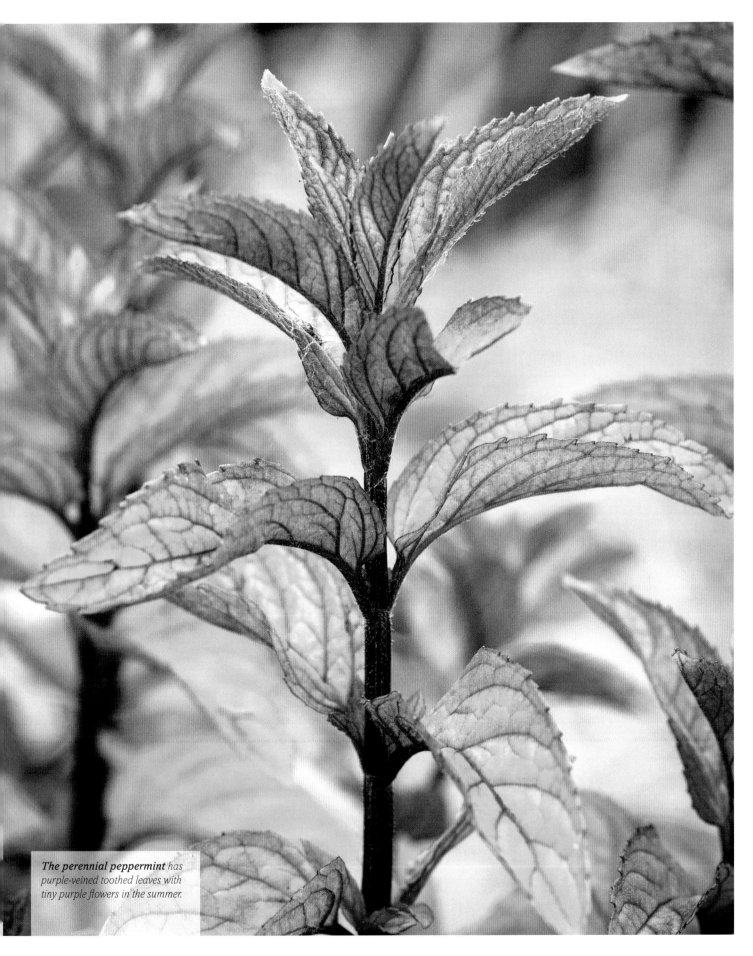

The perennial peppermint has
purple-veined toothed leaves with
tiny purple flowers in the summer.

MOUTHWASH

BATH OIL

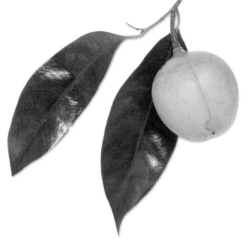

Nutmeg
Myristica fragrans

This **warming** oil with anti-inflammatory properties is useful for relieving muscle and joint pain. It helps **balance** the nervous system, **stimulating** or **calming** as needed, and also has a **detox** action that can improve digestion.

What is it **good for?**

Tooth and gum health Used well diluted as a mouthwash, nutmeg oil has an antiseptic and deodorant action that attacks the bacteria that cause bad breath and tooth decay.

Eases aches and pains A warming massage with a nutmeg oil blend can relieve inflammation and muscle pain, and boost circulation. Its mild analgesic action gives localized pain relief.

Aids sleep A well-known sedative, nutmeg helps relieve stress and can improve the quality of sleep.

Enhances wellbeing When suffering from anxiety or exhaustion, nutmeg can lift the spirits and help you regain focus.

Eases digestion Nutmeg stimulates appetite and digestion, reducing wind and soothing upsets.

Best **uses**

In a mouthwash Dilute 2–3 drops of the essential oil in 1 teaspoon of glycerin or calendula tincture and add to half a cupful of water. Do not swallow.

As a bath oil Add 5–6 drops to 1 tablespoon base oil or full-fat milk and disperse in a bath to relieve muscle aches and indigestion, and aid sleep.

Safe usage *Use well diluted (less than 1 per cent).*

The plant

A native of the Banda Islands *of Indonesia, the evergreen nutmeg tree produces a fruit similar to a peach. This fruit is the source of two spices: nutmeg and mace. Nutmeg (the spice and oil), comes from the seed itself, while mace comes from the covering of the seed.*

The essential oil

Nutmeg essential oil *is obtained by steam-distilling the dried seeds of the nutmeg. This produces a clear oil with a sharp, spicy, musky aroma. West Indian nutmeg is milder and more suitable for aromatherapy than East Indian.*

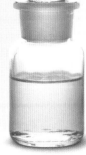

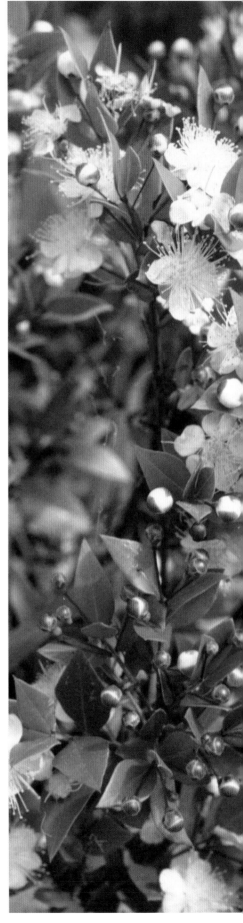

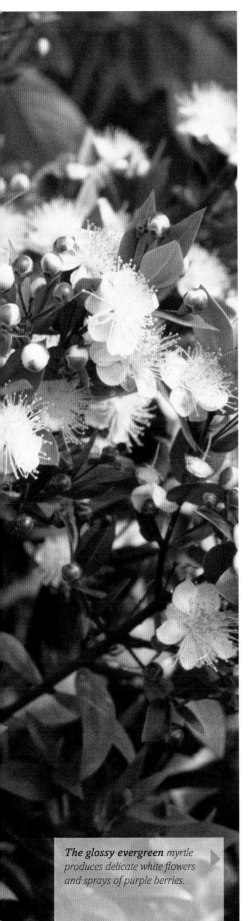

The glossy evergreen myrtle *produces delicate white flowers and sprays of purple berries.*

DIFFUSER

Myrtle

Myrtus communis

Myrtle oil gained its popularity because of its **antimicrobial,** astringent, antiseptic, anti-inflammatory, expectorant, decongestant, and **stimulant** properties. Today, the oil is commonly used for skin health and respiratory ailments.

What is it **good for?**

Tones skin Its astringent properties work on oily skin, open pores, and sagging skin, as welll as on spider veins and haemorrhoids.

Relieves congestion A mild expectorant, myrtle can ease asthma, coughs, and bronchitis. Its anti-inflammatory properties also calm respiratory inflammation caused by allergic reactions.

Acts as an antiseptic The oil can be applied to wounds, spots, and boils, and has been shown to inhibit the growth of several types of bacteria including *Escherichia coli, Staphylococcus aureus, Bacillus subtilis, Salmonella*, and *Listeria*.

Acts as a mild sedative Myrtle calms nerves and its sedative action can relieve depression and insomnia.

Supports the thyroid Myrtle's balancing action helps it to regulate over- and under-active thyroid glands.

Acts as an insect repellent Used in a room spray or diffuser, the oil can help to ward off insects.

Best **uses**

In a diffuser Add 4–5 drops to a diffuser, vaporizer, or oil burner (or add to a steam inhalation) to help clear sinus congestion.

Safe usage *Use well diluted (less than 1.5 per cent).*

The plant

Myrtle is an evergreen shrub *with fragrant white or pink flowers. Native to North Africa, it is commonly found in the southern Mediterranean region. It belongs to the same plant family as tea tree and eucalyptus, and has similar medicinal characteristics.*

The essential oil

Myrtle oil is *steam-distilled from the leaves. It is a pale yellow to green oil with a stimulating, slightly camphorous aroma somewhere between eucalyptus and frankincense.*

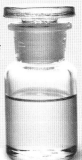

COMPRESS

DIFFUSER

BATH OIL

MASSAGE OIL

Basil

Ocimum basilicum

The name basil comes from the Greek word **"basilikon phuton"** meaning "king". Basil is highly valued in traditional Ayurvedic medicine as a protector of both mental and physical **wellbeing.** Its crisp aroma clears and refreshes the mind and helps to **calm** anxiety.

What is it **good for?**

Enhances wellbeing Basil balances, revives, and strengthens to help combat exhaustion, anxiety, or depression.

Tones and balances skin The oil refreshes skin and helps to control acne.

Supports women's health Basil can help stimulate scanty or delayed periods caused by debility and stress.

Eases digestion Soothing basil can relieve indigestion. Its antiseptic action also helps treat intestinal infections.

Fights cold symptoms The oil helps clear sinuses and soothe coughs.

Eases aches and pains Basil can ease gout and rheumatic pain.

Acts as an insect repellent Its insecticidal properties repel insects. It also relieves the irritation of insect bites.

Best **uses**

In a compress Add a few drops to warm water and make a compress with a cloth to ease pain and congestion.

In a diffuser Add 3–4 drops to a diffuser, vaporizer, or oil burner to clear headaches and refresh the mind.

Safe usage *Potentially toxic over time. Dilute extremely well (less than 0.5 per cent) and do not use for prolonged periods. Avoid in pregnancy, when breasfeeding, and in children under 15 years old.*

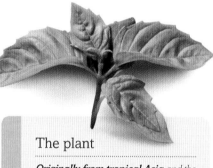

The plant

Originally from tropical Asia *and the Pacific Islands, basil is now cultivated worldwide. The flowers range from white to pink in colour, and are popular with bees and other garden pollinators.*

The essential oil

The oil is steam-distilled *from the leaves and the flowering tops of the plant. It has a sweet, spicy, fresh and slightly balsamic odour, and is clear to pale yellow in colour.*

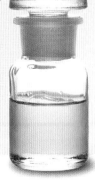

Marjoram

Origanum majorana

This aromatic, **warming**, and **relaxing** oil is known for its ability to aid digestion and relieve stomach and menstrual cramping. It has a gently **sedative** effect that can lower blood pressure and heart rate, ease anxiety, and promote restful sleep.

What is it **good for?**

Relieves anxiety A gentle sedative, the oil can treat nervous tension, anxiety, panic attacks, and insomnia.

Improves circulation The oil has a toning effect on circulation that makes it useful for treating high blood pressure.

Eases cold and flu symptoms The oil's warming decongestant action can fight off chills and help clear sinus and lung congestion.

Acts as a painkiller The oil's analgesic action can ease tension headaches and migraines. Massage into muscles, joints, and tender areas for local relief from muscle pains, sprains, strains, rheumatism, and arthritis.

Supports women's health Its warming action relieves period pains and pre-menstrual symptoms such as anxiety, weariness, and irritability.

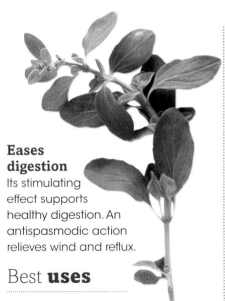

Eases digestion
Its stimulating effect supports healthy digestion. An antispasmodic action relieves wind and reflux.

Best **uses**

As a bath oil Add 15 drops to 1 tablespoon base oil or full-fat milk for a reviving soak.

In a massage oil For abdominal pain, add 10 drops to 1 tablespoon base oil and massage the tummy in a clockwise direction.

Safe usage Non-toxic, non-irritant in dilution.

The plant

Mediterranean sweet marjoram has a long history of use as a medicinal herb.

Spanish marjoram (Thymus masticina) has some similar properties, but is harsher and should be avoided in children under seven years old.

The essential oil

The essential oil, steam-distilled from the dried flowering herb, is a pale yellow or pale amber hue with a warm, spicy, slightly camphorous smell.

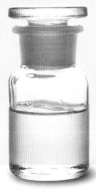

HAND WASH

DIFFUSER

Oregano
Origanum vulgare

Prized for centuries for its **healing** qualities, oregano has a powerful **antibacterial** action. The essential oil is traditionally used to treat complaints as diverse as indigestion and diarrhoea, insect bites, earaches, rheumatism, and coughs.

What is it **good for?**

Has an antibacterial action
Oregano contains compounds that have been shown to inhibit the growth of bacteria such as *Pseudomonas aeruginosa* and *Staphylococcus aureus*. The oil can also help to relieve urinary tract infections.

Helps fight fungal infections
The essential oil has been shown to inhibit the growth of *Candida albicans*, the fungus that causes oral thrush, canker sores, skin rashes, and athlete's foot, and also inhibits the fungi that cause nail infections.

Relieves menstrual cramps
Its analgesic action can ease menstrual cramps and other abdominal pains.

Clears sinuses
A few drops of the oil on a tissue or in a steam inhalation can help to clear blocked sinuses and loosen phlegm.

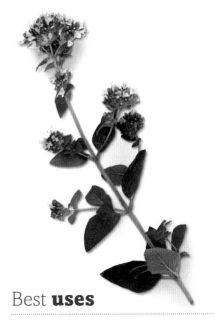

Best **uses**

As an antibacterial wash Add 8–10 drops to an unscented liquid soap for an antibacterial handwash.

In a diffuser Add 2–4 drops to a diffuser to ease congestion.

Safe usage Dilute well before use (less than 1 per cent). Avoid using in pregnancy, when breastfeeding, and in children under seven years old.

The plant

A member of the mint family, this aromatic, culinary herb, sometimes called wild marjoram, originates from hilly, Greek countryside, but is now grown around the world.

The essential oil

The pale yellow oil is produced by steam-distillation of the fresh oregano leaves. It has a spicy, peppery aroma with a hint of camphor.

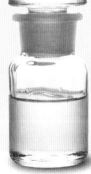

BATH OIL

DIFFUSER

Geranium

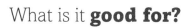
Pelargonium graveolens

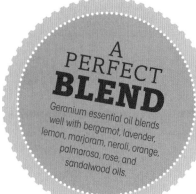

A PERFECT BLEND

Geranium essential oil blends well with bergamot, lavender, lemon, marjoram, neroli, orange, palmarosa, rose, and sandalwood oils.

A **cheerful** oil, appreciated by both adults and children, geranium essential oil has a balancing, cooling, and **reviving** effect on skin, especially when it is weather-damaged or irritated. The oil is also a mild diuretic, making it a useful aid to **detox**, and it can help to soothe urinary tract infections.

What is it **good for?**

Aids detox The oil's gentle diuretic effect helps the body to eliminate excess water and reduce puffiness.

Balances emotions Both calming and uplifting, geranium makes a natural antidepressant. It can reduce restlessness and help to treat anxiety in children and adults.

Acts as a painkiller Geranium has mild analgesic properties that can relieve the pain of neuralgia and conditions such as shingles.

Tones the scalp Geranium oil helps to balance the secretion of sebum on the scalp, making it a useful treatment for flaky dandruff.

Tones skin This balancing oil is suitable for all skin types. Its antiseptic and anti-inflammatory properties help to control acne, and it is cooling for

dry, inflamed skin. Its reviving effect helps to reduce the appearance of wrinkles, scars, and blemishes.

Supports women's health Geranium's cooling and balancing properties can relieve menopausal symptoms such as hot flushes and vaginal dryness. The oil can also soothe painful urinary tract infections.

Best **uses**

As a bath oil To relieve cystitis or pruritis, add 5 drops of geranium and 5 drops of lavender to 1 tablespoon base oil or full-fat milk and disperse in a shallow bath.

In a diffuser To ease anxiety and lift the spirits, add 5 drops of geranium and 5 drops of orange to a diffuser, vaporizer, or oil burner.

Safe usage Non-toxic, non-irritant in dilution. Sensitization possible.

The plant

A native of South Africa originally, geranium is now grown mainly in Réunion, China, and Egypt. Of the 700 different varieties of the Pelargonium plant, only 10 can be used to make the essential oil. Plants are harvested shortly after flowering to capture the highest concentrations of the oil, which comes from the plant's leaves, and not from the flowers as many assume.

The essential oil

The green to amber-coloured essential oil has a powerful, sweet, floral aroma with distinct minty undertones. Once the plant has been harvested, the oil is steam-distilled from the glands found in the leaves and from the green stems of the plant.

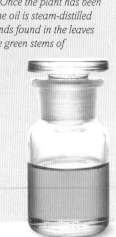

This balancing oil keeps emotions on an even keel.

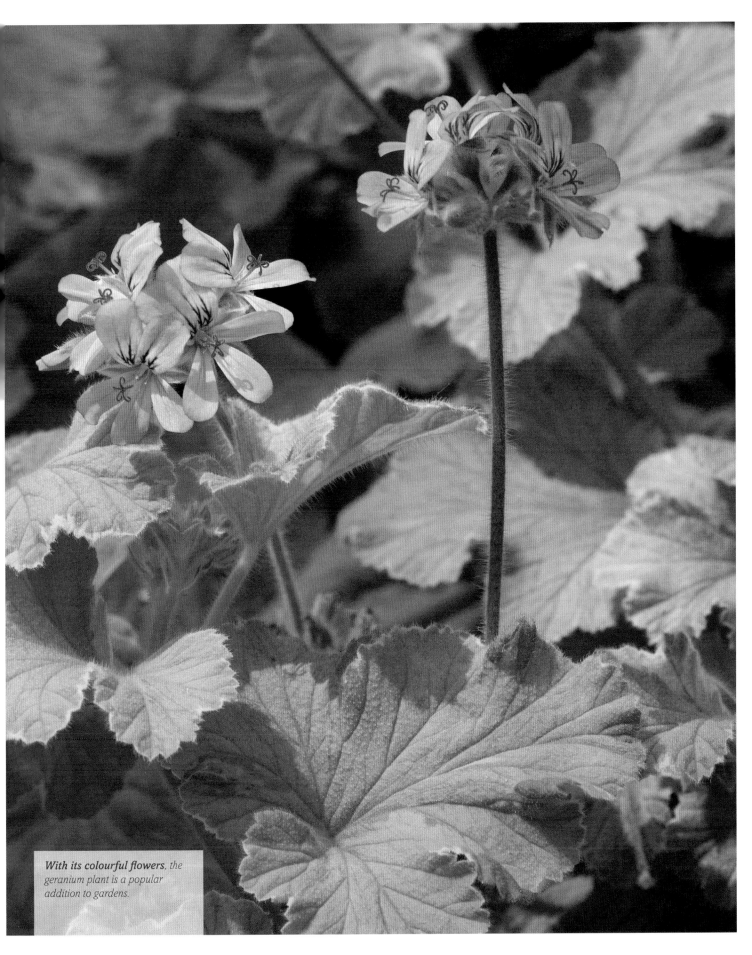

With its colourful flowers, the geranium plant is a popular addition to gardens.

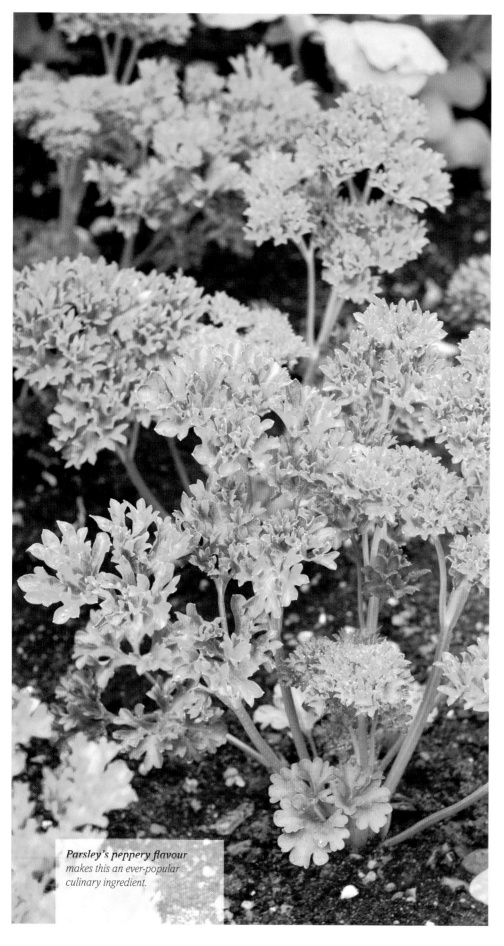

Parsley's peppery flavour *makes this an ever-popular culinary ingredient.*

This well-known herb has a multitude of therapeutic benefits that are present in its essential oil.

SKIN CARE

BATH OIL

Parsley seed

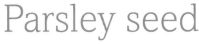
Petroselinum crispum

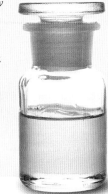

A
PERFECT
BLEND
Try blending parsley essential oil with clary sage, orange, rose, tea tree or ylang-ylang essential oils.

More than just a garnish on your plate, parsley produces an essential oil that is **antibacterial** and has valuable **detoxing** properties that can help to reduce water retention and strengthen digestion. Its **spicy** aroma is much prized as an ingredient in soaps and perfumes – in particular, men's colognes.

What is it **good for?**

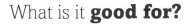

Boosts circulation The oil has a strengthening effect on blood vessels, making it useful for toning varicose veins and slowing down the spread of broken facial capillaries.

Tones skin Its antibacterial and antifungal properties help to treat pimples, acne, and skin infections, as well as disinfect pores.

Stimulates hair growth Diluted in a scalp massage, parsley essential oil encourages hair growth.

Has an antibacterial action Parsley oil helps to inhibit and kill microbes, protecting against various infections and diseases.

Acts as a painkiller By helping to boost the circulation and in turn prevent the accumulation of uric acid in the muscles and joints, parsley can act as a mild pain reliever for sufferers of arthritis and rheumatism.

Aids detox Parsley essential oil supports the healthy function of the kidneys and bladder. It has a diuretic action that can help to reduce fluid retention, and is also a mild laxative. It has an overall strengthening and tonic effect on the digestive system.

Aids digestion Like the fresh herb, the essential oil has carminative properties that can help relieve and treat indigestion, nausea, flatulence, vomiting, and stomach aches.

Calms the mind Parsley is a great de-stresser as it soothes the nerves and has a grounding and calming effect on the mind and emotions.

Enhances wellbeing The aromatherapeutic properties of parsley are purported to help strengthen confidence in overcoming difficulties and to enhance focus and provide a strong sense of purpose.

Best **uses**

As a facial elixir To help combat spider veins, mix 1 tablespoon base oil, 1 drop of parsley essential oil and 2 drops of rose essential oil. Massage very gently into the affected areas.

As a bath oil Add 6–9 drops of parsley essential oil to 1 tablespoon base oil or full-fat milk and add to a warm bath for a soothing soak.

Safe usage *Use well diluted (less than 1 per cent). Avoid using during pregnancy and when breastfeeding.*

The plant

Parsley is native *to the Mediterranean region, but is now grown in gardens worldwide as a versatile culinary herb. The seeds contain most of the essential oil, although the entire plant can be used for making the oil.*

The essential oil

Parsley oil is *steam-distilled from the seeds of the plant. It is a colourless to pale yellow oil with a surprising sweet, warm, woody–spicy, herbaceous aroma.*

DIFFUSER

OINTMENT

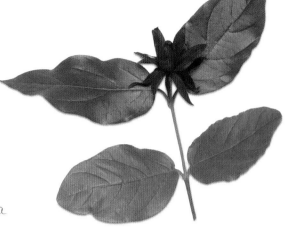

Allspice
Pimenta dioica

A stimulating, potent, **spicy** oil that many associate more with cooking than spa days. Yet small amounts of allspice oil added to an aromatherapy blend help **relieve** muscle and menstrual cramps, and provide **warming** localized pain relief for sprains or strains.

What is it **good for?**

Acts as a painkiller The oil has a local numbing effect that is useful for treating pain caused by neuralgia, muscular injuries, and joint strain, as well as pain from insect bites and stings.

Relieves muscle cramps Allspice has a warming, calming effect that soothes muscle cramps and spasms.

Acts as a mild sedative Its relaxing effect on the body and mind makes the oil useful for treating tension and anxiety. The oil's gently soothing action can help induce sleep.

Relieves indigestion Add to a massage oil blend to relieve indigestion, nausea, and trapped wind.

Eases cold symptoms Use in an inhalation to help relieve congestion.

Best **uses**

In a diffuser Diffuse 3–4 drops to ease anxiety.

As a rub A very small amount of the oil in a base oil or ointment can be used in a warming chest massage to help clear catarrh, congested coughs, and bronchitis.

Safe usage Non-irritant in dilution, sensitization possible. Potentially toxic with prolonged use. Dilute extremely well (less than 0.25 per cent). Avoid in pregnancy, when breastfeeding, and in children under 15 years old.

The plant

Native to the *Caribbean Islands and South America, the pimento tree produces small berry-like fruits, which are ground for use as a cooking spice. Both the leaves and berries are aromatic and are used to make the essential oil.*

The essential oil

Sometimes called pimento oil, *the light to pale brown oil is steam-distilled from the leaves and fruits. The oil's warm, spicy aroma is akin to that of clove and cinnamon essential oils.*

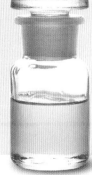

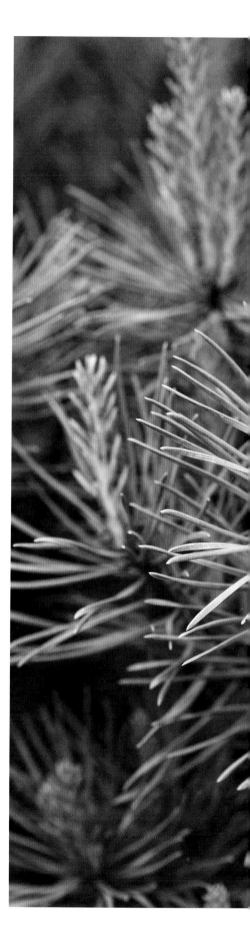

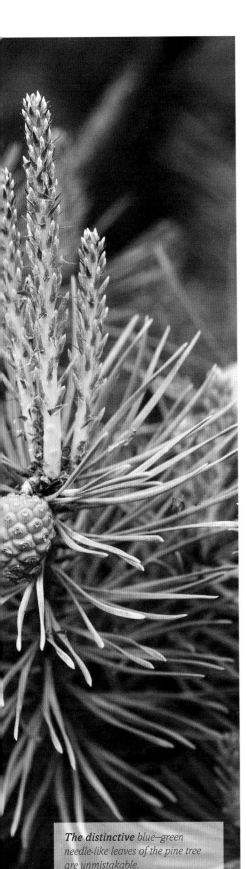

The distinctive blue–green needle-like leaves of the pine tree are unmistakable.

FRAGRANCE

Pine

Pinus sylvestris

Uplifting pine has a **warming** effect on sore joints and muscles, and its **clearing** action helps to unblock sinuses and **ease** breathing. The oil is valued by perfumers for the sweetness it adds to fragrance blends.

A PERFECT BLEND

Blends well with cedarwood, eucalyptus, lavender, lemon, rosemary, sage, and juniper.

What is it **good for?**

Eases breathing Decongesting and antiviral, pine oil protects against viruses, helps to clear catarrh, and eases hay fever symptoms.

Acts as a painkiller A warming oil, pine's analgesic and anti-inflammatory properties soothe muscular aches and painful joints. It can be applied locally to boost circulation to affected areas.

Acts as an antiseptic The oil can be used to treat infectious skin problems such as impetigo and boils.

Acts as an insect repellent Add a few drops to a strip of fabric or piece of wood and place with clothes to protect them from moths.

Supports urinary health The oil is effective for soothing cystitis, prostate problems, and urinary infections.

Enhances wellbeing A grounding oil, pine's aroma revitalizes mind and spirit, relieving exhaustion, tension, and other stress-related symptoms.

Freshens air Pine is ideal for clearing stale smells and eliminating odours.

Best **uses**

As an air freshener Add 20–30 drops to 60ml (2fl oz) each of vodka and water. Pour into a spray bottle and use to clear the air, avoiding furniture.

Safe usage Non-toxic, non-irritant in dilution. Ensure you use the variety Pinus sylvestris as other varieties may be toxic or irritant.

The plant

There are 90 species *of pine tree. The essential oil comes from the Scots, or forest, pine, grown in Europe and Asia. Oil is distilled from the evergreen needles and twigs year round.*

The essential oil

The pale yellow *oil is steam-distilled from the twigs and buds of the tree. It has the distinctive fresh, sweet, resinous aroma of a pine forest.*

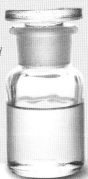

DIFFUSER

MASSAGE OIL

Black pepper
Piper nigrum

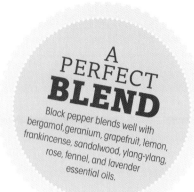
A
PERFECT
BLEND
Black pepper blends well with bergamot, geranium, grapefruit, lemon, frankincense, sandalwood, ylang-ylang, rose, fennel, and lavender essential oils.

A warming, spicy oil, black pepper has strong **antiseptic** properties. Its **stimulating** aroma has a clearing effect on the **mind,** making this a useful oil for improving **focus,** while its ability to boost circulation can **revive** tired muscles and joints and speed the healing of bruises.

What is it **good for?**

Eases aches and pains Black pepper's main constituent, piperine, is an anti-inflammatory, which makes this essential oil a potent ingredient in ointments and salves for aching limbs and sore muscles. The oil also has a warming action that is effective for relieving sports injuries and improving muscle tone.

Stimulates circulation Black pepper essential oil helps to encourage circulation to the extremities, so use for cold hands and feet. Regular use may also help to improve the appearance of cellulite.

Aids detox The oil encourages perspiration and can be used in small doses to support the effective functioning of the lymphatic system. It also has a mild diuretic effect.

Boosts immunity If you are feeling run down, this essential oil is a good choice as it bolsters the body's defences against infections.

Eases breathing A penetrating oil, black pepper can help loosen and clear congestion in the lungs.

Helps to quit smoking Studies have shown that inhaling black pepper vapours can help reduce cravings for cigarettes.

Enhances alertness The oil imbues a general feeling of warmth that can enhance the senses, and it also helps to clear the mind and bring a sense of clarity that can aid focus, motivation, and stamina, while combating mental fatigue.

Best **uses**

In a diffuser If your "can do" attitude is feeling a little worn out, add 3–4 drops of black pepper essential oil to a diffuser, vaporizer, or oil burner to improve motivation and help your levels of concentration.

As a massage oil For a general massage, black pepper essential oil is best used as part of an oil blend. To make a quick oil blend to reduce bruising and relieve sore muscles and joints, add 15 drops of black pepper oil to 1 tablespoon of base oil, and apply locally.

Safe usage Non-toxic, non-irritant in dilution.

The plant

Black peppercorns are actually the dried fruits of a climbing vine-like shrub native to Indonesia, where the spice is still mainly cultivated today. Best known as a cooking spice, black pepper also has a long established history of use as a medicinal spice in India and China. Black pepper essential oil is valued by perfumers for adding a warming spicy note to perfume blends.

The essential oil

The essential oil of the black peppercorn is steam-distilled from the dried, crushed unripe fruit. The thinly textured oil is an amber to yellow–green colour and has a distinctive pungent, spicy aroma that is both warming and fresh.

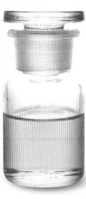

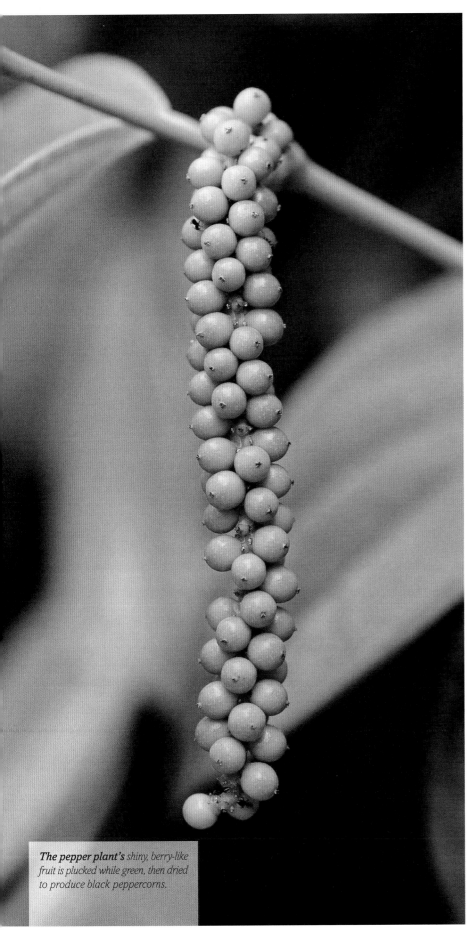

Soothing and warming, black pepper essential oil eases aches and pains and stimulates the circulation.

The pepper plant's *shiny, berry-like fruit is plucked while green, then dried to produce black peppercorns.*

FRAGRANCE

MASSAGE OIL

Patchouli

Pogostemon cablin

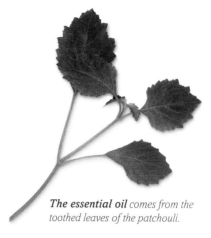

The essential oil comes from the toothed leaves of the patchouli.

A tried and tested aromatherapy favourite, patchouli oil **soothes** and **heals** the skin, improving the appearance of scar tissue and stretch marks. It also **revitalizes** ageing complexions, and its **antiseptic** properties help to treat pimple-prone skin.

What is it **good for?**

Repairs, tones, and cleanses skin Patchouli oil regenerates skin cells, helping scars and stretch marks to fade, and moisturizes dry skin. An astringent, the oil balances sebum secretions to normalize oily and acne-prone skin. It helps to control acne, and to treat sores and impetigo. Its antifungal action is useful for treating athlete's foot.

Repels insects The oil can ward off insects. Use neat on bites and stings.

Aids detox Patchouli oil has a diuretic effect, making it useful in anti-cellulite skincare products and massage oils.

Enhances wellbeing The oil acts as an anti-depressant, and is useful for treating exhaustion, stress, and anxiety. It's also used as an aphrodisiac.

Aids digestion Its balancing effect relieves diarrhoea and constipation.

Best **uses**

As a perfume Patchouli and rose makes a classic scent. Add 10 drops of patchouli and 20 drops of rose absolute to 2 tablespoons base oil or vodka.

As a massage oil Add patchouli oil to a base oil for an uplifting and relaxing massage that relieves tension and anxiety, and can also help to boost a sluggish digestion.

Safe usage *Non-toxic, non-irritant in dilution.*

The plant

The patchouli bush*, native to India and Malaysia, is called "puchaput". To produce the oil the leaves are lightly fermented or scalded to break the cell walls and release the aroma.*

The essential oil

The leaves are steam-distilled *to produce a pale yellow to pale green oil with a spicy, woody, musky scent prized by perfume makers. The smell is rather "love it or hate it", so it's best used in small amounts and in blends.*

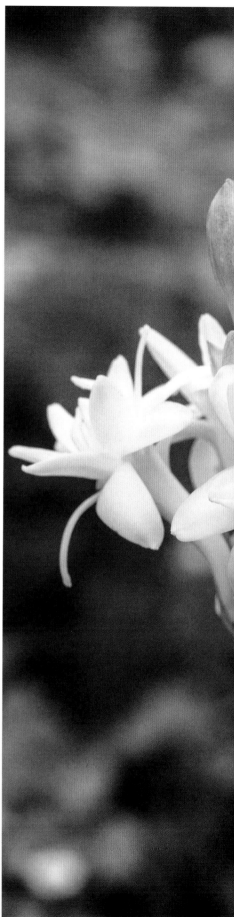

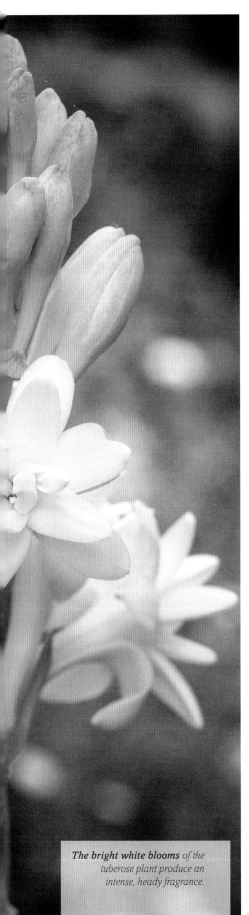

The bright white blooms of the tuberose plant produce an intense, heady fragrance.

MASSAGE OIL

DIFFUSER

Tuberose
Polianthes tuberosa

Tuberose helps to **calm** the nervous system and is widely used to provide **relief** from depression, anger, nervous exhaustion, stress, and tension. The same calming and uplifting properties make it a natural **aphrodisiac** for both men and women.

What is it **good for?**

Acts as a mild sedative Calming on the nervous system, the oil acts like a sedative to help promote restful sleep.

Boosts circulation This warming oil can help to improve circulation and chase away winter chills.

Balances emotions Tuberose is a grounding oil. It increases emotional stamina, relieving stress, tension, anxiety, depression, and anger, and also inspires creativity and calm.

Acts as an aphrodisiac A relaxing oil, the heady, sensual aroma helps to release inhibitions and lift a low libido, especially when due to stress.

Combats body odour A strong, long-lasting, floral aroma combined with antibacterial properties helps to eliminate body odour.

Best **uses**

As a massage oil Make a warming massage oil by adding 10–20 drops of tuberose to 2 tablespoons base oil. As it has a strong, heady aroma, a little goes far, so it's best to dilute well.

In a diffuser Spice up the atmosphere in a room by adding 3–4 drops of the oil to a diffuser, vaporizer, or oil burner.

Safe usage *Use well diluted (less than 1 per cent). Avoid use on hypersensitive skin and on children under seven years old.*

The plant

The night-blooming tuberose *is also known as the "Night Queen". It takes around 1550kg (3000lb) of handpicked flowers to extract 0.5kg (1lb) of the absolute oil. Tuberose is related to narcissus and jonquil and has distinctive tubular flowers.*

The essential oil

The dark orange–brown viscous *absolute is solvent-extracted from the flowers. It has a strong, spicy–sweet, creamy aroma.*

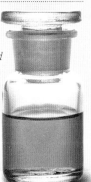

STEAM
INHALATION

OINTMENT

Ravensara, Ravintsara

Ravensara aromatica, Cinnamomum camphora

A warming, stimulating oil with **antiviral** and **antiseptic** properties, this oil is a natural choice during the cold and flu season. Confusion around the oil's source (see box, below), means the oil is now commonly called ravintsara, though the name ravensara is still seen.

What is it **good for?**

Provides cold and flu relief
The oil's decongestant and antiviral properties can ease cold and flu symptoms such as coughs and sinusitis, and cleanse air in sick rooms.

Combats viruses
Its antiviral properties are useful for treating cold sores, shingles, and herpes.

Enhances wellbeing
Stimulating and reviving, ravintsara eases nervous exhaustion and stress, and helps to lift depression and negative thoughts.

Boosts immunity
Ravintsara has immunostimulant properties, which means it can help support immunity, especially when defences are low due to stress and overwork.

Aids digestion
Gently massaged into the abdomen, the oil stimulates digestion, while its antiseptic properties make it a useful treatment for tummy upsets and gastric flu.

Relieves pain
The oil has a relaxing and analgesic action on aching muscles and joints, and can be used in a compress to soothe and treat sprains and strains.

Best **uses**

In a steam inhalation
To relieve sinus or respiratory tract infections, add 3–4 drops to a bowl of hot water, cover your head and the bowl with a towel, and breathe deeply for 15 minutes. Blend with oils that have similar decongestant properties, such as eucalyptus, thyme, or pine.

As a cold-sore treatment
The oil can be used neat to treat cold sores. Dab on with a cotton swab as needed.

Safe usage Non-toxic, non-irritant in dilution.

The plant

There is confusion *around this oil. In the past, the name ravensara was used for oil from the Agatophyllum aromaticum tree. However, ravensara is used in perfumery; the aromatherapy oil ravintsara is from the leaf of a variety of camphor tree in Madagascar.*

The essential oil

The essential oil *is steam-distilled from the young, leafy twigs. It is a thin, clear to yellow oil with a camphor-like aroma that is somewhere between lavender and tea tree essential oils.*

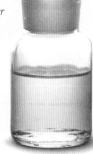

This immune-boosting oil offers protection in the winter months.

SKIN CARE

MASSAGE OIL

Rose

Rosa damascena, R. centifolia

Roses have been used as **medicinal** plants since antiquity, and are celebrated for their calming, **uplifting** aroma. The oil has a toning, **anti-inflammatory**, and **rejuvenating** effect, and its mild detoxifying and antiseptic properties can relieve pain and nausea.

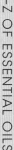

What is it **good for?**

Rejuvenates skin Rose oil supports cell and tissue regeneration, which helps to maintain the skin's elasticity and reduce the appearance of fine lines. It makes an excellent choice for minimizing the appearance of broken capillaries on the skin.

Heals skin The oil helps to repair sun-damaged skin and damage from burns and scalds, as well as reduce the appearance of stretch marks. Its skin-calming and anti-inflammatory properties can soothe dry, hot, itchy skin.

Fights bacteria Rose oil has been shown to have antimicrobial properties. In one study, Damask rose demonstrated antibacterial activity against 15 strains of bacteria.

Enhances wellbeing The oil creates a sense of relaxed wellbeing and can help to increase feelings of vitality. This calming property makes it useful for taking the edge off stress-related conditions.

Supports women's health Rose oil has a toning effect on the uterus, which can help to ease heavy, clotted or painful periods. It is also used to limit the effects of, and provide relief from, premenstrual tension.

Relieves digestive discomfort A mild detoxifying and antiseptic effect, combined with nerve-soothing properties, help relieve tummy upsets, nausea, and constipation. The oil has a fortifying effect on the gallbladder and liver, supporting efficient digestion and absorption of nutrients.

Best **uses**

As a skin toner Make a toner by combining 2 tablespoons witch-hazel and 4 tablespoons rose flower water with 4 drops of rose absolute oil. Put in a plain bottle or spray bottle and use as needed. Shake well before use.

As a massage oil Rose can relieve feelings of depression, anxiety, and grief. Blend 4 drops of rose, 4 drops of geranium and 4 drops of orange essential oils with 2 tablespoons base oil for an uplifting body massage.

Safe usage *Non-irritant. Absolute is non-toxic; use essential oil in dilutions of less than 1 per cent due to its methyl eugenol content.*

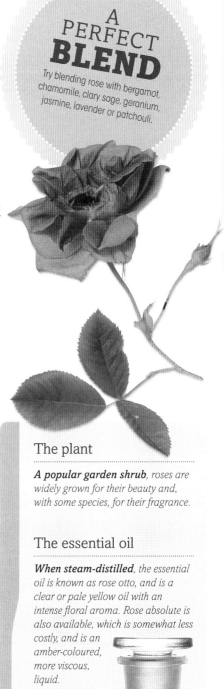

A PERFECT **BLEND**

Try blending rose with bergamot, chamomile, clary sage, geranium, jasmine, lavender or patchouli.

The plant

A popular garden shrub*, roses are widely grown for their beauty and, with some species, for their fragrance.*

The essential oil

When steam-distilled*, the essential oil is known as rose otto, and is a clear or pale yellow oil with an intense floral aroma. Rose absolute is also available, which is somewhat less costly, and is an amber-coloured, more viscous, liquid.*

SHOWER

MASSAGE OIL

Rosemary

Rosmarinus officinalis

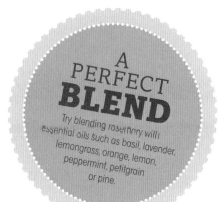

A PERFECT **BLEND**

Try blending rosemary with essential oils such as basil, lavender, lemongrass, orange, lemon, peppermint, petitgrain or pine.

Toning and **cleansing** rosemary oil helps to clear the mind. It contains potent **antibacterial** and antifungal substances that can fight infection, and has a warming **anti-inflammatory** action that helps relieve pain. Its **stimulating** effect on the lymphatic system aids detox and improves circulation.

What is it **good for?**

Helps fight germs Rosemary essential oil contains rosmarinic acid, which in addition to being anti-inflammatory, is also antiviral and antibacterial. This makes rosemary useful for fighting off respiratory infections and for using topically on skin infections. The oil can be dabbed neat on sores, bites, and scabies to reduce inflammation and aid healing.

Acts as a hair tonic The oil helps to stimulate the circulation, which in turn combats hair loss and dandruff.

Aids detox The oil stimulates both the circulation and lymphatic systems, aiding the removal of waste products and relieving water retention, which in turn helps to fight cellulite.

Boosts circulation Rosemary is useful for treating low blood pressure and warming cold hands and feet. Its boost to circulation also brings some relief to sprains and strains, and soothes sore muscles after exercising.

Improves focus Rosemary essential oil stimulates the nervous system and increases circulation to the brain, which in turn helps to improve memory, concentration, and mental alertness. The oil has a reviving effect when you are feeling tired, debilitated, or lethargic, which also makes it an especially useful remedy for jet lag.

Relieves menstrual cramps The oil's warming and anti-inflammatory properties help to relieve painful period cramping.

Best **uses**

As a shower gel To revive both body and mind, try this after-sport scented shower gel. Add 55 drops of rosemary, 30 drops of peppermint, and 40 drops of lemon essential oils to a 250-ml (9-fl oz) bottle of unfragranced shower gel, and enjoy a refreshing and stimulating shower.

As a massage oil Add 10 drops of the essential oil to 1 tablespoon base oil to create a simple, warming, pain-relieving, and detoxifying massage oil.

Safe usage Non-irritant in dilution. Avoid use near the nose in children under seven years old.

The plant

Rosemary is a popular aromatic herb *with silvery green leaves and pale blue flowers. The plant is a Mediterranean native and today is still produced mainly in France, Spain, Croatia, Tunisia, and Morocco. This ubiquitous herb has been used widely in food, medicine, and during religious ceremonies for thousands of years.*

The essential oil

The virtually colourless oil *that is extracted from rosemary is steam-distilled from the fresh flowering tops of the herb. The essential oil has a pungent, fresh, and pleasant herbaceous aroma.*

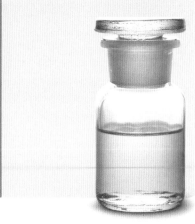

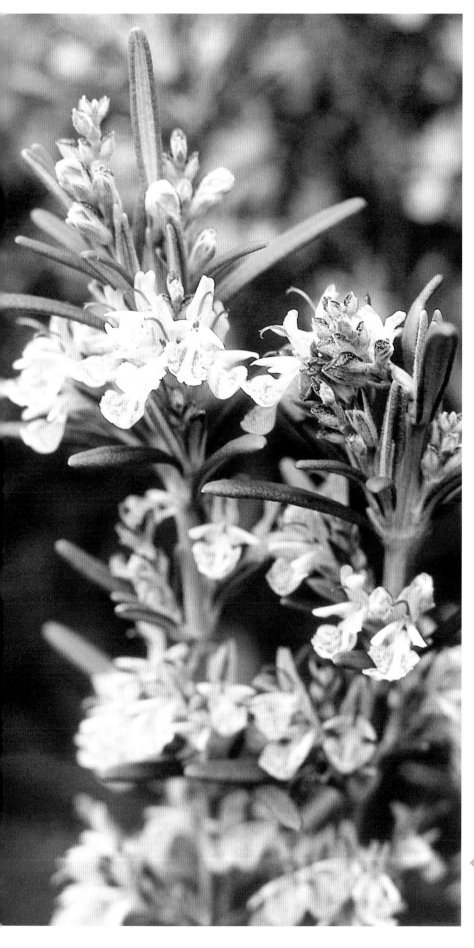

This refreshing and cleansing oil is a popular addition to hair treatments, adding shine to lacklustre hair.

Rosemary has *highly fragrant needle-shaped leaves with delicate lavender blue to purple blooms.*

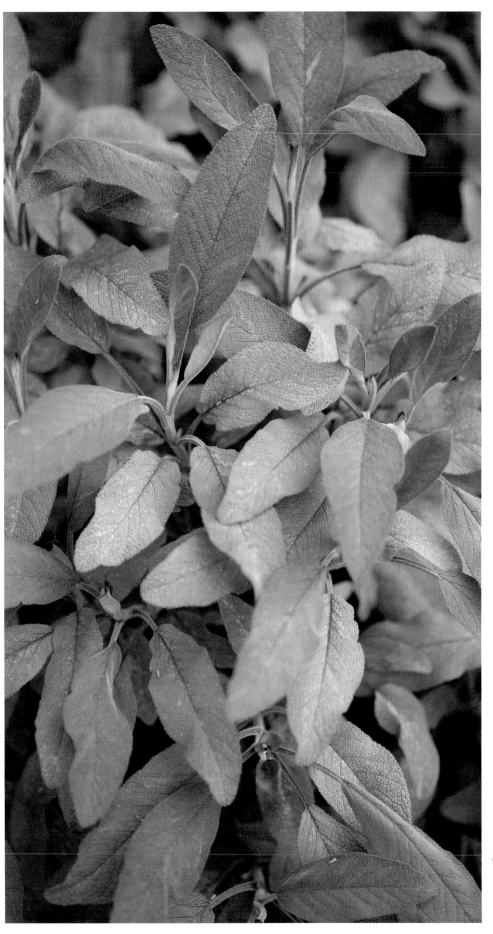

This warming, antibacterial oil has a potent effect and should be diluted well before use.

The finely veined, distinctive leaves *of this evergreen shrub are highly aromatic.*

MOUTHWASH   FOOT BATH

Sage (Dalmatian)

Salvia officinalis

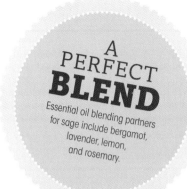

A PERFECT BLEND
Essential oil blending partners for sage include bergamot, lavender, lemon, and rosemary.

An extremely stimulating oil, sage is primarily used as a warming oil that can help to relieve aching muscles. The oil also has an **astringent** quality that makes it a useful skin toner. Use it to **relieve** stress and improve mental **focus** when you are tired or under pressure.

What is it **good for?**

Acts as an antiseptic Sage essential oil has a particular affinity to the gums, and its antibacterial properties can help to eliminate the bacteria that can harbour in the mouth and cause bad breath and gum disease.

Brightens the complexion Sage has circulation-boosting properties that help to improve skin tone and minimize the appearance of open pores. Its antioxidant action reduces the harmful effects of free radicals, which can make skin look dull, so can help to brighten tired-looking complexions.

Acts as a hair and scalp tonic Sage has an effective anti-fungal action and so is a useful oil to help control dandruff.

Calms nerves During periods of stress and exhaustion, sage can have a tonic effect on the nervous system. It revives and stimulates, bringing renewed vitality.

Acts as a deodorant Sage essential oil has a naturally deodorizing effect that can help to fight body and foot odour. It's useful for relieving excessive sweating, particularly during the menopause.

Best **uses**

As a mouthwash Make an antiseptic mouthwash to treat inflamed gums or combat bad breath by adding 1 drop of sage essential oil to 1 teaspoon glycerine or calendula tincture, then dilute the mixture in half a glass of water. Rinse the mouthwash around the mouth and gums and then spit it out.

In a foot bath To fight foot odour, add 4–5 drops of sage essential oil to a shallow basin of warm water. Soak the feet for 10–15 minutes, then dry them thoroughly.

Safe usage Use very well diluted (less than 0.5 per cent). Avoid using during pregnancy and when breastfeeding, and avoid using on children under 15 years old. Toxic if ingested.

The plant

Another popular culinary herb, with an established history of medicinal use, the name "sage" is derived from the Latin word "salvare", which means "heal" or "save". The plant, which has silver–grey leaves and blue to purplish flowers, is a native of the Mediterranean region, but now grows throughout much of the world.

Spanish sage (Salvia lavandulifolia) is often preferable to use rather than Dalmatian sage as it is considerably less harsh, although should still be avoided during pregnancy and when breastfeeding.

The essential oil

Steam-distillation of the dried leaves of the sage plant produces a thin, clear essential oil that has a sharp, slightly spicy, fresh, and herbaceous aroma.

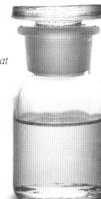

BATH OIL

MASSAGE OIL

Clary sage

Salvia sclarea

Renowned for **uplifting** the mind and emotions, clary sage also has a **tonic** effect on many body systems, including the digestive and circulatory systems. It can **revive** tired muscles, relieve menstrual and labour pains, and is considered an **aphrodisiac**.

What is it **good for?**

Lifts mood Clary sage lifts depression and calms nerves, creating a sense of peace and, in some, euphoria. It is used to return vitality after an illness.

Relieves aches and pains A powerful muscle relaxant, clary sage can ease muscular aches and pains.

Aids digestion Massaged over the abdomen, the oil can aid digestion and relieve tummy upsets and wind.

Boosts circulation Its tonic effect is partly due to it boosting the circulation. It can help lower high blood pressure.

Supports women's health The oil can be used to treat the symptoms of PMS, ease period cramps, and relieve anxiety and hot flushes in menopause.

Acts as an aphrodisiac Clary sage can help restore libido and vitality.

Best **uses**

As a bath oil For menstrual pain or stress, add 5–6 drops to 1 tablespoon base oil or full-fat milk and disperse in a bath. Soak for at least 10 minutes.

In a massage oil Add 1–2 drops of clary sage and 2 drops of lavender oils to 1 tablespoon base oil for a massage to aid digestion and boost circulation.

Safe usage *Use well diluted to avoid potential skin irritation (less than 0.5 per cent). Avoid on hypersensitive skin and on children under seven years old.*

The plant

Related to sage*, but with tall, dramatic flower stems, clary sage is a native of southern Europe. The herb has long been prized as a medicinal plant and is also a popular ingredient in perfumes.*

The essential oil

The oil is a colourless *to pale green liquid with a herbaceous, sweet, slightly nutty aroma. It is steam-distilled from the flowering tops and leaves.*

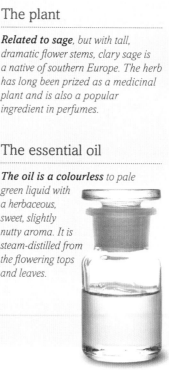

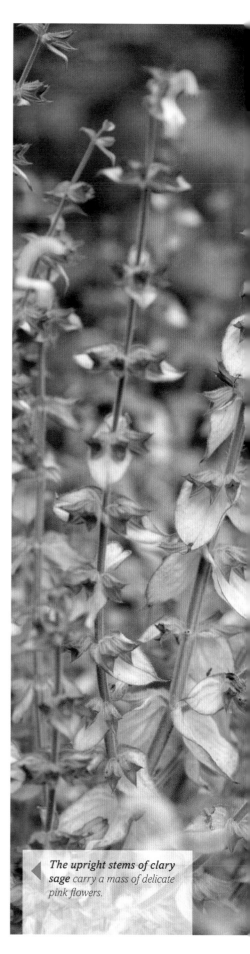

The upright stems of clary sage carry a mass of delicate pink flowers.

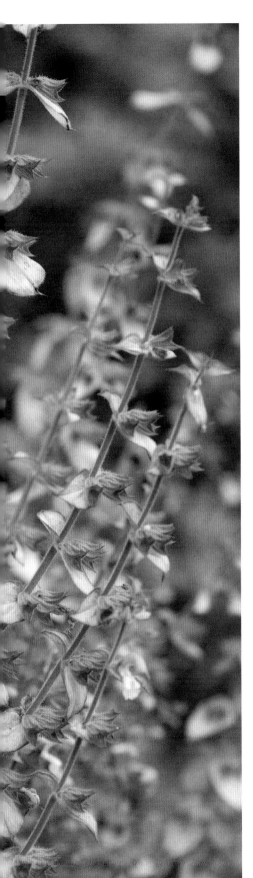

DIFFUSER

FRAGRANCE

Sandalwood

Santalum album

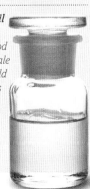

Aromatic sandalwood has elegant, oval-shaped leaves.

Sandalwood has a long history in Ayurvedic and Chinese medicine. Its **anti-inflammatory** and antiseptic properties **revive** and **heal** dry and damaged skin. It has a **restorative** effect on mind and emotions, and calms respiratory conditions.

What is it **good for?**

Protects and balances skin The oil's anti-inflammatory and astringent effects help to balance skin. It treats oily skin effectively, while also soothing dry, itchy, or inflamed skin. It can reduce the appearance of scars and blemishes and soothe razor burn.

Restores vitality Sandalwood can dispel anxiety and lift depression, aiding sleep and helping to reignite a passion for life. The oil is considered an aphrodisiac, especially for men.

Acts as an antiseptic Its mild antiseptic action is used to ease the effects of genito-urinary tract infections.

Eases breathing Sandalwood has a cooling and anti-inflammatory effect on the mucous membranes and can help calm chronic coughs. A mild decongestant and antiseptic, it can help to treat bronchitis, laryngitis, and respiratory tract infections.

Best **uses**

In a diffuser Add 3–4 drops to a diffuser or to water in a room spray to perfume air and promote calm.

As an aftershave balm For a reviving and calming aftershave balm, add 1 drop of sandalwood essential oil to 1 teaspoon almond base oil. Warm the oil between the palms and then use to soothe skin after shaving.

Safe usage *Non-toxic, non-irritant in dilutions of less than 2 per cent.*

The plant

***The sandalwood tree**, a native of India, was for many years such a popular source of essential oil that it became seriously endangered. When buying the oil, it is important to check that it comes from a sustainable source.*

The essential oil

***The essential oil** is steam-distilled from the heartwood of the tree. It is pale yellow to pale gold in colour and has a subtle, sweet, and soothing woody aroma.*

FIRST AID

MASSAGE OIL

STEAM
INHALATION

Summer savory

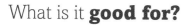
Satureja hortensis

Once believed to be a powerful **aphrodisiac,** monks of the Benedictine order were banned from growing summer savory in their gardens. Today it is recognized for its **calming** effect on the digestive system, helping to ease trapped wind. It is helpful for **boosting strength and resolve** in times of stress.

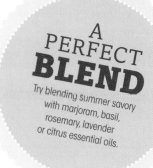
A
PERFECT
BLEND
Try blending summer savory with marjoram, basil, rosemary, lavender or citrus essential oils.

What is it **good for?**

Helps fight infection Savory has effective antiseptic properties that help to combat the bacteria that can cause skin infections. This makes it a useful remedy to have on hand for first-aid applications. Research has shown that savory essential oil can inhibit the growth of *Candida albicans*, the fungus responsible for athlete's foot and thrush.

Aids digestion The gentle aromatic, carminative, and digestive properties of savory essential oil make it a useful treatment for digestive problems such as flatulence, nausea, and diarrhoea.

Relieves stress Savory essential oil has a bolstering effect when you are feeling stressed to the point of giving up. It is also helps to motivate when you feel exhausted at the prospect of a difficult task.

Soothes sore throats Using the oil in a diffuser or steam inhalation helps ease coughs, colds, and sore throats.

Treats bites and stings Dab the diluted oil on to skin for instant relief from insect bites and stings.

Promotes hair growth Summer savory is a traditional remedy for encouraging hair growth. The diluted oil can be massaged into the scalp.

Best **uses**

For first aid Mix 3–4 drops of the essential oil in 1 tablespoon St John's wort macerated oil or 2 tablespoons vodka and dab onto insect bites, or patches of athlete's foot or other fungal infections.

In a massage oil For a soothing massage after you've over-indulged, mix 2–3 drops of the essential oil in 1 tablespoon base oil. Massage the abdominal area gently in a clockwise motion.

In an inhalation Add a few drops to a bowl of warm water and inhale to relieve congestion and cold symptoms.

Safe usage Use well diluted (less than 1.5 per cent). Avoid using on hypersensitive skin and on children under seven years old.

The plant

The Saxons named savory after its spicy, pungent taste. A member of the mint family, summer savory is a Mediterranean native, with small leathery leaves and light purple flowers. It is widely used in cooking.

Winter savory (Satureja montana) is thought to have a stronger antiseptic action and aroma that makes it less popular in aromatherapy, but useful in small quantities to boost the medicinal properties of other oils.

The essential oil

Steam-distilled from the leaves and stems, the essential oil is pale yellow to pale orange with a spicy, herbaceous aroma.

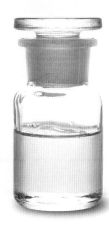

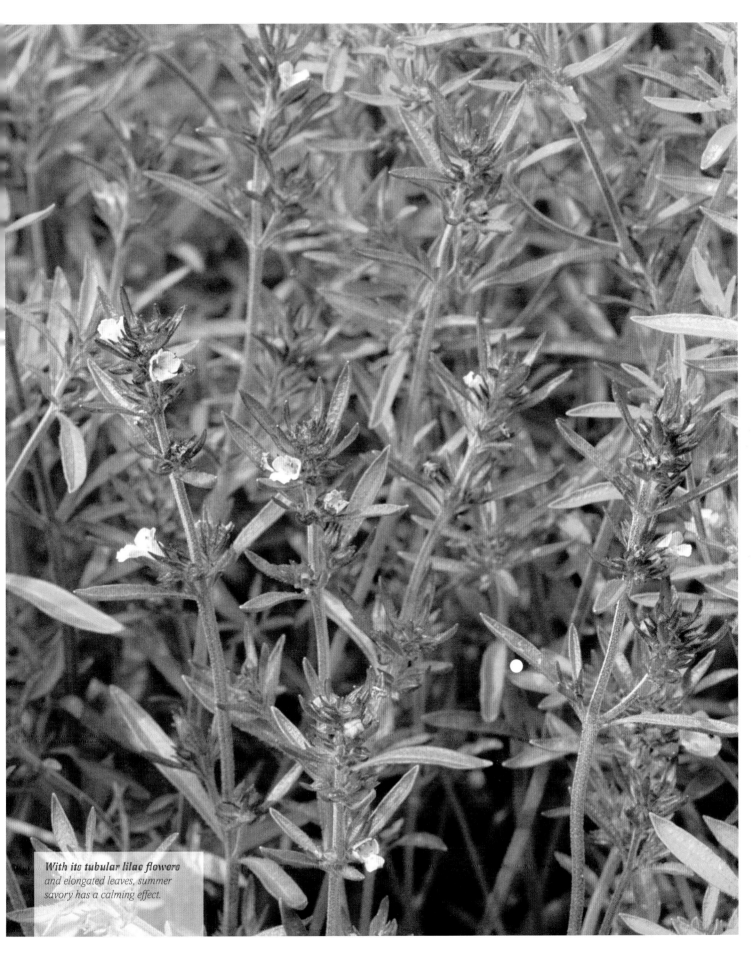

With its tubular lilac flowers and elongated leaves, summer savory has a calming effect.

HAIR CARE   DIFFUSER   STEAM INHALATION

DIFFUSER   OINTMENT

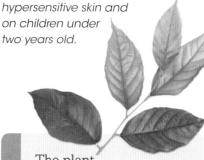

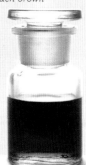

Benzoin

Styrax benzoin

Benzoin, also known as gum benzoin, is a traditional ingredient in **incense.** Today the oil is added to skin creams for its antiseptic, **healing,** and **calming** properties. In scents, it is a popular fixative, slowing the evaporation of the perfume to help it last longer.

What is it **good for?**

Calms itchy skin Benzoin is an effective remedy for a range of dry, irritable, and itchy skin conditions, including sun- and wind-damaged skin and conditions such as eczema and psoriasis. The oil gives mature skin a boost by increasing elasticity.

Heals wounds The oil has useful antibacterial properties that help heal cuts and wounds. It can be used to treat acne and other skin eruptions.

Eases aches and pains Benzoin essential oil has a local stimulating effect that improves circulation. Used in a massage blend, it can help to loosen stiff muscles and relieve the soreness of arthritis and rheumatism.

Enhances wellbeing Soothing and warming, benzoin is known to have a calming effect on the mind and to help ease depression.

Best **uses**

For hair For an itchy scalp, add 5 drops to a mild unscented shampoo.

In a diffuser Add to a diffuser, vaporizer, or oil burner, for a sweet scent.

In an inhalation A steam inhalation helps clear congestion.

Safe usage Use well diluted (less than 2 per cent). Avoid on hypersensitive skin and on children under two years old.

The plant

***This large tropical tree** is native to Thailand and its adjacent islands. Benzoin resin is collected by making an incision in the trunk that allows the sap to escape. As it flows, the fresh gum is yellowish, but becomes a darker red–brown colour as it dries.*

The essential oil

***Benzoin oil** is golden brown with a sweet, vanilla-like scent. Too thick and sticky to be used undiluted, it is sold as an oleoresin or tincture to be used like an essential oil.*

Clove

Syzygium aromaticum, Eugenia caryophyllata

Clove yields a **warming** oil that can be used in small amounts to add **antiseptic** and **analgesic** properties. It is a useful mouthwash for oral infections, and its spicy aroma is comforting and relaxing.

What is it **good for?**

Cares for teeth and gums Widely used in both conventional and complementary dental health products, clove is both an antiseptic and anaesthetic, helping to fight the germs that cause bad breath and relieve swollen gums and toothache.

Calms and treats skin Added to acne treatments, clove oil helps to reduce red, painful inflammation and kill the bacteria that causes acne. It can also be used to treat warts.

Clears congestion Expectorant properties make the oil useful for respiratory infections, such as coughs, colds, sinusitis, and asthma. As a room scent, it clears and disinfects the air.

Relieves anxiety Clove oil has a relaxing, comforting aroma that can reduce anxiety and enhance focus on the task at hand.

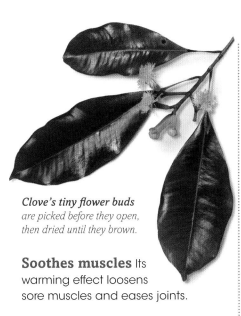

Clove's tiny flower buds are picked before they open, then dried until they brown.

Soothes muscles Its warming effect loosens sore muscles and eases joints.

Best **uses**

In a diffuser Diffuse 2–3 drops to clear or disinfect air.

As a muscle rub Add 3 drops to 1 tablespoon base oil for a warm rub.

Safe usage Use very well diluted (less than 0.5 per cent). Avoid on hypersensitive or damaged skin and on children under seven years old.

The plant

We tend to think of clove *as a spice, but it is actually a herb derived from the dried flower buds of the tree.*

The essential oil

The essential oil *can be steam-distilled from the leaves, stems, and buds. This yields a clear to pale yellow liquid with a rich and appealing spicy aroma.*

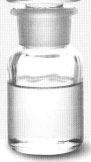

DIFFUSER

OINTMENT

Tagetes
Tagetes erecta

Tagetes is traditionally used to treat infections and wounds, **repel** insects, and to clear congestion. The oil also has a **mild sedative** effect that **calms** anxiety and nerves. With its **uplifting** aroma, it is a popular perfumery ingredient, especially in men's fragrances.

What is it **good for?**

Heals wounds The oil has an antiseptic action that can help to treat infection in wounds, cuts, and abscesses, as well as fungal infections.

Relieves cramping Tagetes calms digestive irritation and inflammation and its antispasmodic action relieves menstrual and muscle cramps.

Clears congestion The oil helps to open up the bronchial passages and encourage the removal of phlegm from the sinuses and lungs.

Calms nerves With its mild sedative effect, tagetes eases anxiety, panic, and stress, lifts depression, dispels anger, and can induce relaxation.

Acts as an insect repellent The oil's insecticidal properties can help to repel flies and mosquitoes. Pop some in your bag for holidays.

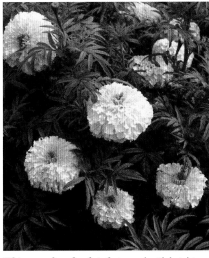

This popular shrub is festooned with bright yellow and orange blooms in summer and autumn.

Best **uses**

In a diffuser Add 3–4 drops to a diffuser, vaporizer, or oil burner to ease coughs, bronchitis, and chest infections, or to use as an insect repellent.

In an ointment To treat fungal infections, add 10–15 drops to an ointment base. Apply as needed.

Safe usage Use well diluted (less than 2 per cent). Highly photo-toxic even in low dilutions so avoid on the skin for 24 hours before exposure to the sun.

The plant

Also called Southern marigold, *this member of the marigold family, a popular border shrub, has bright yellow–orange flowers.*

The essential oil

The essential oil *is steam-distilled from the flowers. It has a golden colour and an aromatic, earthy, floral aroma with hints of citrus.*

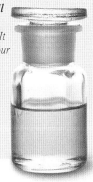

BATH OIL

SKIN CARE

Thyme

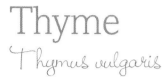

Thymus vulgaris

A popular oil for baths and ointments, thyme **boosts** circulation and **relieves** tired and sore muscles and joints. The oil is an effective **antiseptic**, helping to clear fungal infections, as well as fight colds and loosen stubborn phlegm. Its **stimulating** aroma can help clear and **refresh** the mind.

A PERFECT BLEND

Try blending thyme essential oil with bergamot, clove, eucalyptus, lavender, tangerine, lemon or pine essential oils.

What is it **good for?**

Soothes coughs The antiseptic and antispasmodic properties of thyme essential oil make it a great remedy for easing the symptoms of colds, such as coughs and sore throats, and for soothing the symptoms of chronic bronchitis.

Fights fungal infections Try adding thyme essential oil to hair rinses, or massaging the diluted oil into the scalp, nails, or feet to help clear conditions such as dandruff and seborrheic dermatitis, athletes foot, and fungal nail infections.

Eases aches and pains The oil has a warming effect that helps to loosen tight muscles and ease aching joints.

Helps clear acne Studies show that constituents in thyme can be more effective than benzoyl peroxide, the active ingredient in most anti-acne creams or washes, at killing propionibacterium – the bacterium that causes acne.

Enhances wellbeing Thyme essential oil brings relief when you are feeling anxious, stressed or low.

Treats urinary infections Thyme essential oil's antiseptic and antifungal properties make this oil an ideal choice to help deal with uncomfortable urinary tract infections, such as cystitis.

Improves circulation Thyme essential oil has a stimulating and general toning effect on the circulatory system, which makes it a useful treatment for low blood pressure, weakness, and anaemia.

Best **uses**

As a bath oil Add 5–6 drops of thyme essential oil to 1 tablespoon base oil or eggcupful of milk and disperse in a warm bath to help treat urinary tract infections.

As a skin toner Try blending 2 drops each of thyme and mandarin essential oils in a base of 2 teaspoons aloe vera juice to 90ml (3fl oz) witch hazel. Shake the blend well and apply with a cotton wool ball, or pour the blend into a spray bottle and use as a refreshing facial spritzer.

Safe usage Use well diluted (less than 2 per cent).

The plant

This is a low, creeping aromatic herb that is a member of the mint family. Thyme is native to the Mediterranean region where it thrives in the hot, sunny locations and the well-drained soil. Thyme is widely used as both a culinary and medicinal herb.

The essential oil

The flowering tops and leaves of the popular herb, thyme, can be steam-distilled to create the essential oil. Several different chemotypes are used in the aromatherapy essential oil. Thyme linalol (Thymus vulgaris ct linalol) is more gentle and the most suitable essential oil for general aromatherapy use.

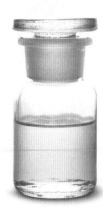

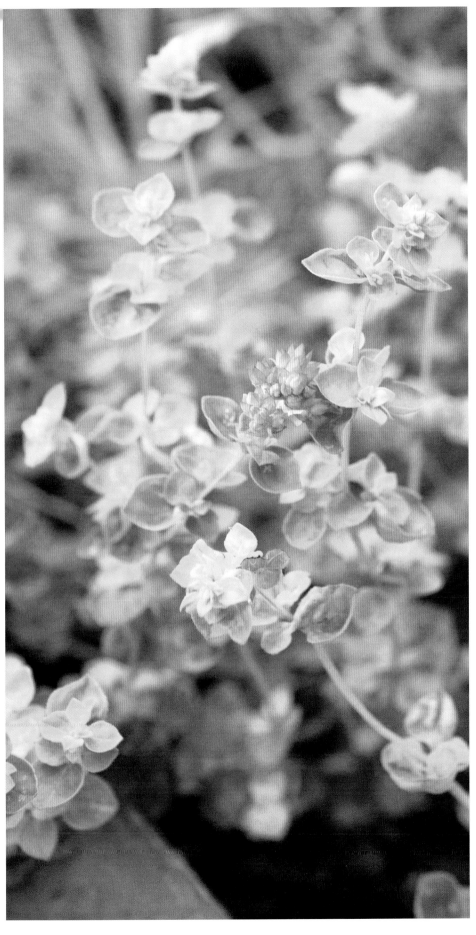

With its antiseptic properties, thyme essential oil is a useful oil for fighting winter colds.

This evergreen shrub has tiny oval-shaped leaves with white or pink flowers in early summer.

SKIN CARE

MASSAGE OIL

Fenugreek

Trigonella foenumgraecum

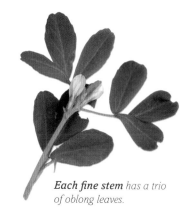

Each fine stem *has a trio of oblong leaves.*

A well-known **digestive aid** and laxative, fenugreek also has a **relaxing** effect on the nerves and an **antiseptic** and expectorant action on respiratory infections. It **stimulates** the circulation and can treat bruises and swelling when applied to the skin.

What is it **good for?**

Clears and soothes skin The oil's antibacterial and antifungal properties help treat skin infections such as boils. It also has an anti-inflammatory quality that relieves itchy, dry skin conditions.

Aids relaxation The oil has a relaxing effect on the nerves that can soothe anxiety and help lower blood pressure.

Eases congestion Fenugreek acts as an expectorant and soothes and relaxes inflamed respiratory tissues.

Aids detox Its tonic and antioxidant properties encourage perspiration and boost the metabolism. A mild laxative, it helps the body to remove waste.

Aids digestion Fenugreek soothes digestive upsets and aids digestion.

Supports women's health The oil can help to ease period pains, regulate cycles, and calm hot flushes.

Best **uses**

As a facial oil Add 4–6 drops of the oil to 1 tablespoon of a light base oil for use on inflamed or acne-prone skin.

In a massage oil Make a relaxing and skin-soothing massage blend by adding 15 drops of fenugreek essential oil to 1 tablespoon base oil. You can also use this to ease indigestion, gently massaging the oil into the abdomen in a clockwise motion.

Safe usage *Non-irritant in dilution.*

The plant

Native to the Middle and Near East*, the spice is also known as methi. Fenugreek produces distinctive, triangular, oil-rich seeds. Its round leaves can be dried and used as herbs.*

The essential oil

The essential oil *is actually an absolute extracted from the seeds. This produces a yellow–brown waxy liquid with a potent, sweet–spicy, earthy scent.*

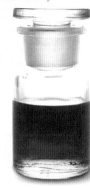

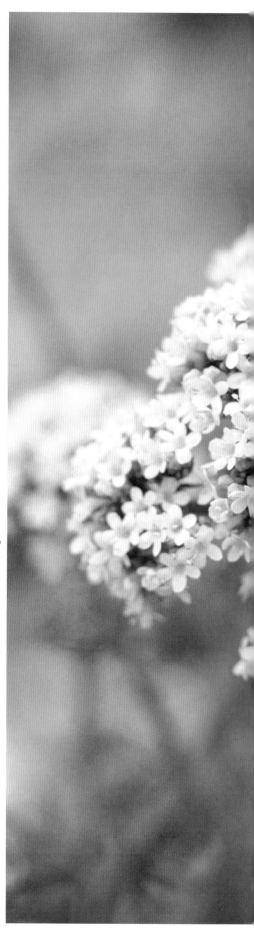

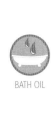
BATH OIL

MASSAGE OIL

Valerian
Valeriana officinalis

The most widely used herbal **sedative**, valerian is a recognized treatment for **insomnia** and tension. Its other psychological benefits include **lifting depression** and anxiety. It can help regulate blood pressure, slow palpitations, and settle digestion.

What is it **good for?**

Promotes restful sleep A powerful sedative, valerian can treat insomnia and improve sleep quality.

Balances emotions The oil can help to soothe nerves, and calm anxiety, depression, and restlessness. A good treatment for stress and tension.

Lowers blood pressure Valerian can help to regulate blood pressure and calm a rapid heartbeat.

Aids detox The oil's mild laxative effect encourages healthy bowel movements, and its diuretic action promotes urination. It can also calm an upset stomach, especially when this is linked to stress, and aid the effective metabolism of nutrients.

Supports women's health Valerian soothes stomach cramps and can ease pre-menstrual tension.

Best **uses**

In a bath oil Add 2 drops each of rose, valerian, and sandalwood essential oils to 1 tablespoon base oil or full-fat milk and disperse in a bath.

In a massage oil Added to an oil blend, valerian essential oil can be used to help encourage a state of deep relaxation. Try blending 4 drops each of valerian, lavender, and cedarwood essential oils to 2 tablespoons base oil.

Safe usage *Non-toxic, non-irritant in dilution.*

The plant

Native to parts of Europe and Asia, *the plant has distinctive leathery leaves and clusters of pink or white flowers. The name valerian is derived from the Latin "valere", which means "to be well" or "to feel good".*

The essential oil

Steam-distilled from the root, *the yellow to yellow–green oil has an earthy, musky, woody aroma that can be overpowering. For the best effect, blend with softer, sweeter oils.*

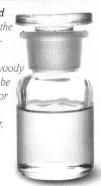

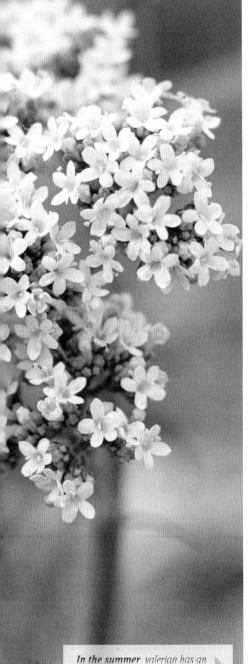

In the summer valerian has an abundance of sweetly scented delicate flower heads.

HAIR CARE

DIFFUSER

Vanilla

Vanilla planifolia

A relative newcomer to aromatherapy, vanilla is familiar to most as a flavouring for desserts and baked goods. Its **soothing** and softening properties can help **repair** rough or **damaged** skin. It is a mild **pain-reliever** and has antiseptic properties.

What is it **good for?**

Soothes dry skin Vanilla essential oil has skin- and hair-softening and soothing properties. It is also rich in antioxidants that can help protect the skin from the damage caused by environmental pollutants and toxins.

Acts as a painkiller The main aromatic chemical in vanilla is vanillin, which has similar pain-relieving properties to the capsaicin found in chilli peppers. When vanilla oil is diluted, it can be used on the skin to provide temporary, localized relief from general aches and pains and from toothache.

Helps relieve stress Vanilla can be used to help dispel general feelings of negativity as well as feelings of anxiety. This uplifting property is also thought to contribute to its aphrodisiac effect.

Helps to treat acne A mild antibacterial action enables vanilla essential oil to help fight the bacteria that cause acne and to reduce the occurrence of more minor pimples, blackheads, and spots.

Best **uses**

As a hair conditioner Add 10 drops of vanilla essential oil to 1 tablespoon coconut oil to make a hair mask that will condition and add shine to hair. Coat hair thoroughly and wrap in a towel for 10–15 minutes before shampooing and rinsing.

In a diffuser To help relieve stress and ease anxiety, add 1–2 drops of vanilla absolute to a diffuser, vaporizer, or oil burner.

Safe usage *Non-toxic and non-irritant.*

With its strong scent, just small amounts of vanilla are needed.

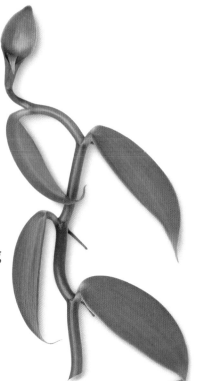

The green vanilla pods are dried prior to use.

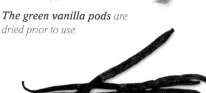

The plant

The vanilla bean *is actually the fruit pod from a type of orchid. The green pods are dried slowly until they turn black. Once they start to curl, the pods are ready to use either as a culinary flavouring or to produce an essential oil absolute.*

The essential oil

A thick, dark brown oil*, vanilla absolute is solvent-extracted from the cured seed pods. Its familiar, sometimes overwhelming, scent, should be used sparingly in any blend.*

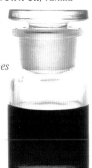

BATH OIL

DIFFUSER

Vetiver

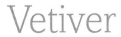
Vetiveria zizanioides

Working mostly on an emotional level, vetiver has a profoundly **grounding** effect for those who are distressed or panicky. The essential oil can help to improve circulation and is a useful **antiseptic** and **astringent** in the treatment of oily and combination skin.

A PERFECT **BLEND**

Vetiver blends well with clary sage, cedarwood, jasmine, lavender, patchouli, rose, ginger, ylang ylang and citrus oils.

What is it **good for?**

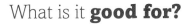

Soothes sore muscles Vetiver oil makes a warming and pain-relieving remedy for muscular aches and pains, sprains, general stiffness, and for rheumatism and arthritis.

Helps heal wounds Its antiseptic and slightly astringent properties make this oil a good treatment for cuts, grazes, wounds, and sores.

Helps fade scars and marks By promoting skin-healing and the growth of new tissue, vetiver is ideal for reducing the appearance of stretch marks, scars, and burns.

Has a cooling action Add vetiver to a cold compress to cool fever, sunstroke, and soothe headaches.

Promotes emotional balance Vetiver is grounding and calming when you are feeling emotionally overwhelmed, weepy, under pressure, and uncertain which direction to take. It can help relieve distress, anger, and hysteria in both adults and children.

Acts as an aphrodisiac Vetiver is thought to enhance libido and is often used to awaken sexual desire in men and women, especially when libido has been dampened by overwork and mental fatigue.

Promotes restful sleep A natural sedative, the oil is often used to promote relaxation and restful sleep.

Best **uses**

As a bath oil Make a relaxing bath oil by mixing 4–6 drops in 1 tablespoon base oil or full-fat milk. Disperse in a warm bath and have a quiet soak for at least 15 minutes.

In a diffuser Promote a peaceful, grounding atmosphere in your home or office by adding 3–4 drops of the essential oil to a diffuser, vaporizer, or oil burner.

Safe usage *Non-toxic, non-irritant in dilution.*

The plant

A tall perennial grass *native to India, vetiver is a relative of other fragrant grasses such as citronella, lemongrass, and palmarosa. Roots over 24 months old have the highest oil content, but take longer to distil, making this an expensive oil.*

The essential oil

The oil is steam-distilled *from the chopped up rootlets, which are soaked in water prior to distillation. The resulting oil is a thick, dark amber liquid with a spicy, earthy fragrance that has a hint of lemon.*

STEAM
INHALATION

SKIN CARE

Violet

Viola odorata

Violet is renowned for its **relaxing,** soothing, and inspiring properties. It is a traditional remedy for calming irritations to the respiratory tract, **rejuvenating** mature or weather-damaged skin, and **soothing** sensitive skin conditions. Its elegant floral aroma is **calming** on the mind and emotions.

A PERFECT BLEND

Ideal blending partners for violet essential oil include tuberose, clary sage, lavender, benzoin, cumin, basil, sandalwood, geranium, and citrus essential oils.

What is it **good for?**

Soothes dry skin Violet essential oil has a gentle and reviving effect on the skin and is well-known for its ability to help hydrate and soothe dry and sun- or wind-damaged skin. It is used to help minimize the appearance of spider veins and enlarged pores.

Acts as a painkiller The oil contains anti-inflammatory compounds that can relieve pain and inflammation in muscles and joints; applied locally, it can encourage circulation to an affected area. It can also provide relief for headaches and migraines.

Helps treat anxiety The oil is comforting and calming when you are feeling nervous, anxious, or exhausted. This grounding effect can also help to ease feelings of dizziness brought on by anxiety and stress.

Eases congestion Violet has expectorant properties that help to shift phlegm and relieve the pressure caused by blocked sinuses.

Best **uses**

As an inhalation Make a steam inhalation by adding 5–6 drops of violet essential oil to a bowl of hot water. Place a towel over your head and inhale deeply to loosen catarrh or relieve anxiety. This is also an effective way to condition and cleanse the skin.

As a facial elixir Make a quick, but luxurious, facial oil by adding 2 drops of violet absolute and carrot seed oil to 1 tablespoon rosehip seed oil.

Safe usage Non-toxic, non-irritant in dilution.

The plant

The essential oil of violet is an absolute, concentrated in the downy heart-shaped leaves rather than in the purple flowers. It takes around 1000kg (2200lb) of violet leaves to produce just 1kg (2¼lb) of the absolute, which is why true violet absolute is so expensive, and mostly used in high-end perfume products.

The essential oil

The absolute essential oil of violet is solvent-extracted from the crushed leaves of the plant. This process produces a thick oil that is a green to brown colour. It has an earthy aroma with intense, elegant floral notes that make it a valuable ingredient in perfumes.

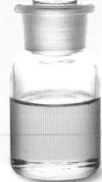

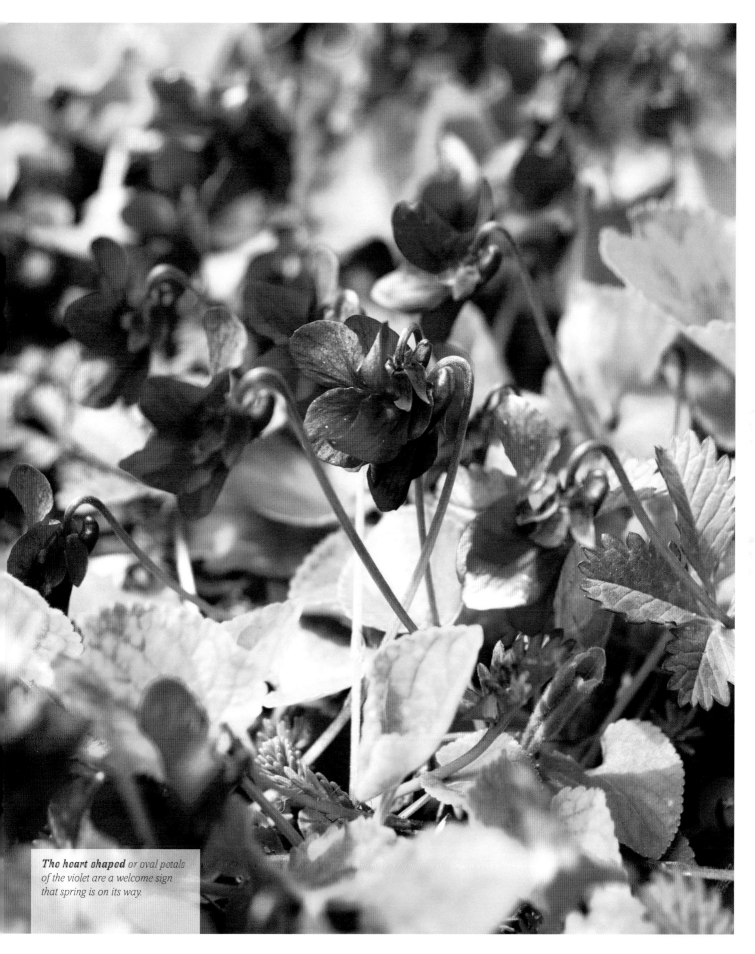

The heart shaped or oval petals
of the violet are a welcome sign
that spring is on its way.

COMPRESS

DIFFUSER

Plai

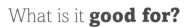
Zingiber cassumunar, Z. montanum

Although plai is related to ginger, it is a **cooling,** rather than a warming, oil, making it ideal for feverish conditions and inflammation. It has a general **tonic** effect on the body and is highly valued for its ability to **relieve** the pain of arthritis and rheumatism and even post-operative pain. Plai is also a traditional Thai treatment for stretch marks.

A
PERFECT
BLEND

Plai essential oil blends well with marjoram, black pepper, helichrysum, rosemary, cypress, lavender, and neroli essential oils.

What is it **good for?**

Acts as an antihistamine With its cooling, anti-inflammatory action, plai makes a natural antihistamine that can be helpful for managing conditions such as hay fever. Its soothing action has the potential to reduce the severity of asthma attacks in some individuals, where it can be used as a complementary treatment alongside prescribed medication.

Acts as a painkiller Plai essential oil is a popular analgesic that helps to ease many types of pain, including pain caused by injury, strained muscles, arthritis, and rheumatism. Some evidence suggests it may help relieve post-operative pain and inflammation.

Fades scars and stretch marks In Thailand, plai is a traditional remedy used to reduce the appearance of stretch marks and scars.

Relieves abdominal cramps Plai essential oil has antispasmodic and analgesic properties that can help to relieve menstrual cramping as well as the pain that is caused by irritable bowel syndrome.

Best **uses**

As a compress To help soothe and relieve sprains and strains, add 4–5 drops of plai essential oil to a shallow bowl of cool water, then soak a small, clean cloth in the mixture, wring it out well, and apply the cloth to the affected area.

In a diffuser To relieve the misery of hay fever and help reduce the severity of asthma attacks, try adding 3–4 drops of plai essential oil to a diffuser, vaporizer, or oil burner to disperse in a room.

Safe usage Non toxic, non-irritant in dilution.

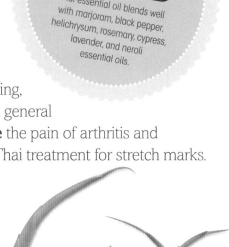

The plant

The therapeutic properties of the plai plant are concentrated in its distinctive root. It is also an ornamental plant with its distinctive blade-shaped leaves and brightly coloured "pseudo-stem" that resembles a pine cone.

The essential oil

Steam-distilled from the fresh roots of the plai plant, the colourless to pale yellow oil has an uplifting herbaceous, spicy aroma with hints of eucalyptus.

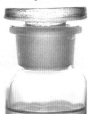

MOUTHWASH

MASSAGE OIL

Ginger

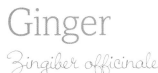
Zingiber officinale

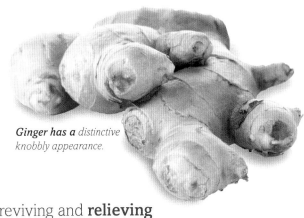

Ginger has a distinctive knobbly appearance.

Most of us know ginger as the remedy of choice for reviving and **relieving** the nausea that often accompanies pregnancy or travel sickness. In addition, it is also a useful **antiseptic** in cases of cold or flu, and it has an **analgesic** property that can help to ease tension headaches and muscular pain.

What is it **good for?**

Eases digestion Ginger has a wonderfully calming effect on the digestive system, helping to soothe unsettled digestion caused by stress or over-indulgence. It also relieves pregnancy-related nausea and nausea caused by motion sickness or the side effects of medication.

Revives a tired mind Comforting and warming, ginger essential oil helps to lift feelings of general fatigue and is also reviving when you are suffering from nervous fatigue or mental confusion.

Helps to combat colds Antiseptic and pain-relieving, ginger essential oil can help to ward off cold viruses, and once a cold has set in, it can soothe the pain and discomfort of sore throats, and ease congestion.

Relieves muscle pain Applied locally, ginger oil boosts circulation and provides warmth that revives and eases the pain of sore, tired muscles.

Relieves headaches Its anti-inflammatory and analgesic properties make ginger a natural choice for relieving headaches and migraines.

Best **uses**

For a gargle Add 2 drops of ginger essential oil to 1 teaspoon vodka and dilute in a small tumblerful of hot water. When sufficiently cooled, use as a gargle to treat sore throats.

In a massage oil For quick relief from headaches, migraines, and/or nausea, blend 2 drops of ginger essential oil with 1 teaspoon base oil. Massage gently into the temples and pulse points as needed.

Safe usage Non-toxic, non-irritant in dilution.

The plant

The ginger plant produces a distinctive, knobbly root that has been used as a culinary and medicinal ingredient for thousands of years, especially by the Chinese. Its enduring popularity is testament to the plant's therapeutic healing properties and its widespread culinary appeal.

The essential oil

Ginger essential oil is steam-distilled from the fleshy root of the ginger plant. The oil can vary in colour from pale yellow to dark amber and has a warm, spicy, woody scent with a hint of lemon and pepper.

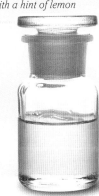

Naturally soothing, ginger is the go-to remedy for digestive upsets.

Base
Oils

Base, or carrier, oils provide a medium for **diluting and dispersing** concentrated essential oils, which can otherwise irritate skin. Derived from **vegetable, nut, or seed sources**, or made by macerating a **herb** in a plant oil, base oils have their own benefits.

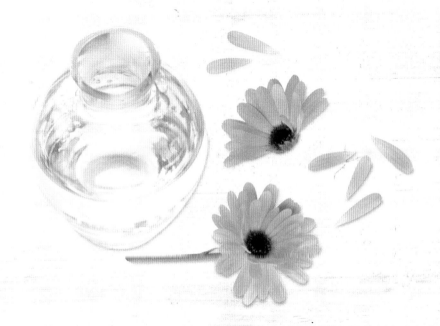

Argan

Argania spinosa

Argan oil comes from a tree found growing only in Morocco. With high levels of antioxidant **vitamin E** and essential fatty acids, it's a soothing oil for all skin types, and for hair and nails. It is **moisturizing** and protective against environmental factors, such as weather and pollutants.

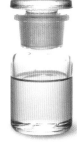

The kernels of the Moroccan argan fruit produce the rich, skin-nourishing, golden–yellow argan oil.

Argan oil has a characteristic nutty aroma.

What is it **good for?**

Makes an all-round moisturizer
A non-greasy, dry oil that can be used under make-up during the day and for skin repair at night, argan can minimize the appearance of scars and stretch marks and help to soften sun- or wind-damaged skin. Apply sparingly to lips before bedtime to aid healing and repair skin overnight.

Acts as a hand conditioner
Warm a few drops of the oil in the palms, then massage well into the hands, taking extra time to work into the nails and cuticles.

Conditions hair For damaged or dry hair, argan oil conditions and restores shine. Use as a pre-wash deep treatment, or for frizzy hair, rub a few drops into the hair just after washing for light control.

Tones skin With regular use, the oil helps to balance oily skin and reduce inflammation around spots and acne.

Borage

Borago officinalis

This oil is pressed from the seeds of the borage, or starflower, plant. Added to a base oil blend, it has a **beneficial effect** on mature, damaged, **sensitive skin**, or skin prone to breakouts due to hormonal fluctuations.

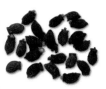

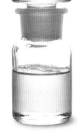

Borage seeds are mainly grown commercially for their oil.

This pale yellow, almost odourless, oil has strong anti-inflammatory properties.

What is it **good for?**

Rejuvenates skin Borage is a great choice for mature or damaged skin. It contains the fatty acid gamma linolenic acid (GLA), which helps to tone and rejuvenate skin. It has a hydrating effect and is regenerating, increasing skin-cell strength and improving elasticity.

Reduces inflammation Its anti-inflammatory properties make borage a good choice for skin prone to eczema, psoriasis, seborrheic

The borage herb is native to the Mediterranean region.

dermatitis, and breakouts due to hormonal fluctuations.

Keeps nails healthy Use the oil regularly on nails to maintain strength and keep cuticles healthy.

Enriches skin Just a small amount of this oil enriches a base oil blend. In blends and serums, borage is used at 2–10 per cent of the total base oil mix.

Canola

Brassica napus

Also known as rapeseed oil, canola has the benefits of being **widely available**, relatively **inexpensive**, and effective on dry, sensitive, or mature skin. However, it's often genetically modified and highly processed so choose organic brands.

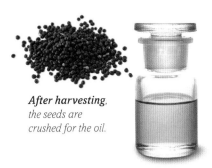

After harvesting, the seeds are crushed for the oil.

This golden oil is virtually odourless so works well in aromatherapy blends.

What is it **good for?**

Moisturizes skin Light and easily absorbed, canola helps to maintain the moisture balance of dry skin.

It is a widely available base oil You don't need to go to a specialist shop to find canola. Good, food-quality canola is available in the supermarket. Canola is also very stable so keeps for a long time.

Provides a neutral base The oil is almost odourless, so works well with most blends. Enrich it with avocado, borage or rosehip seed oil, or enhance its skin-soothing properties by adding a healing macerate such as calendula or St John's wort.

From the brassica family, canola has delicate yellow blooms.

Safe usage *Ideally, choose organic oil to avoid possible pesticide residues that can be present in some genetically modified organisms (GMOs).*

Shea nut butter

Butyrospermum parkii

Extracted from the nuts of African karite trees, shea butter has a long history in cooking, but has more recently found its way into cosmetic formulations where its thick, **waxy texture** acts like an **emulsifier** and provides **skin-enriching** properties.

Shea nut butter ranges from bright yellow in its raw state to white.

The oil has a nutty, sweet aroma. The less odour and colour, the more refined it is.

What is it **good for?**

Repairs damaged skin Rich in fatty acids, antioxidant carotenoids, and vitamin E, shea nut butter helps to improve the condition of dry and mature skin and soothes eczema, psoriasis, skin allergies, and blemishes. It can also be used to treat dry, itchy scalp conditions.

Hydrates skin The fatty acids in shea nut butter are a good match for those in human skin. By helping to form a thin protective layer on the skin, the oil helps prevent moisture loss and encourages healing of chapped lips. It also helps to soften cracked, dry skin on heels, elbows, and knees.

Can be used as a shaving balm Adding shea nut butter to shaving cream formulations helps to achieve a smoother shave.

Calendula macerated oil

Calendula officinalis

Calendula macerated oil is made by infusing marigold flowers into an oil such as sunflower. The result is a **rich** herbal oil with recognized **healing** properties. Calendula is especially popular for sensitive and dry skin due to its ability to **soothe** irritated skin quickly and **repair** skin tissue.

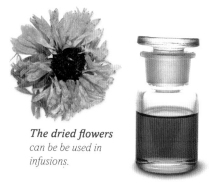

The dried flowers can be be used in infusions.

This macerated oil, made from the fresh flowers, is a rich golden colour.

What is it **good for?**

Repairs skin Calendula is mildly antiseptic so it can help ulcers, skin eruptions, cuts, and dermatitis to heal more quickly.

Can be used as after-sun skin care Calendula oil helps to condition and restore skin, and reduces inflammation after sun exposure.

Acts as a healing massage oil Calendula makes a good choice when a large area of skin requires attention as the oil spreads more easily over a large surface area than a cream-based product does.

Can be used for first aid Hypercal cream, which is a mainstay of most natural first-aid kits, is a mixture of hypericum (St John's wort) and calendula. If you are making a skin salve or ointment, add calendula macerate to help speed healing time.

Coconut

Cocos nucifera

This is a light, **moisturizing**, and **nourishing** semi-solid that quickly melts at body temperature. Coconut oil is suitable for all skin and hair types, but is especially beneficial for dry skin and hair. Raw, unrefined, unbleached organic coconut oil is best and adds a **pleasant aroma** to blends.

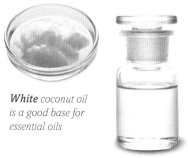

White coconut oil is a good base for essential oils

Coconut oil is a semi-solid that melts at body temerpature to produce a liquid that can be used in aromatherapy blends.

What is it **good for?**

Conditions hair Coconut oil helps combat dandruff and can restore lustre and shine to dry or damaged hair. Use the oil as a pre-shampoo conditioner or, for deeper conditioning, leave in overnight and wash the oil out in the morning.

Acts as a make-up remover Warm a little bit of coconut oil between the palms, then gently massage over the face and use a tissue or a damp facecloth to remove make up.

Heals rough, irritated skin The oil has an anti-inflammatory effect that can help to heal wounds, blisters, and rashes and to soothe razor burn after shaving. Use in place of mineral oil for chapped lips and for eczema and dermatitis.

Cares for teeth and gums The practice of "oil pulling" – swishing around 1 tablespoon coconut oil in the mouth for 20 minutes – helps to reduce bacteria, control plaque, and fight decay and infection. Don't swallow; there's also no need to rinse afterwards.

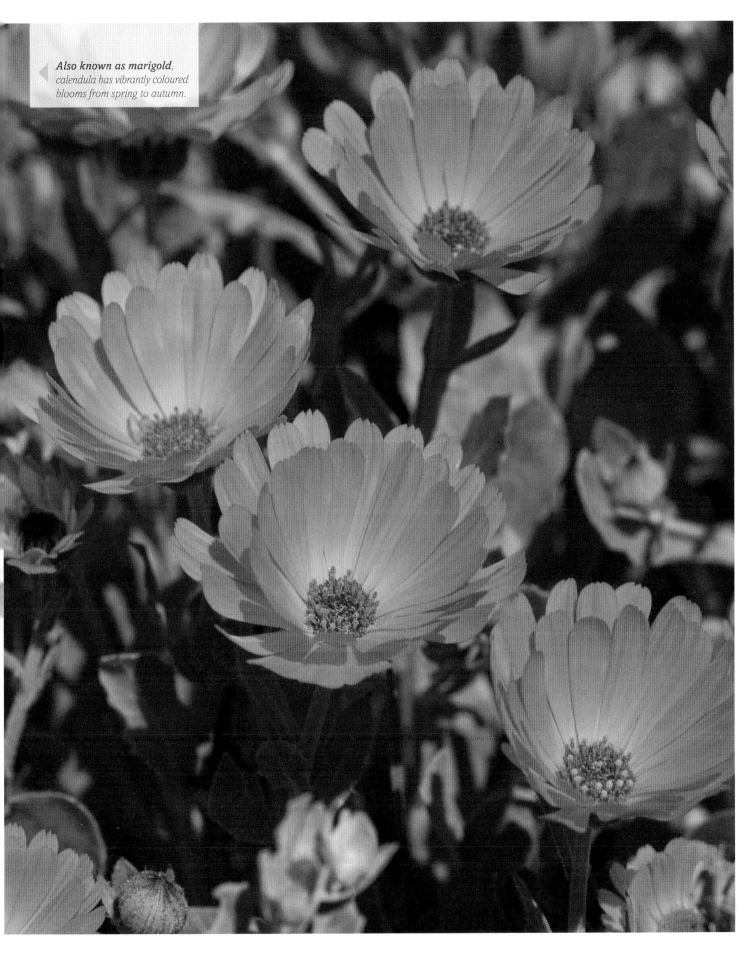

Also known as marigold, calendula has vibrantly coloured blooms from spring to autumn.

Hazelnut

Corylus avellana

A light oil with a fine texture and mild, nutty aroma, hazelnut is **rich in nutrients**, including vitamin E and linoleic acid, an essential fatty acid that protects the outer layer of skin. A **nourishing** oil, it is ideal for **reviving** dull, damaged, or dry skin. Its gentle **astringent** action improves skin tone.

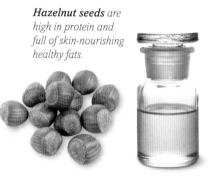

Hazelnut seeds are high in protein and full of skin-nourishing healthy fats.

This pale yellow oil is rich in vitamins and minerals.

What is it **good for?**

Balances skin Hazelnut oil is an excellent choice for a facial massage oil, especially for oily or acne-prone skin types. Its astringent action helps to tone and balance skin, while its emollient properties provide moisture and protection for skin. The oil can also be used to balance and condition oily hair.

Protects skin Its light texture makes this oil a good choice for wind- and sun-damaged skin. It can be added to skin creams to take advantage of its mild SPF factor, and to after-sun treatments to help repair and condition skin.

Works in a blend Hazelnut can be used on its own or as an enriching oil for a base-oil blend. For example, if skin is very dry but still needs toning, try blending this oil with a deeply moisturizing oil such as rosehip seed or avocado oil to create the combination that's right for your skin.

Sunflower

Helianthus annuus

A popular and affordable all-purpose oil, sunflower blends easily with other bases and essential oils. It is very high in **vitamin E**, which repairs and protects skin, and is easily absorbed into the skin.

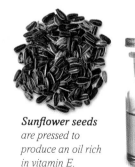

Sunflower seeds are pressed to produce an oil rich in vitamin E.

A pale golden colour, sunflower oil has a delicate, nutty aroma and is a natural emulsifier.

What is it **good for?**

The cheery sunflower produces edible seeds.

Hydrates skin There is evidence that sunflower oil can help to improve the barrier function of the skin, helping skin to retain moisture and fight off infection. This effect is due to the presence of light waxes, which help form a protective emollient barrier on the skin.

Heals skin The oil is protective and helps to repair sun-damaged skin. Healing vitamin E and carotenoids (a vegetable form of vitamin A) can reduce scarring and smooth the appearance of existing wrinkles and fine lines. In addition, the oil contains omega-6 linoleic acid, which helps decrease skin inflammation in acne, eczema, and sunburn, and helps to generate new skin cells.

Treats acne The carotenoids in the oil are excellent for cleansing and moisturizing acne-prone skin.

St. John's wort macerated oil

Hypericum perforatum

The well-known **sedative** effects of St John's wort herb also exist in the macerated oil, which is made by infusing a base oil with the fresh or dried herb. It has a **pain-relieving** effect, and its **anti-inflammatory** properties have a calming action on red, sore or inflamed skin conditions.

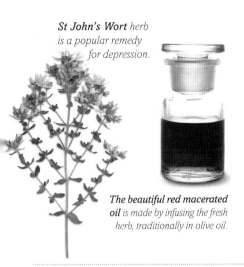

St John's Wort herb is a popular remedy for depression.

The beautiful red macerated oil is made by infusing the fresh herb, traditionally in olive oil.

What is it **good for?**

Calms inflammation Try using this oil to treat dry, painful inflamed skin conditions, such as eczema, psoriasis, and some types of lupus. It can also be used at the first sign of a tingle to treat cold sores and viral skin lesions.

Acts as a painkiller The oil can help calm nerve pain and soothe inflamed joints and tendonitis, as well as reduce inflammation in sunburn, minor scalds, cuts, and grazes. It can also relieve muscle and nerve pain.

Is a good massage base St John's wort adds a grounding, earthy aroma to a massage. It can be used on its own or added to massage oil blends to boost the effects of a relaxing massage. It also works well added to blends intended to treat nervousness, depression, and premenstrual or menopausal symptoms.

Safe usage *Do not apply before sun exposure as the oil may increase the photo-sensitivity of the skin.*

Flaxseed oil

Linum usitatissimum

Pressed from the tiny seeds of the plant, flaxseed oil is **rich in omega-3 fatty acids** and vitamin E, making it a **rejuvenating** oil for tired, dry or mature skin. Also known as linseed oil, it has **antioxidant** and **anti-inflammatory** qualities that can benefit acne-prone skin.

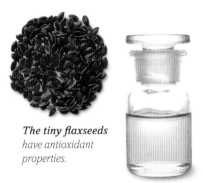

The tiny flaxseeds have antioxidant properties.

For the best-quality oil, look for cold-pressed and unfiltered products.

What is it **good for?**

Fades scars and stretch marks The high vitamin E content of flaxseed oil helps to reduce the appearance of scarring and stretch marks.

Hydrates skin Flaxseed oil seals in moisture, making a reviving remedy for dry skin conditions. Its anti-inflammatory action calms eczema and psoriasis.

Has anti-ageing effects The omega-3 fatty acids in flaxseed oil help protect and rejuvenate skin cells,

brightening dull-looking skin and smoothing the appearance of lines.

Treats acne Use the oil to cleanse and condition oily or acne-prone skin and rosacea. It contains omega-3 alpha-linolenic acid (ALA), a powerful anti-inflammatory that reduces the soreness and redness around acne.

Enriches base oil blends Flax seed generally isn't used on its own, but is added to other base oils, creams, and lotions to add skin-strengthening properties.

Macadamia

Macadamia ternifolia

This **protective silky oil** is pressed from the native Australian nut. It has a sweet, nutty aroma and contains naturally high amounts of **palmitoleic acid**, also found in human sebum. This acid helps to protect skin from premature ageing and weather damage.

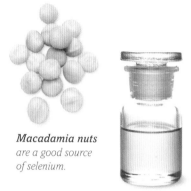

Macadamia nuts are a good source of selenium.

The pale yellow oil produced from the macadamia has a nutty aroma and a similar texture to human sebum.

What is it **good for?**

Protects skin Macadamia oil contains nourishing fatty acids and sterols, or plant hormones, that help to moisturize and repair skin. It is a great choice for healing skin after too much exposure to the sun, wind, or cold weather conditions. The oil is also great for conditioning hair.

Has anti-ageing effects Macadamia is rich in omega-7 palmitoleic acid, which has been shown to help delay skin ageing.

The oil has a particularly regenerating, moisturizing, and hydrating effect on mature skin. It is also non-irritating to the skin around the eyes – try patting the tiniest amount around the eyes to fight bags and sagging skin.

It is long-lasting Macadamia will keep longer than most nut and seed oils (up to 12 months), but it needs to be stored in a cool dark place to keep it at its best.

Neem

Melia azadirachta

Pressed from the fruit and seeds of the tree, neem oil is highly **antiseptic** – a little goes a long way. It has a strong, pungent odour so is best used to **enrich** other oils. It is particularly good at helping to **heal** infections and for dry skin conditions, and makes an effective **insect repellent**.

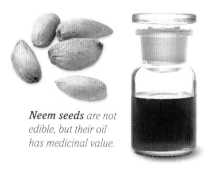

Neem seeds are not edible, but their oil has medicinal value.

The distinctive-looking oil has a strong aroma and should be used in small quantites only.

What is it **good for?**

Treats dandruff Neem is a useful dandruff remedy. Try blending with coconut oil for a pre-wash hair mask. Leave in for 10 minutes, then rinse off.

Works well in blends Neem is effective even in small amounts and blending it helps to counter its strong aroma. To find what works for you, start with just a few drops diluted in a neutral base oil, such as sunflower or almond, and gradually increase the amount to no more than 5 per cent of the blend.

Acts as an insect repellent Neem is a powerful insecticide that has become a staple of many natural head-lice treatments and mosquito repellents. For head lice, apply neat from root to tip and comb through with a nit comb, then wash out.

Heals skin The oil can be dabbed neat on to cold sores and contains anti-inflammatory compounds that help ease eczema and psoriasis. Its skin-softening properties can improve the appearance of scaly, dry skin.

Moringa

Moringa oleifera

Also known as ben oil, moringa is pressed from the seeds of the plant. It contains high levels of the fatty **oleic acid** and is a deeply penetrating oil with skin-softening properties. It is rich in **antioxidants**, which help to protect skin from premature ageing due to free radicals.

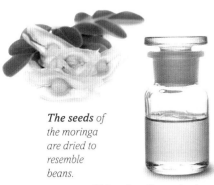

The seeds of the moringa are dried to resemble beans.

This pale yellow, odourless oil is rich in fatty acids that soften and moisturize skin.

What is it **good for?**

It makes a good massage base Highly lubricating and similar in composition to olive oil, but much lighter and odourless, moringa oil makes an ideal oil base for aromatherapy massage blends. Its light texture in particular helps to make a pleasant facial massage or elixir.

Conditions skin Moringa can help to reduce the appearance of large pores, as well as fine lines, wrinkles, stretch marks, and scars.

Moisturizes skin Its high fatty-acid content nourishes skin and helps prevent moisture loss. The oil provides instant hydration for dry, damaged, or mature skin. Blend with coconut oil to make a hair and scalp treatment that restores shine and fights dandruff.

Helps controls acne With antibacterial and anti-inflammatory properties, the oil is useful for acne-prone skin. Studies show that moringa can help to kill off the germs that can cause skin infections.

Evening primrose

Oenothera biennis

Cold-pressed from the oil-rich seeds, evening primrose is an **enriching** oil that contains **skin-loving fatty acids**, such as omega-6 linoleic acid, which strengthens membranes around the skin, and **anti-ageing** gamma linolenic acid (GLA).

The fragrant flowers of the evening primrose are edible.

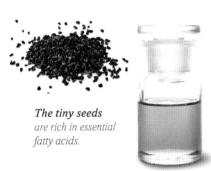

The tiny seeds are rich in essential fatty acids.

Golden evening primrose oil is pressed from the seeds of the plant, but has a short shelf life.

What is it **good for?**

Has anti-ageing effects Light and easily absorbed, the oil has anti-inflammatory and skin-rejuvenating properties that can improve tone and elasticity in mature skin.

Conditions skin Evening primrose helps skin retain moisture and increases skin cells' ability to absorb oxygen and fight off infection. The oil penetrates deep into the skin, helping to heal conditions such as eczema and acne. To help soften brittle and easily breakable nails, rub in 1–2 drops daily.

Can be added to cosmetics If you are adding evening primrose oil to home-made cosmetics, it should make up 5–10 per cent of the blend. The oil has a short shelf life, so once opened, it should be stored in the fridge and used within 6–9 months. If you need just a small amount for a massage blend or cream, add from capsules, rather than open a bottle.

Olive

Olea europea

Rich in skin-nourishing **fatty acids**, **antioxidants**, and **vitamin E**, over the years olive oil has earned its reputation as an affordable, but also superior, **moisturizing** and healing treatment. Use it neat or in a multitude of cosmetic formulations for skin and hair.

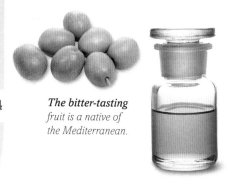

The bitter-tasting fruit is a native of the Mediterranean.

This heavy, viscous green oil is widely used for both culinary and cosmetic purposes.

What is it **good for?**

Conditions skin This deeply penetrating oil helps to keep skin soft and well-conditioned. A naturally occurring compound, squalene, provides a barrier against water loss. Rub a few drops into the nails and cuticles to protect and condition them.

Has anti-ageing effects Its antioxidant properties help maintain the integrity of skin cells and fight off the effects of free radicals, which cause premature skin ageing.

Can be used as a hair tonic Olive oil can be used as a pre-treatment before shampooing, or as an overnight hair mask to treat dry and damaged hair and irritated, sensitive scalps.

Acts as a make-up remover Olive oil makes an effective and simple make-up remover, helping to lift all traces of grime and dirt and leave skin well moisturized and conditioned.

Avocado

Persea gratissima

Avocado is one of the best oils for **soothing** dry skin and softening rough skin patches, such as those on the elbows and heels. Naturally high in vitamins, minerals, and **antioxidants**, the rich oil is cold-pressed from the fruit and used in small amounts to **enrich** lighter oil bases.

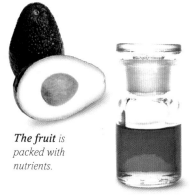

The fruit is packed with nutrients.

Avocado oil is pressed from the fruit (not the skin) and is a distinctive dark green colour.

What is it **good for?**

Conditions and soothes skin Avocado helps to hydrate parched skin and aid the regeneration of skin cells. A high fatty acid content means this is a great oil for conditioning rough skin on the feet, knees, or elbows, and also for reviving hair damaged by styling or the sun.

Repairs and protects skin If used regularly, the oil can help to prevent or minimize the appearance of stretch marks.

Acts as an anti-ageing oil Avocado oil gives lustre and shine to tired or dull complexions. It contains fatty acids and phytosterols (plant hormones) that help to replenish and revitalize mature skin.

Acts as a natural SPF While it can't be used as a sunscreen on its own, avocado oil does contain a natural SPF factor at a low level that can help to protect skin and hair from sun exposure. The oil also relieves the pain of sunburn.

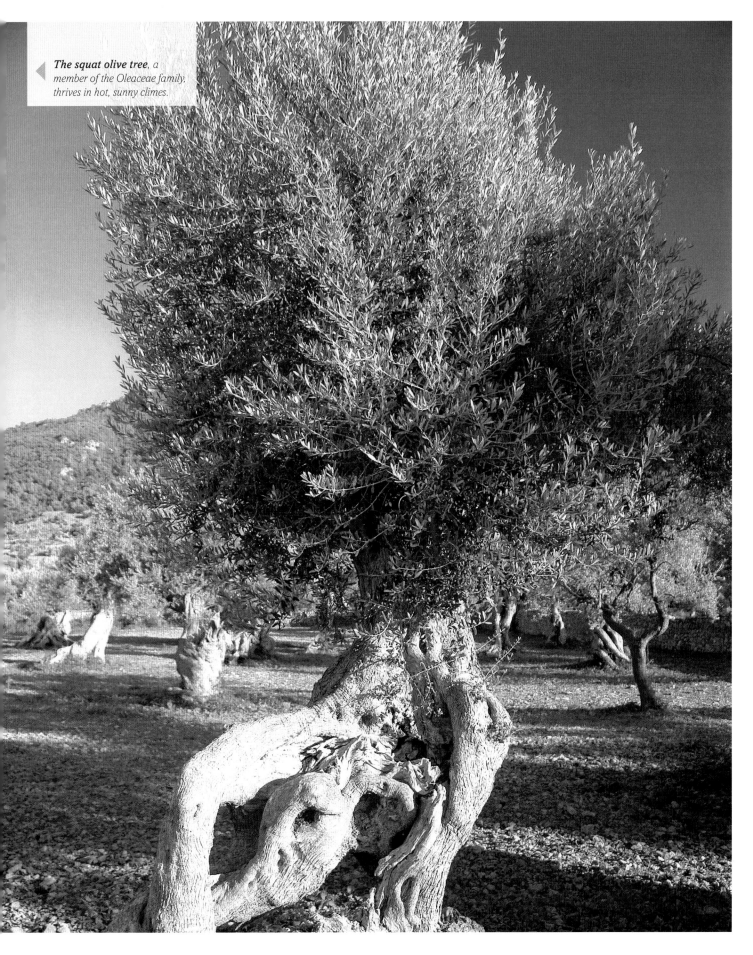

The squat olive tree, a member of the Oleaceae family, thrives in hot, sunny climes.

Almond

Prunus amygdalus dulcis

This light general-purpose oil is cold-pressed from the seeds of the sweet almond tree. Vitamin rich, the oil is suitable for **all skin types**, but especially for **sensitive skins**, and it is gentle enough to be used on children. It helps **soothe** dry, irritated skin and prevent moisture loss.

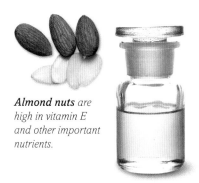

Almond nuts are high in vitamin E and other important nutrients.

Almond oil, pressed from the seeds of the tree, is a light oil with a subtle aroma.

What is it **good for?**

Acts as a natural moisturizer
Almond oil provides a long-lasting barrier against the elements that helps prevent moisture loss, soothes and encourages the healing of dry, irritated skin, and relieves inflamed skin conditions, such as eczema.

It is suitable for babies and young children
Almond oil is gentle enough to use on babies and young children, for example to treat nappy rash or cradle cap. Other gentle oils, such as olive and sunflower are also recommended for babies.

Helps lubricate massage blends
The oil is absorbed slowly, which makes it a popular choice as a massage oil base. It also has a delicate aroma that will not compete with the essential oils in a blend.

Acts as a make-up remover
Almond oil removes dirt and make-up effectively, leaving the skin feeling soft and supple.

Apricot kernel

Prunus armeniaca

Apricot kernel oil is a **light cold-pressed oil**, rich in the fatty acid known as gamma linoleic acid, or GLA, which helps skin to maintain its moisture balance. Light enough to leave no greasy residue, the oil is particularly suitable as a base for facial serums and light **moisturizing** lotions.

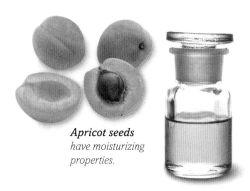

Apricot seeds have moisturizing properties.

Apricot kernel oil is an emollient oil that helps to soften skin. A pale to dark yellow, it has a nutty aroma.

What is it **good for?**

Helps restore moisture
If skin feels dry, itchy, or tight after bathing or cleansing, this is the perfect oil to apply lightly to damp skin before towelling off. For mature skin, it is softening and improves skin elasticity, helping to smooth out fine lines.

It is suitable for sensitive skin
Apricot oil soothes sensitive skin and provides a thin barrier against irritants. It makes an ideal substitute for petroleum-based baby oils.

Acts as a massage base
Apricot kernel absorbs more slowly than some oils, which makes it a great base for massage blends and night-time skin treatments. A little goes a long way, so buy the best you can afford.

Conditions hair
The oil makes an effective treatment for flyaway hair and also minimizes the appearance of split ends. Work a few drops into damp hair and allow it to dry naturally to seal in moisture all day long.

Rosehip seed

Rosa cannina

The oil from the seeds of the rose plant is a luxurious source of **skin-nourishing** fatty acids. Renowned for its **soothing** anti-inflammatory effect, it is suited to dry, mature, and weather-damaged skin.

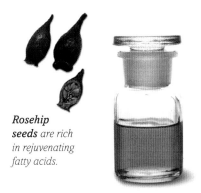

Rosehip seeds are rich in rejuvenating fatty acids.

The golden oil can be used neat on small areas of skin, or added to blends to enrich other oils.

The rose plant produces clusters of bright red seeds.

What is it **good for?**

Has anti-ageing effects Rosehip contains the essential fatty acids omegas 3 and 6 that support cell and tissue regeneration, helping to keep skin supple and reduce the appearance of fine lines around the eyes. It is great for treating spider veins.

Prevents scarring The oil can be added to body lotions and creams to minimize the appearance of stretch marks. It can also help reduce scarring from wounds, burns, and after surgery.

Treats acne The oil is a source of trans-retinoic acid, a form of vitamin A, which is a recognized treatment for acne-prone skin. Rosehip helps balance the skin's oils and its toning action minimizes pores. It is also good for calming pimples and boils.

Eases itching Soothing and easily absorbed, when the skin is dry and itchy rosehip seed's cooling, anti-inflammatory action brings quick relief.

Sesame

Sesamum Indicum

Pressed from the familiar sesame seed, this oil is **packed with nutrients**, including vitamin E and potassium, both of which help to **rejuvenate** and **protect** the skin. The oil also has inherent **anti-inflammatory** properties, making it especially suited to healing dry skin conditions.

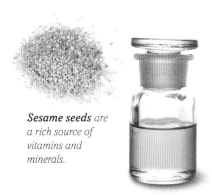

Sesame seeds are a rich source of vitamins and minerals.

The slightly thick, pale yellow oil was used traditionally as a healing salve and is a popular cooking oil.

What is it **good for?**

Tones skin This deeply penetrating oil helps to repair damaged cells and improve circulation, which in turn gives tired or weather-damaged skin a healthy glow.

Useful for head and face massage Ayurvedic practitioners believe that even without the addition of essential oils, sesame oil produces a calming and warming effect that boosts circulation and aids detox, while relieving stress and promoting sleep.

Moisturizes skin Sesame helps to keep skin hydrated, and is particularly well suited to those with dry to normal skin. The oil also relieves itchy, burning, and inflamed skin conditions.

Acts as a sunscreen While sesame oil can't be used on its own to protect the skin against the sun's damaging rays, adding some of the oil to facial and body preparations will boost their SPF factor, while also helping to protect skin from the harmful effects of free radicals that are generated by the sun's rays.

Jojoba

Simmondsia chinensis

Jojoba is actually a **liquid wax** rather than an oil, and because it is so similar to human sebum, it is considered one of the main treatments for dry and mature skin. Its waxy nature adds a **protective** layer that helps skin retain moisture. Readily absorbed, it can be used on all skin types.

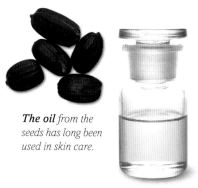

The oil from the seeds has long been used in skin care.

Jojoba oil is a long-lasting oil which is actually a liquid wax that has a bright golden appearance.

What is it **good for?**

Conditions skin and hair Jojoba can be used to soften hard, dry or rough skin and to relieve the symptoms of skin conditions such as eczema and psoriasis. Just a little added to hair gives instant shine and it can also be used to treat dry scalp conditions and dandruff.

Has anti-ageing effects Jojoba is a good oil for dry, chapped, weather-worn, and mature skins. It helps to reduce water loss and improves suppleness and elasticity, helping to reduce the appearance of fine lines, wrinkles, and scars.

Acts as a make-up remover Jojoba oil is suitable for all skin types, and can be used to lift and dissolve the dirt and oil that clogs pores, leaving skin instantly moisturized. Its thick texture makes it a great substitute for soap when shaving. A little applied to the legs or face helps to lubricate the skin, enabling an extra close shave that also helps to prevent razor irritation.

Cocoa butter

Theobroma cacao

A natural and effective **emollient** with a distinctive chocolate–vanilla aroma, cocoa butter can be added to body and face creams and balms to **provide a barrier** against moisture loss and environmental damage. It is good for dry and damaged skin, and helps to fade stretch marks.

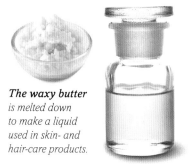

The waxy butter is melted down to make a liquid used in skin- and hair-care products.

When melted down, the oil can be used as an emulsifier to hold oil- and water-based products together.

What is it **good for?**

Prevents moisture loss Cocoa butter acts as a barrier to prevent water loss and keep skin hydrated. The oil aids skin elasticity and tone by supporting collagen production, helping to prevent premature wrinkles and reduce stretch marks. It also helps soften and hydrate the hair.

Thickens creams and acts as an emulsifier Solid and pale yellow at room temperature, cocoa butter can be gently melted into face and bodycare formulations to thicken them and add benefits. Cocoa butter is a natural emulsifier, helping oil- and water-based lotions to hold together.

Best for clear skin and dry complexions Cocoa butter can be occlusive, which means it can clog pores. For this reason it may not be suitable for skin that is prone to acne or pimples.

Wheatgerm

Triticum vulgare

A **nurturing** and **skin-protecting** oil, wheatgerm oil has the highest vitamin E content of any vegetable oil and is also rich in betacarotene. While too sticky and thick to use on its own, the oil adds multiple **skin-conditioning** benefits to base oil blends and lotions and creams.

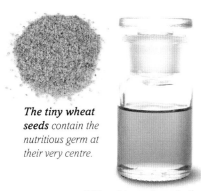

The tiny wheat seeds contain the nutritious germ at their very centre.

This golden-coloured oil has a dense texture and a distinctive aroma.

What is it **good for?**

Repairs skin Wheatgerm oil moisturizes and heals dry or cracked skin, and also helps to fade scarring and stretch marks. It is an especially rich source of vitamin E, which helps to protect skin from the effects of the weather, to moisturize and heal dry or cracked skin, and to maintain an even skin tone.

Has anti-ageing effects Vitamin E helps fight the effects on the skin of damaging free radicals and supports cellular regeneration and collagen formation. Vitamin E-rich wheatgerm has a revitalizing effect on mature or weather-worn skin, helping to rejuvenate and prevent the development of premature fine lines around the eyes and mouth.

Works well in a blend With its thick, sticky consistency and distinctive grassy–nutty aroma, wheatgerm oil is best used to enrich the powers of other lighter base oils. It should make up 5–10 per cent of the final base oil blend.

Grapeseed

Vitis vinifera

This light, odourless, and inexpensive all-purpose oil can be used in a wide array of applications from massage to skin care. High in **antioxidants**, it is mild, but very nourishing. It has good **emollient** properties and a gentle **toning** effect that benefits both mature and acne-prone skin.

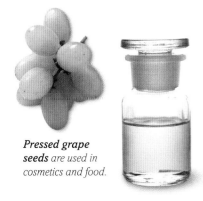

Pressed grape seeds are used in cosmetics and food.

This smooth, pale oil has a short shelf life of around six months and keeps best in a cool, dark place.

What is it **good for?**

Has anti-ageing effects Rich in the emollient linoleic acid (omega-6), grapeseed oil leaves the skin with a satiny finish. The oil is easily absorbed and has a mildly astringent effect that helps to tone and condition tired or dull-looking skin.

Is suitable for allergenic and sensitive skin This non-allergenic oil is suitable for those who cannot use nut oils. It is mild enough to use on infants and on sensitive skin.

Treats acne Grapeseed's astringent properties help to balance oily and acne-prone skin, refreshing the complexion and reducing redness and irritation.

Is a good massage base Grapeseed oil makes a great non-greasy base oil for massage blends. It also has the added benefit of dispersing in water, making it an ideal choice for bath-oil blends.

Healing
Remedies

Harness the **healing powers** of essential oils to provide relief from a range of **common complaints**. Learn how to use oils in **therapeutic massages** and baths, clearing inhalations, **soothing compresses**, and skin-healing ointments and creams.

Digestive problems

Lifestyle factors such as diet, as well as **stress** and emotional upset, can all impact on the **healthy functioning** of the digestive system, leading to blockages and other problems. Essential oils treat digestive upsets **holistically**, addressing both the root causes, such as anxiety, and providing relief for symptoms. If a condition persists or is acute, consult your doctor.

Bloating and constipation

The unpleasant feeling of being bloated occurs when your abdomen is stretched, puffy, and uncomfortable. It's common to feel this way during a festive period or celebrations. You can avoid feeling overfull by cutting down on fizzy drinks, monitoring portion sizes, sitting down to eat, and taking regular exercise. Constipation can be caused by poor diet and stress, and symptoms can be relieved by making dietary and lifestyle changes. Try increasing your daily intake of fibre to at least 18–30g ($^3/_4$–1oz) a day. Fresh fruit, vegetables, and cereals are all high in fibre. You can also try including some bulking agents in your diet, such as oat bran, which helps to make stools softer and easier to pass. Drink plenty of water, too, exercise regularly, and keep active. The following remedies can help to ease digestive complaints.

Settling carrot and orange compress

The combination of carrot seed, orange, and fennel in this warming compress has a tonifying and soothing effect on the digestive system. Orange essential oil calms unsettled digestion and helps food move through the digestive tract, in turn relieving constipation, trapped wind, and easing indigestion. Carrot seed is mildly diuretic so helps to reduce fluid retention, and soothing fennel eases nervous indigestion caused by emotional upset, or indigestion after a rushed meal. This remedy is not suitable in pregnancy.

Ingredients

Makes 1 compress
Almond oil 1 tsp
Orange essential oil 3 drops
Fennel essential oil 2 drops
Carrot seed essential oil 2 drops

How to **make**

1 Fill a bowl with hot water. Add the essential oils to the base oil, then add to the water.

2 Soak a flannel in the bowl, then remove the flannel and squeeze out the excess water.

3 Wrap the flannel in a towel or cling film to insulate it. Place the compress on the abdomen. Leave the flannel in place while it cools to body temperature, then repeat 3 times.

Stimulating spearmint massage

Abdominal massage is an effective way to treat constipation and is easily self-administered. Cooling spearmint essential oil is extremely soothing for digestion as it helps to calm nausea and indigestion and can also improve a sluggish system.

Ingredients

Makes 30ml (1fl oz)
Grapeseed oil 2 tbsp
Spearmint essential oil 5 drops
Pine essential oil 5 drops
Rosemary essential oil 5 drops

How to **make**

1 Combine all the ingredients together in a bowl. Transfer to a sterilized dark glass bottle and seal with a cap or dropper.

2 Massage clockwise into the abdomen. Allow the oil to absorb into the skin before you get dressed. Store the remaining oil in a cool, dark place. Keeps for up to 3 months.

Soothing dill bath soak

This tummy-settling bath blend makes use of the antispasmodic properties of marjoram, together with the stimulating effect of black pepper and soothing dill to relieve trapped wind and pep up a sluggish digestion. It helps food to move along the digestive tract.

Ingredients

Makes 15ml (½fl oz)
Base oil or full-fat milk 1 tbsp
Black pepper essential oil 3 drops
Dill essential oil 3 drops
Marjoram essential oil 3 drops

How to **make**

1 Combine all the ingredients together in a bowl.

2 Disperse the blend immediately in a warm bath and enjoy a relaxing and soothing soak.

Indigestion

Indigestion can be felt as pain or discomfort in the upper abdomen, or as a burning sensation behind the breastbone. The symptoms of indigestion often appear shortly after eating or drinking, and may be caused by stomach acid coming into contact with the sensitive stomach lining. The stomach acid breaks down the lining, leading to irritation and inflammation. In most cases, indigestion is related to eating and is often followed by heartburn, or reflux (see below), although it can be triggered by other factors such as smoking, drinking alcohol, pregnancy, stress or taking certain medications. Try the massage below to ease symptoms.

Cardamom massage

Essential oils that are antispasmodic, calming, and warming, such as coriander, mandarin, and cardamom, can help to relieve indigestion.

Ingredients

Makes 30ml (1fl oz)
Almond oil 2 tbsp
Mandarin essential oil 5 drops
Coriander essential oil 3 drops
Cardamom essential oil 2 drops

How to **make**

1 Combine all the ingredients together in a bowl. Transfer to a sterilized dark glass bottle and seal with a cap or dropper.

2 Gently massage into the chest and abdomen. Allow the oil to absorb into the skin before you get dressed. Store the remaining oil in a cool, dark place. Keeps for up to 3 months.

Reflux

Acid reflux is a condition where stomach acid comes back up into the mouth and causes an unpleasant, sour taste. It can also be accompanied by symptoms such as wind and bloating, and indigestion and heartburn. Reflux can be caused by a number of things, such as eating big portions and high-fat meals, eating too many acidic foods, and chronic stress. Try this soothing massage to help calm the symptoms.

Peppermint and ginger massage

Essential oils can help relieve the symptoms of reflux when massaged onto the chest and abdomen. You may also find that a slice of lemon or fresh ginger, or a sprig of fresh peppermint infused in a glass of hot water is helpful.

Ingredients

Makes 30ml (1fl oz)
Sunflower oil 2 tbsp
Peppermint essential oil 7 drops
Ginger essential oil 5 drops
Dill essential oil 3 drops

How to **make**

1 Combine all the ingredients together in a bowl. Transfer to a sterilized dark glass bottle and seal with a cap or dropper.

2 Gently massage into the abdomen, chest, and upper back. Allow the oil to absorb into the skin before you get dressed. Store the remaining oil in a cool, dark place. Keeps for up to 3 months.

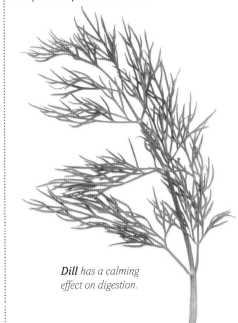

Dill *has a calming effect on digestion.*

Nausea and sickness

Nausea is the unpleasant sensation that can precede vomiting, or the feeling can be there without vomiting. Vomiting occurs when the stomach contents are forcefully expelled through the mouth. Nausea and vomiting may be due to a variety of causes, such as eating or drinking too much, hormonal changes in the first trimester of pregnancy, or an infection. These causes may need little or no treatment. However, if there is no obvious cause for prolonged bouts of sickness, talk to your doctor as it is important to identify the underlying cause. Try the remedies here to ease nausea.

Warming cardamom compress

If the abdomen is tender and painful to touch, gently applying a warm compress can be soothing and just as effective as an abdominal massage.

Ingredients

Makes 1 compress
Almond oil 1 tsp
Cardamom essential oil 2 drops
Black pepper essential oil 2 drops

How to **make**

1 Fill a bowl with warm water. Add the essential oils to the base oil and then to the water.

2 Soak a flannel in the bowl, then remove the flannel and squeeze out the excess water.

3 Wrap the flannel in a towel or piece of cling film to insulate it. Place the compress on the abdomen. Leave the flannel in place while it cools to body temperature, then repeat the process 3 times.

Ginger diffusion

Ginger is a classic remedy for overcoming nausea and tummy upsets, whether caused by over-indulgence, pregnancy hormones, or travel sickness. Here, ginger essential oil is partnered with Roman chamomile. A slightly gentler oil than German chamomile, Roman chamomile is suitable for young children and for those who have a delicate constitution.

Ingredients

Makes enough for 1 diffusion
Ginger essential oil 6 drops
Roman chamomile essential oil 3 drops
Peppermint essential oil 3 drops

How to **make**

1 Add the essential oil blend to a diffuser, vaporizer or oil burner.

2 Gently fragrance your chosen environment.

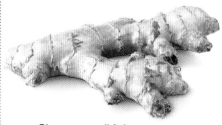

Ginger *can quell feelings of nausea.*

Diarrhoea

Diarrhoea is frequent, watery bowel movements. It can be caused by eating foods that irritate the gut, by a bowel infection, or by nerves and stress. Keep well hydrated if you have diarrhoea. These remedies can soothe intestinal lining.

Tummy-calming massage blend

Blend antispasmodic essential oils, such as cypress and ginger, with pain-relieving lavender for this therapeutic blend.

Ingredients

Makes 30ml (1fl oz)
Sunflower oil 2 tbsp
Cypress essential oil 6 drops
Ginger essential oil 5 drops
Lavender essential oil 3 drops

How to **make**

1 Combine all the ingredients together in a bowl. Transfer to a sterilized dark glass bottle and seal with a cap or dropper.

2 Massage clockwise into the abdomen. Allow the oil to absorb into the skin before you get dressed. Store the remaining oil in a cool, dark place. Keeps for up to 3 months.

Mandarin and geranium compress

Mandarin can settle digestion and is effective for overcoming feelings of nausea. Here it's combined with geranium and black pepper, which help to stimulate and support the digestive system. This compress will help to soothe an unsettled stomach and restore normal bowel movements. The heat also relaxes the abdominal muscles.

Ingredients

Makes 1 compress
Almond oil 1 tsp
Mandarin essential oil 3 drops
Geranium essential oil 2 drops
Black pepper essential oil 2 drops

How to **make**

1 Fill a bowl with hot water. Add the essential oils to the base oil, then to the water.

2 Soak a flannel in the bowl, then remove the flannel and squeeze out the excess water.

3 Wrap the flannel in a towel or piece of cling film to insulate it. Place the compress on the abdomen. Leave the flannel in place while it cools to body temperature, then repeat the process 3 times.

Appetite loss

There are a number of reasons why you might lose your appetite. Some conditions are temporary, or sometimes, appetite loss can indicate a serious condition such as anorexia nervosa, which is an eating disorder where a person keeps their body weight as low as possible. A condition such as anorexia requires specialist treatment. Always consult your doctor if you experience an unexplained loss of appetite. The bath soak below can help to stimulate appetite.

Peppermint soak

Ginger and peppermint stimulate the appetite. Added to a warm bath, they are absorbed into the skin and their scent inhaled. Peppermint and ginger herbal teas also help to stimulate appetite.

Ingredients

Makes 15ml (½fl oz)
Base oil or full-fat milk 1 tbsp
Peppermint essential oil 5 drops
Ginger essential oil 2 drops

How to **make**

1 Combine all the ingredients together in a bowl.

2 Disperse the blend immediately in a warm bath and enjoy a relaxing soak.

Mouth, gum, and tooth problems

Most oral disease is caused by bacterial infection. When bacteria forms in the mouth it produces a sticky, colourless film on the teeth called plaque, which hardens into tartar. Plaque and tartar irritate and inflame gums, which can destroy the gums and tissues. Research has linked gum disease to cardiovascular health and diabetes so a healthy mouth is thought to promote good health.

Bad breath (halitosis) has many causes, but is usually down to poor oral hygiene. If bacteria builds up in the mouth, it breaks down pieces of food lodged in the teeth and creates an bad odour. The following remedies help to improve oral hygiene.

Soothing gum oil

Myrrh essential oil, helps to reduce gum inflammation, while clove has a numbing effect to help relieve pain and soreness.

Ingredients

Makes 15ml (½fl oz)
Olive oil 1tbsp
Clove essential oil 1 drop
Myrrh essential oil 1 drop
Peppermint essential oil 1 drop

How to **make**

1 Combine all the ingredients together in a bowl. Transfer to a sterilized small glass jar.

2 Gently rub the oil blend into the gums, then rinse out with water.

Oregano gargle

To combat halitosis, try a gargle with antibacterial oils.

Ingredients

Makes 15ml (½fl oz)
Sunflower oil 1 tbsp
Peppermint essential oil 1 drop
Oregano essential oil 1 drop

How to **make**

1 Mix the oil blend with cold water.

2 Wash the solution around the mouth for 3–5 minutes, then spit it out. Rinse with water. Use 3 times daily.

Safe usage Do not swallow. Not suitable in pregnancy.

Respiratory complaints

While it is hard to avoid all cold viruses, there are steps you can take to **boost** immunity. Once a cold has set in, early treatment can also help to minimize its severity. Chronic conditions, such as asthma, require careful medical management, but there are ways to help control them. Essential oil's **decongesting**, **antiviral**, and **calming** properties can ease respiratory complaints.

Colds and sinusitis

A cold is a mild viral infection of the nose, throat, sinuses, and upper airways. This viral infection is very common and usually clears up on its own within a week or two. The main symptoms of a cold include an initial sore throat, blocked or runny nose, sneezing, and coughing.

Sinusitis is another common condition in which the lining of the sinuses becomes inflamed, and this usually follows a viral infection such as a cold. Symptoms of sinusitis include a green or yellow nasal discharge, blocked nose, pain and tenderness around the cheeks, eyes or forehead, a sinus headache and a temperature. The symptoms often improve within two to three weeks. While you can't "cure" a cold virus, there are several ways in which you can use essential oils to bring relief to colds and blocked sinuses.

Frankincense throat and chest rub

Frankincense essential oil helps to soothe the mucous membranes, calm breathing, and can also ease coughs, sore throats, and bronchitis. It is blended here with other soothing oils to create a warming upper-body rub to help combat colds and congestion.

Ingredients

Makes 30ml (1fl oz)
Sunflower oil 2 tbsp
Frankincense essential oil 7 drops
Sandalwood essential oil 5 drops
Lavender essential oil 3 drops

How to **make**

1 Mix all the ingredients together in a bowl. Pour into a sterilized dark glass bottle. Seal with a cap or dropper.

2 Gently massage into the chest, throat, and upper back. Allow the oil to absorb before you get dressed.

Clearing eucalyptus diffusion

Eucalyptus has wonderful clearing properties that help to relieve blocked sinuses. Using a diffuser to disperse this essential oil in the air is an effective way to ease congested sinuses. Sit near the diffuser for the most direct effect.

Ingredients

Makes enough for 1 diffusion
Cedarwood essential oil 4 drops
Eucalyptus essential oil 4 drops
Ravensara essential oil 4 drops

How to **make**

1 Add the essential oil blend to a diffuser, vaporizer or oil burner.

2 Gently fragrance your chosen environment.

Cajuput and tea tree inhalation

Steam inhalations are very effective at treating sore throats and relieving congestion.

Ingredients

Makes enough for 1 inhalation
Cajuput essential oil 6 drops
Tea tree essential oil 4 drops
Lavender essential oil 4 drops

How to **make**

1 Add the essential oils to a bowl of hot water. Cover your head with a towel, making a tent over the bowl, lean over the bowl, and inhale deeply.

2 Allow the steam to soothe the throat for 5–10 minutes, taking a break from the steam if needed.

Asthma

Asthma is a common long-term condition that can cause coughing, wheezing, breathlessness, and tightness in the chest. The severity of the symptoms varies from person to person. In most people, the condition can be controlled well for most of the time, although some experience more persistent problems.

Occasionally, asthma gets gradually or suddenly much worse. This is known as an asthma attack, and these more severe attacks may require urgent hospital treatment and can even be life-threatening, although this is unusual.

No single cause for asthma has been identified, however there are several factors that may trigger an asthma attack. Inhaled or ingested allergens, such as dust mites and certain foods, can trigger an attack. Exercise and emotional stress can also produce asthmatic symptoms. Learning to manage the condition and avoid potential allergens is key to preventing attacks. The following remedies use oils to help calm mild symptoms so can be used alongside usual medical treatments. Consult your doctor before using these remedies, and always seek urgent medical help if you experience a severe asthma attack.

Eucalyptus and lemon inhalation

Sometimes asthma symptoms can be triggered by the presence of an infection such as a cold or flu virus. An inhalation using clearing essential oils can be useful to help ease asthma symptoms in these circumstances.

Ingredients

Makes enough for 1 inhalation
Lemon essential oil 4 drops
Eucalyptus essential oil 4 drops
Peppermint essential oil 4 drops

How to **make**

1 Place the oil drops directly on a tissue or handkerchief.

2 Keep the tissue with you and inhale by wafting the tissue under the nose. Do not cover the nose with the tissue.

Frankincense diffusion

Asthma symptoms can sometimes worsen if a person has had an emotional upset or specific trauma. In these circumstances, a diffusion with calming

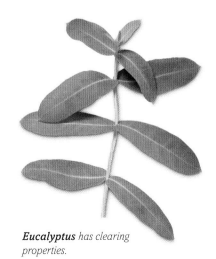

Eucalyptus has clearing properties.

essential oils such as frankincense, sandalwood, and lavender can be effective in easing the symptoms.

Ingredients

Frankincense essential oil 7 drops
Sandalwood essential oil 5 drops
Lavender essential oil 3 drops

How to **make**

1 Add the essential oil blend to a diffuser, vaporizer or oil burner.

2 Gently fragrance your chosen environment.

Calming chamomile massage

If asthma symptoms are typically brought on by exposure to allergens, such as dust mites or certain foods, have a ready-prepared massage blend to hand, made up of soothing essential oils such as chamomile, and an oil such as helichrysum, which has an antispasmodic action.

Ingredients

Makes 30ml (1fl oz)
Sunflower oil 2 tbsp
Helichrysum essential oil 4 drops
Lavender essential oil 4 drops
Roman chamomile essential oil 4 drops

How to **make**

1 Combine all the ingredients together in a bowl. Transfer to a sterilized dark glass bottle and seal with a cap or dropper.

2 Gently massage into the chest, throat, and upper back. Allow the oil to absorb into the skin before you get dressed. Store the remaining oil in a cool, dark place. Keeps for up to 3 months.

Circulatory problems

Circulatory problems can be caused by poor diet, smoking, having a sedentary lifestyle, and stress. Improving **lifestyle factors** such as diet and building a regular **exercise regime** can help to address problems. Essential oils can **stimulate** sluggish circulation and may help to provide the **motivation** to change your lifestyle.

Varicose veins and haemorrhoids

Varicose veins develop when the small valves inside the veins stop working properly. In a healthy vein, blood flows smoothly to the heart and the blood is prevented from flowing backwards by a series of tiny valves that open and close to enable it to pass through. If these valves weaken or are damaged, the blood can start to flow backwards and then collect in the vein, eventually causing the vein to become swollen and enlarged (known as varicose). Pregnancy, being overweight, and old age are all factors that can increase the chances of developing varicose veins.

Haemorrhoids, also known as piles, are related to varicose veins. These are swellings containing enlarged blood vessels that are found inside or around the rectum and anus. In many cases, haemorrhoids don't cause symptoms, and some people don't even realise that they have them. The compress below can help to ease and relieve symptoms such as pain or itching.

Soothing cypress compress

Cypress essential oil has a toning effect on the veins and is a useful oil for circulatory problems as it helps to regulate the flow of blood, making it particularly useful for conditions such as varicose veins. Here it is combined with detoxifying lemon and geranium essential oils, and juniper essential oil, which has an astringent action that is helpful for shrinking varicose veins and haemorrhoids.

Ingredients

Makes 1 compress
Sunflower oil 2 tsp
Cypress essential oil 3 drops
Lemon essential oil 3 drops
Juniper essential oil 3 drops
Geranium essential oil 1 drop

How to **make**

1 Fill a bowl with cold water. Add the essential oils to the sunflower oil, then add to the water.

2 Soak a flannel in the bowl, then remove the flannel and squeeze out the excess water.

3 Place the compress over the varicose veins, or for haemorrhoids, sit on the compress with a towel underneath. Leave in place for 10 minutes.

High blood pressure

Hypertension is another term for high blood pressure. Blood pressure is measured in millimetres of mercury (mmHg) and it is recorded as two figures: systolic pressure – the pressure of the

Essential oils can be used to stimulate or calm circulation.

blood when your heart pushes blood out, and diastolic pressure – the pressure of the blood when your heart rests in between beats, which reflects how strongly your arteries are resisting blood flow.

It is perfectly normal for the systolic blood pressure to increase on exertion or during emotional stress, but in a healthy body it will return to normal quite quickly. A number of lifestyle and dietary changes can be made to help reduce the risk of hypertension, for example increasing exercise, reducing salt intake, stopping smoking, and reducing stress and stimulants. A relaxing massage can help to combat the cumulative effects of stress and tension.

If you have been diagnosed with high blood pressure, talk to your doctor before using any complementary remedy to make sure that your condition is being monitored medically. Continue to take your usual prescribed medication alongside remedies unless directed otherwise by your doctor.

Lavender and marjoram massage

Essential oils that have a hypotensive action (meaning they help to lower blood pressure), as well as calming and sedating effects, can be used to alleviate mild hypertension. Here, lavender, marjoram, and ylang ylang essential oils are combined to make a therapeutic massage blend that can be used to help combat mild hypertension.

Ingredients

Makes 30ml (1fl oz)
Almond oil 2 tbsp
Lavender essential oil 6 drops
Marjoram essential oil 6 drops
Ylang ylang essential oil 3 drops

How to **make**

1 Combine all the ingredients together in a bowl. Transfer to a sterilized dark glass bottle and seal with a cap or dropper.

2 Gently massage into the body. Allow the oil to absorb into the skin before you get dressed. Store remaining oil in a cool, dark place. Keeps for up to 3 months.

Sluggish circulation

There are many different symptoms that can indicate poor circulation. For example, cold extremeties such as the feet and toes and fingers and hands, water retention, and cramps, all suggest that general circulation is sluggish. Apart from the daily discomfort that poor circulation can cause, there are some potentially more serious consequences. Simple dietary and lifestyle changes can help to improve the circulation. For example, if you sit at a desk all day, ensure that you take regular breaks and move around, stop eating convenience foods, and try to give up smoking. The massage below can help to stimulate circulation.

Stimulating rosemary massage

Some essential oils are stimulating and can help to improve circulation. These warming oils dilate the capillaries to increase blood flow. This in turn stimulates the flow of lymph, which helps control the passage of fluids around the body. Poor lymphatic drainage results in a build-up of fluid in the tissues.

Ingredients

Makes 30ml (1fl oz)
Almond oil 2 tbsp
Rosemary essential oil 3 drops
Thyme essential oil 3 drops
Black pepper essential oil 3 drops
Ginger essential oil 3 drops
Clove essential oil 1 drop

How to **make**

1 Combine all the ingredients together in a bowl. Transfer to a sterilized dark glass bottle and seal with a cap or dropper.

2 Gently massage into the body. Allow the oil to absorb into the skin before you get dressed. Store remaining oil in a cool, dark place. Keeps for up to 3 months.

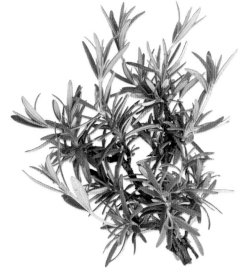

Rosemary *helps improve poor circulation.*

Fluid retention and urinary tract infections

Swelling and puffiness, known as oedema, indicate **fluid retention**, which can have a number of causes. Infections in the urinary system can cause bladder inflammation. Certain essential oils have **diuretic**, anti-inflammatory, and **antiseptic** properties that can help to ease symptoms.

Swelling

Swelling is typically the result of inflammation or a buildup of fluid that can occur internally or that can affect your outer skin and muscles. Using essential oils that have detoxifying properties helps to flush out excess fluids and reduce inflammation. Consult your doctor if you have any unexplained swelling.

Geranium compress

A number of essential oils work as circulatory tonics that can help to reduce swelling and fluid retention and are effective used in massage, in the bath or as a compress, as in the remedy here.

Ingredients

Makes 1 compress
Almond oil 1 tbsp
Geranium essential oil 5 drops
Cypress essential oil 4 drops
Yarrow essential oil 3 drops
Lemon essential oil 3 drops

How to **make**

1 Fill a bowl with cold water. Add the essential oils to the almond oil, then add to the water.

2 Soak a flannel in the bowl, then remove the flannel and squeeze out the excess water.

3 Place the compress on the affected area. Leave the flannel in place while it reaches body temperature, then repeat the process 3 times.

Detox massage

The lymphatic system is responsible for removing the waste products created by the body's organs and tissues. The blend of detoxifying essential oils used in this massage supports the action of the lymphatic system. Grapefruit specifically encourages lymphatic drainage and acts as a diuretic when it is massaged directly into the skin, helping to combat areas of puffiness caused by water retention. Rosemary helps to stimulate lymphatic circulation, helping the body to remove waste products and also relieving water retention. These two potent oils are combined here with black pepper, which works as a mild diuretic. To maximize the effect of this detox massage, use the oils in combination with a body brush to stimulate the circulation.

Ingredients

Grapeseed oil 2 tbsp
Grapefruit essential oil 5 drops
Rosemary essential oil 5 drops
Black pepper essential oil 5 drops

How to **make**

1 Combine all the ingredients together in a bowl. Transfer to a sterilized dark glass bottle and seal with a cap or dropper.

2 Gently massage into the skin in upwards circular movements. Allow the oil to absorb into the skin before you get dressed. Store the remaining oil in a cool, dark place. Keeps for up to 3 months.

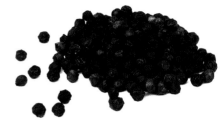

Black pepper *helps to flush out waste products.*

Urinary tract infection

Urinary tract infections (UTIs) are very common. They can be painful and uncomfortable, but they usually pass within a few days, though sometimes you may need a course of antibiotics. UTIs are more common in women than in men. Children can also get UTIs, but this is less common.

A UTI develops when part of the urinary tract becomes infected, usually by bacteria, which can enter the urinary tract through the urethra or, more rarely, through the bloodstream. There is usually no obvious reason why the urinary tract becomes infected, although some women find they develop a UTI after having sex. As UTIs are far less common in men than in women these need investigating to find an underlying cause.

Cystitis is inflammation of the bladder, usually caused by an infection. Most cases are thought to occur when bacteria that live harmlessly in the bowel or on the skin enter the bladder through the urethra. It's a common type of UTI, particularly in women, and is usually more of a nuisance than a cause for serious concern. Mild cases will often get better by themselves within a few days. However, some people experience episodes of cystitis frequently and may need regular or long-term treatment. There's also a chance that cystitis could lead to a more serious kidney infection, so it's important to seek medical advice if your symptoms don't improve over a few days, or if you have a fever, severe pain, or blood or pus in the urine. Try the following remedies to help ease symptoms and bring relief.

Bergamot sitz bath

As UTIs are caused by infection, essential oils with antibacterial activity are recommended to help fight the infection and support your recovery. Here, antiviral and antibacterial bergamot is combined with astringent chamomile and soothing lavender. The oils are added to a shallow "sitz" bath, which is waist height only and ideal for treating UTIs.

Ingredients

Makes enough for 1 sitz bath
Bergamot essential oil 4 drops
German chamomile essential oil 3 drops
Lavender essential oil 2 drops

How to **make**

1 Fill the bath to waist height. Adjust the temperature depending on how long you wish to remain in the bath. For a bath of up to five minutes, run hot water at a temperature of 40–45°C (104–113°F). If you want to stay in the bath for up to 15 minutes, keep the water at 33–35°C (91–95°F). Alternatively, fill a bowl with warm water, add the essential oils, then soak a clean flannel in the water. Remove the flannel and squeeze out the excess water, then gently wash the affected area with the flannel. After washing, pat dry the area carefully.

2 If using the oils in a shallow bath, add the essential oils to the bath once run, then soak as required.

Tea tree wash

The antiseptic properties of tea tree essential oil are especially useful for treating UTIs. Try this simple wash to ease discomfort. Always ensure your flannels and towels are clean before using and are washed immediately after every use.

Ingredients

Makes enough for 1 wash
Almond oil 1 tsp
Tea tree essential oil 3 drops
Bergamot essential oil 3 drops

How to **make**

1 Fill a large bowl with warm water. Add the essential oils to the almond oil, then add to the water.

2 Soak a clean flannel in the water, then remove the flannel and wring it out.

3 Gently wash the affected area with the flannel, patting the area dry carefully afterwards.

Antiseptic and soothing essential oils are useful for easing the symptoms of UTIs.

Muscle and joint problems and general aches and pains

Healthy muscles and joints help ensure strength and manoeuvrability. Old age can put a strain on joints and muscles, but **activity** helps maintain **flexibility**. Aches and pains can be due to muscle tension or other causes. Try oils that are **anti-inflammatory**, detoxifying, and **pain-relieving**.

Backache, neck pain, and sciatica

Back pain is a common problem that affects most people at some point in life. It may be triggered by bad posture, by bending awkwardly, or by lifting heavy loads and objects incorrectly. In most cases, back pain improves over a period of weeks or months, although some experience recurrent long-term pain.

Neck pain, or a stiff neck, is a common problem and usually nothing to worry about. You can get a painful or stiff neck if you sleep awkwardly, use a computer for a prolonged period of time, or strain a muscle because of bad posture. The pain and stiffness usually get better after a few days or weeks. Anxiety and stress can also cause tension in the neck muscles that can lead to neck pain. If pain is acute or long-lasting, consult your doctor.

A stiff neck accompanied by other symptoms such as fever, headache, or intolerance to bright lights, should be investigated immediately.

Sciatica is the name for pain that is caused by irritation or compression of the sciatic nerve, which is the longest nerve in the body. It runs from the back of the pelvis, through the buttocks, and all the way down the legs, ending at the feet. When this nerve is compressed or irritated, it can cause pain, numbness, and a tingling sensation that radiates from the lower back down one leg to the foot and toes. While sciatica pain can also be accompanied by general back pain, the pain of sciatica usually affects the buttocks and legs more than the back. Try the following pain-relieving remedies.

Muscle-relaxing massage

Essential oils and massage can be extremely effective in treating backache and neck pain where the pain is due to tension or muscular fatigue. Regular massage with oils and essential oil baths can help to prevent backache by reducing stress, relaxing tight muscles, and improving general wellbeing, which helps to relieve held-in tension. The following massage blend can also be added to a bath for a relaxing soak, combining the essential oils with just a tablespoon of arnica oil, or alternatively with a tablespoon of full-fat milk or vodka.

Ingredients

Makes 30ml (1 fl oz)
Arnica macerated oil 2 tbsp
Rosemary essential oil 5 drops
Marjoram essential oil 5 drops
Ginger essential oil 5 drops

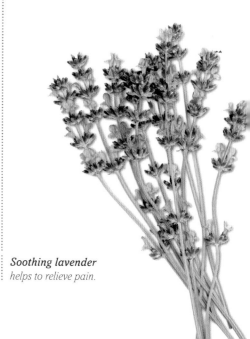

Soothing lavender
helps to relieve pain.

How to **make**

1 Combine the ingredients in a bowl. Transfer to a sterilized dark glass bottle. Seal with a cap or dropper.

2 Massage into the back and neck. Allow the oil to absorb into the skin before you get dressed. Store the remaining oil in a cool, dark place. Keeps for up to 3 months.

Soothing lavender compress

Lavender is mildly analgesic and antispasmodic so can soothe sciatic pain.

Ingredients

Makes 1 compress
Almond oil 1 tsp
Lavender essential oil 5 drops
Coriander essential oil 2 drops
Black pepper essential oil 5 drops

How to **make**

1 Fill a bowl with warm water. Add the essential oils to the almond oil, then add to the water.

2 Soak a flannel in the bowl, then remove the flannel and squeeze out the excess water.

3 Wrap the flannel in a towel or cling film to insulate it. Place the compress on the affected area. Leave it in place while it cools to body temperature, then repeat the process 3 times.

Headaches and migraines

Headaches are one of the most common health complaints. In many cases they can be easily treated with small lifestyle changes, such as getting more rest and drinking enough fluids so that you stay well hydrated. Tension headaches are often described as a constant ache that affects both sides of the head, and these are commonly linked to stress, poor posture, skipping meals, and dehydration. Migraines are less common than headaches. They're usually felt as a severe, throbbing pain at the front or side of the head. Other symptoms of migraines may include nausea, vomiting, and increased sensitivity to light or sound. A soothing compress or head massage can bring relief.

Calming peppermint and lavender compress

With its gently stimulating and analgesic properties, peppermint is an established treatment in aromatherapy for tension headaches, working in a similar way to drugs such as paracetamol. Its cooling action clears and refreshes the mind. Relaxing lavender helps to bring relief to headaches caused by anxiety and stress.

Ingredients

Makes 1 compress
Almond oil 1 tsp
Peppermint essential oil 3 drops
Lavender essential oil 2 drops

How to **make**

1 Fill a bowl with warm water. Add the essential oils to the almond oil, then add to the water.

2 Soak a flannel in the bowl, then remove the flannel and squeeze out the excess water.

3 Place the compress on the forehead. Leave the flannel in place while it cools to body temperature, then repeat the process 3 times.

Warming marjoram compress

Marjoram essential oil has both a sedative and analgesic effect, so as well as relieving pain, it can also help to reduce the anxiety and tension that lead to headaches and migraine.

Ingredients

Makes 1 compress
Almond oil 1 tsp
Lavender essential oil 3 drops
Marjoram essential oil 2 drops

How to **make**

1 Fill a bowl with warm water. Add the essential oils to the almond oil, then add to the water.

2 Soak a flannel in the bowl, then remove the flannel and squeeze out the excess water.

3 Wrap the flannel in a towel or piece of cling film to insulate it. Place the compress on the temples. Leave the flannel in place while it cools to body temperature, then repeat the process 3 times.

Rosemary and eucalyptus temple massage

Tension headaches caused by mental effort can be treated with rosemary. Eucalyptus is useful for soothing headaches caused by sinus congestion or allergic reactions. Here, the two oils are combined with refreshing peppermint and relaxing lavender.

Ingredients

Makes 30ml (1fl oz)
Almond oil 2 tbsp
Rosemary essential oil 5 drops
Peppermint essential oil 3 drops
Lavender essential oil 2 drops
Eucalyptus essential oil 2 drops

How to **make**

1 Combine all the ingredients together in a bowl. Transfer to a sterilized dark glass bottle and seal with a cap or dropper.

2 Massage gently into the temples in a circular motion. Store the remaining oil in a cool, dark place. Keeps for up to 3 months.

Arthritis

Arthritis is caused by joint inflammation. The two most common types are rheumatoid arthritis and osteoarthritis. Rheumatoid arthritis is a chronic autoimmune disease that causes swelling, pain, and stiffness in joints, commonly affecting the hands, wrists, and feet. Osteoarthritis makes joints painful and stiff. It occurs when there is damage in and around joints. Most joints can be affected with arthritis, but the condition commonly causes problems in the knees, hips, and the small joints of the hands. Massage and bath soaks can ease the stiffness caused by arthritis.

Circulation-boosting massage

Warming, relaxing, and pain-relieving oils such as marjoram, help to relieve the pain of arthritis. Black pepper and ginger stimulate circulation, in turn revitalizing tired, aching joints. Black pepper also has anti-inflammatory properties, making it an ideal oil for soothing arthritis. Ginger also has an anti-infammatory effect and is naturally reviving and stimulating when applied locally. Try using this massage oil blend locally to bring relief to affected areas.

Ingredients

Makes 30ml (1fl oz)
Almond oil 2 tbsp
Marjoram essential oil 6 drops
Black pepper essential oil 5 drops
Ginger essential oil 4 drops

How to **make**

1 Combine all the ingredients together in a bowl. Transfer to a sterilized dark glass bottle and seal with a cap or dropper.

2 Massage into the affected joints. Allow the oil to absorb into the skin before you get dressed. Store the remaining oil in a cool, dark place. Keeps for up to 3 months.

Soothing yarrow soak

Nutmeg and yarrow oils help to reduce inflammation. Adding these oils to a warm bath combines the soothing effects of warm water with the oils' benefits.

Ingredients

Makes 15ml (½fl oz)
Base oil or full-fat milk 1 tbsp
Nutmeg essential oil 3 drops
Yarrow essential oil 3 drops
Lavender essential oil 5 drops

How to **make**

1 Combine all the ingredients together in a bowl.

2 Disperse immediately in the bath and enjoy a relaxing soak.

Muscular aches and pains

Muscular aches and pains are common and can involve several muscles. Muscle pain can also involve ligaments, tendons, and fascia (the soft tissues that connect muscles, bones, and organs). It's usually related to tension, overuse, or injury from exercise or movement. Muscle pain may be a sign of another condition. For example, certain infections and disorders, such as lupus, affect connective tissues and cause muscle pain. Another cause of muscular aches and pains is fibromyalgia, a condition that causes tenderness in the muscles and surrounding tissue, sleep difficulties, fatigue, and headaches. A targeted massage or compress can reduce pain.

"Unknotting" massage

An essential oil massage can help to stimulate the circulation, relieve pain, and reduce inflammation. The blend here with pain-relieving plai and stimulating black pepper can also be added to a bath with 1 tablespoon of either full-fat milk or base oil.

Ingredients

Makes 30ml (1fl oz)
Arnica macerated oil 1 tbsp
Almond oil 1 tbsp
Plai essential oil 5 drops
Lemongrass essential oil 2 drops
Black pepper essential oil 3 drops

How to **make**

1 Combine all the ingredients together in a bowl. Transfer to a sterilized dark glass bottle and seal with a cap or dropper.

2 Massage into the affected area. Allow the oil to absorb into the skin before you get dressed. Store the remaining oil in a cool, dark place. Keeps for up to 3 months.

Hot ginger compress

Alternating hot and cold compresses can be an effective way to deal with aches and pains. This warming ginger blend boosts circulation and soothes sore, aching muscles.

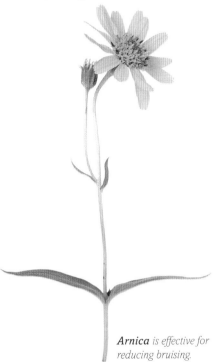

Arnica is effective for reducing bruising.

Ingredients

Makes 1 compress
Almond oil 1 tsp
Ginger essential oil 7 drops
Lavandin essential oil 4 drops
Rosemary essential oil 4 drops

How to **make**

1 Fill a bowl with warm water. Add the essential oils to the almond oil, then add to the water.

2 Soak a flannel in the bowl, then remove the flannel and squeeze out the excess water.

3 Wrap the flannel in a towel or cling film to insulate it. Place the compress on the affected area. Leave it in place while it cools to body temperature, then repeat the process 3 times.

Sprains and strains

Sprains are torn ligaments, which join bone to bone, and strains are injuries to tendons, which connect muscle to bone. Sprains are more serious. They can be inflamed, painful, and hot to touch. The initial treatment for both is PRICE: "protection, rest, ice, compression, elevation". Try the following soothing remedies.

Anti-inflammatory lemongrass compress

Try this cold compress on a sprain. This compress uses pain-relieving lemongrass and the anti-inflammatory oils, ginger and black pepper.

Ingredients

Makes 1 compress
Almond oil 1 tsp
Black pepper essential oil 5 drops
Lemongrass essential oil 2 drops
Ginger essential oil 5 drops

How to **make**

1 Fill a bowl with cold water. Add the essential oils to the almond oil, then add to the water.

2 Soak a flannel in the bowl, then remove the flannel and squeeze out the excess water.

3 Place the compress on the affected area. Leave the flannel while it cools to body temperature, then repeat the process 3 times.

Analgesic rosemary massage

A massage with analgesic and anti-inflammatory oils promotes healing. Here, arnica is also used, a traditional remedy to reduce bruising and swelling.

Ingredients

Makes 30ml (1fl oz)
Arnica oil 1 tbsp
Almond oil 1 tbsp
Marjoram essential oil 5 drops
Rosemary essential oil 5 drops
Thyme essential oil 5 drops

How to **make**

1 Combine all the ingredients together in a bowl. Transfer to a sterilized dark glass bottle and seal with a cap or dropper.

2 Massage into the affected area. Allow the oil to absorb into the skin before you get dressed. Store the remaining oil in a cool, dark place. Keeps for up to 3 months.

Skin and hair

Our skin has a protective function, forming a **barrier** against our external environment. Sometimes, though, skin can become irritated, clogged or affected by hormonal changes, or can become damaged by the weather or by being broken. Essential oils can **tone**, balance, and **soothe** a wide range of skin problems, and can also help to **nourish** and hydrate skin.

Acne

Acne is a common skin condition caused by chronic inflammation of the hair follicles and sebaceous glands. It affects many people at some point, but is most common in adolescence. Acne causes spots to develop usually on the face, back, and chest. The spots can range from blackheads and whiteheads to deep, inflamed, pus-filled pustules and cysts, which can be severe and long-lasting, sometimes leading to scarring. It's very important to keep skin clean using a mild cleanser. Be careful not to scrub the skin too hard as it could cause irritation. These skin-soothing remedies can help calm problem skin.

Lavender massage

Skin-regenerating oils help to promote healing and minimize scarring. Lavender, is antiseptic and calming on the skin. Here it is combined with palmarosa, which is gently astringent and anti-inflammatory, helping to soothe inflamed skin.

Ingredients

Makes 15ml (½fl oz)
Wheatgerm oil 1 tsp
Rosehip seed oil 1 tsp
Calendula macerated oil 1 tsp
Palmarosa essential oil 3 drops
Lavender essential oil 1 drop

How to **make**

1 Combine all the ingredients together in a bowl. Transfer to a sterilized dark glass bottle and seal with a cap or dropper.

2 Massage into the skin on the body or face. Allow the oil to absorb into the skin before you get dressed. Store the remaining oil in a cool, dark place. Keeps for up to 3 months.

Lemon and bergamot facial sauna

Essential oils can help to bring acne and pimples under control by helping to clear infection and reduce inflammation. The oils can also help mentally, reducing the stress and anxiety that can often accompany skin conditions. For a deep-pore cleanse, try this essential oil facial steam. The skin-clarifying and toning effects of lemon are combined with the antiseptic and skin-balancing properties of petitgrain, and soothing and antibacterial bergamot.

Ingredients

Makes 1 facial sauna
Bergamot essential oil 3 drops
Lemon essential oil 2 drops
Petitgrain essential oil 1 drop

How to **make**

1 Add the essential oils to a bowl of hot water. Cover your head with a towel, make a tent over the bowl of hot water, and then lean forwards over the bowl.

2 Allow the steam to act on the face for 5 minutes, taking a break from the steam if necessary. Wash your skin with cool water and pat dry with a clean towel.

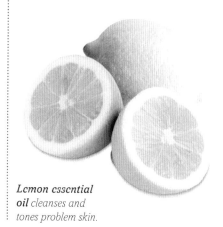

Lemon essential oil cleanses and tones problem skin.

Palmarosa massage

The essential oils geranium and palmarosa have skin-balancing properties that naturally help to reduce the amount of sebum produced by the oil glands. Combining these essential oils with skin-conditioning base oils helps to create a nourishing and toning massage oil that can help to calm outbreaks.

Ingredients

Makes 15ml (½fl oz)
Jojoba oil 1 tsp
Grapeseed oil 2 tsp
Palmarosa essential oil 3 drops
Geranium essential oil 2 drops

How to **make**

1 Combine all the ingredients together in a bowl. Transfer to a sterilized dark glass bottle and seal with a cap or dropper.

2 Massage into the skin on the body or face. Allow the oil to absorb into the skin before you get dressed. Store the remaining oil in a cool, dark place. Keeps for up to 3 months.

Tea tree hot compress

Tea tree essential oil is renowned for its antiseptic properties, making it an excellent choice for treating problem skin conditions. Added to a hot compress, it can help to soothe and cleanse skin. If you wish, you can also apply it neat on spots and pimples as an antiseptic ointment.

Ingredients

Makes 20 to 30 treatments
Grapeseed oil 1 tbsp
Tea tree essential oil 3 drops
Cajuput essential oil 2 drops
Lavender essential oil 1 drop

How to **make**

1 Fill a bowl with warm water. Add a few drops of the essential oil blend. Transfer the remaining blend to a sterilized glass jar and store in a cool, dark place. The blend keeps for up to 3 months.

2 Soak a flannel in the bowl, then remove the flannel and squeeze out the excess water.

3 Wrap the flannel in a towel or piece of cling film to insulate it. Place the compress on the area requiring treatment. Leave the flannel while it cools to body temperature, then repeat the process 3 times.

Athlete's foot

Athlete's foot is caused by fungi growing on the skin. The fungi thrive in warm, dark, moist places such as the feet, usually between the toes. Affected skin may be itchy, red, scaly, dry, cracked, or blistered. It's not usually serious, but should be treated to stop it spreading to other parts of the body or to other people. Keep feet clean, carefully dry the feet, especially between the toes, and go barefoot when possible. Try the massage below to help combat this fungal infection.

Geranium foot massage

Antifungal essential oils, such as tea tree and geranium, are ideal for athlete's foot. Here, these oils are blended with lavender essential oil, which helps to heal skin conditions and rejuvenate skin.

Ingredients

Makes 30ml (1fl oz)
Neem oil 2 tbsp
Geranium essential oil 4 drops
Tea tree essential oil 4 drops
Lavender essential oil 3 drops

How to **make**

1 Combine all the ingredients together in a bowl. Transfer to a sterilized dark glass bottle and seal with a cap or dropper.

2 Massage into clean, dry skin on the feet. Allow the oil to absorb into the skin before you get dressed. Store the remaining oil in a cool, dark place. Keeps for up to 3 months.

Bruising

Bruises are bluish or purple-coloured patches. They appear on unbroken skin when tiny blood vessels under the skin, known as capillaries, break. The blood leaks into the tissues, causing discolouration, which fades through shades of yellow or green. Try these healing remedies.

Cooling lavender compress

Applying an ice-cold compress with healing oils as quickly as possible can help to reduce bruising.

Ingredients

Makes 1 compress
Almond oil 1 tsp
Yarrow essential oil 3 drops
Lavender essential oil 5 drops

How to **make**

1 Fill a bowl with ice and cold water. Add the essential oil blend to the almond oil, then add to the water.

2 Soak a flannel in the bowl, then remove the flannel and squeeze out the excess water.

3 Place the compress on the area requiring treatment. Leave the flannel in place while it reaches body temperature. Repeat 3 times.

Arnica massage

Arnica macerated oil, ideal for bruising, is blended here with regenerative and rejuvenating helichrysum and lavender oils for a massage blend that can help to reduce the appearance of bruises.

Ingredients

Makes 30ml (1fl oz)
Arnica oil 2 tbsp
Helichrysum essential oil 3 drops
Lavender essential oil 3 drops

How to **make**

1 Combine all the ingredients together in a bowl. Transfer to a sterilized dark glass bottle and seal with a cap or dropper.

2 Gently massage the affected area. Allow the oil to absorb into the skin before getting dressed. Store the remaining oil in a cool, dark place. Keeps for up to 3 months.

Body odour

Body odour is the unpleasant smell that can occur when the body sweats. The sweat doesn't smell, but bacteria on the skin break down the sweat into acids that produce the odour. Deodorizing oils help to regulate perspiration and reduce and control unwelcome body odour.

Lemon deodorant

Deodorants work to cover the smell of body odour. The essential oils grapefruit and lemon combine fantastic deodorizing properties with an appealing aroma to keep you smelling fresh throughout the day.

Ingredients

Makes 100ml (3½fl oz)
Witch hazel 90ml (3fl oz)
Glycerine 1 tsp
Aloe juice 1 tsp
Palmarosa essential oil 5 drops
Lemon essential oil 5 drops
Coriander essential oil 3 drops
Grapefruit essential oil 3 drops

How to **make**

1 Mix all the ingredients together in a bowl. Pour into a sterilized bottle with an atomizer.

2 Shake before use. Apply to clean underarms and use whenever it is required.

Safe usage Do not use on freshly shaved skin.

Pine-fresh shower gel

The best way to avoid developing unwelcome body odour is to keep the areas of your body that are prone to sweating, such as the armpits, feet, and genital area, clean and free of bacteria. Changing your clothes regularly and washing daily will also help to avoid a buildup of sweat and bacteria.

Ingredients

Makes 30ml (1fl oz)
Unscented shower gel 2 tbsp
Lemongrass essential oil 7 drops
Pine essential oil 7 drops
Vetiver essential oil 1 drop

How to **make**

1 Make a fresh and revitalizing shower gel by adding the essential oils to an unfragranced shower gel.

2 Use the gel once or twice a day to keep skin clean and odour-free.

Eczema and psoriasis

Eczema is when skin becomes itchy, red, dry, and cracked. It is often long-term (chronic), although it can improve, especially in young children. Atopic eczema ("atopic" means a tendency to develop a sensitivity to allergens), also known as atopic dermatitis, is the most common type

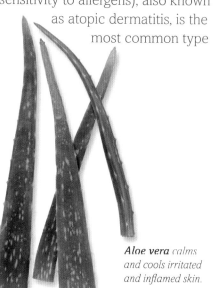

Aloe vera calms and cools irritated and inflamed skin.

of eczema. It mainly affects children, but can affect adults, too. Its exact cause is unknown, but it often occurs in people who are prone to allergic reactions, or who have a family history of allergies, and it can be linked to stress. Psoriasis is an inflammatory skin disease that is linked to stress and diet. Sufferers develop red, crusty patches of skin, usually on the elbows, knees, scalp, and back.

Soothing essential oils can be used to treat eczema and psoriasis to help control itching and reduce inflammation.

Calming chamomile compress

Chamomile has been found to be very effective for treating eczema due to its anti-inflammatory and soothing effects that help to relieve and calm itchy and inflamed skin. Sandalwood and lavender are both soothing essential oils that are especially effective on dry, itchy skin. Apply this compress to affected areas to help balance and soothe the skin.

Ingredients

Makes 1 compress
Sunflower or almond oil 1 tsp
German chamomile essential oil 1 drop
Lavender essential oil 3 drops
Sandalwood essential oil 3 drops

How to **make**

1 Fill a bowl with cold water. Add the essential oils to the base oil, then add to the water.

2 Soak a flannel in the bowl, then remove the flannel and squeeze out the excess water.

3 Place the compress on the area requiring treatment. Leave the flannel in place while it reaches body temperature. Repeat 3 times.

Lavender bath float

Create a relaxing bath float with this mix of skin-soothing oats and bran, dried flowers, and uplifting oils. Helichrysum is calming on itchy breakouts, and cistus is mildy astringent, helping to tone skin.

Ingredients

Makes 45g (1½oz)
Organic jumbo oats 1 tbsp
Bran 1 tbsp
Dried lavender flowers 1 tbsp
Helichrysum 4 drops
Lavender essential oil 4 drops
Cistus essential oil 1 drop

How to **make**

1 Make a herb bag using a muslin cloth. Lay the cloth out and place 1 tablespoon each of organic jumbo oats, bran, and dried lavender flowers on the cloth. Add the essential oils.

2 Gather the cloth around the bath mix and tie a ribbon around the corners to keep all the ingredients together.

3 Place the float in a warm bath and dab on the skin to soothe affected areas.

Stress-busting diffusion

Aromatherapy is especially effective in reducing stress and anxiety, making it helpful for dealing with stress-related cases of psoriasis and eczema. The calming oils in this diffusion will help to soothe the anxiety that can be caused by and exacerbate skin conditions.

Ingredients

Makes 1 diffusion
Cedarwood essential oil 4 drops
Frankincense essential oil 3 drops
Geranium essential oil 2 drops

How to **make**

1 Add the essential oil blend to a diffuser, vaporizer or oil burner.

2 Gently fragrance your chosen environment.

Eczema ointment

Chamomile and rose cool and balance skin. Combined with an unscented base they can be applied to affected areas to take the heat out of itchy skin.

Ingredients

Makes 15ml (½fl oz)
Unfragranced lotion 1 tbsp
Roman chamomile essential oil 3 drops
Rose absolute essential oil 2 drops

How to **make**

1 Mix the essential oils into the lotion or ointment.

2 Dab on to affected areas of skin.

Stretch marks

Stretch marks are caused by excessive and rapid weight gain, for example during pregnancy, which over-stretches skin and causes the fibres in the deeper layers to tear.

This leaves wavy reddish stripes that gradually turn white. The marks usually appear on the thighs, breasts, abdomen, and buttocks. Massage tones skin, which may limit the effects and severity of stretch marks. However, once they appear they are permanent, although they do fade over time.

Skin-toning massage

A massage with nourishing oils improves skin tone, encourages the renewal of skin cells, and makes skin look and feel smoother. Here, moisturizing base oils are blended with toning frankincense and skin-cell regenerating mandarin and neroli essential oils.

Ingredients

Makes 30ml (1fl oz)
Almond oil 1tbsp
Wheatgerm oil 1tsp
Apricot kernel oil 1tsp
Avocado oil 1tsp
Frankincense essential oil 7 drops
Mandarin essential oil 5 drops
Neroli essential oil 3 drops

How to **make**

1 Combine all the ingredients together in a bowl. Transfer to a sterilized dark glass bottle and seal with a cap or dropper.

2 Gently massage the affected area. Allow the oil to absorb into the skin before you get dressed. Store the remaining oil in a cool, dark place. Keeps for up to 3 months.

Sunburn

Sunburn occurs when skin is damaged by the sun's ultraviolet rays. Skin becomes red, sore, warm, tender, and, occasionally, itchy, and starts to flake and peel after a few days. It is extremely important to try to avoid getting sunburnt in the first place as damaging the skin in this way increases the chances of developing serious health problems later on, for example skin cancer. If skin does become burnt, try to keep the affected area cool and moist. Essential oil remedies that are calming and cooling are ideal.

Cooling lavender compress

Skin-healing oils, such as lavender and chamomile essential oils, and cooling peppermint essential oil are combined here to make a cooling compress that can be applied to help bring relief to tender, sunburnt skin.

Ingredients

Makes 1 compress
Aloe vera juice 1 tbsp
Lavender essential oil 4 drops
Peppermint essential oil 1 drop
German chamomile essential oil 2 drops

How to **make**

1 Fill a bowl with cold water. Add the aloe vera juice and essential oil blend.

2 Soak a flannel in the bowl, then remove the flannel and squeeze out the excess water.

3 Place the compress on the affected area of skin. Leave the flannel on the skin while it reaches body temperature. Repeat 3 times.

Cradle cap

Cradle cap, also known as seborrhoeic dermatitis, is a condition that causes greasy, yellow scaly patches on babies' scalps. It's a harmless condition that doesn't usually itch or cause any discomfort. Most cases clear up on their own over a period of weeks or months. The cause of cradle cap is unknown, but may be linked to an excess of sebum. Essential oils blended with base oils, or with an unfragranced baby shampoo, can help it to clear.

Gentle scalp massage

Massaging almond or olive oil into the scalp at night loosens crusts. Patchouli is astringent and tones skin; palmarosa is skin-balancing; and lavender heals and soothes skin if crusts peel off. This blend is suitable for infants over 12 months; for babies 3-12 months, use just one drop of lavender; under 3 months just the base oil.

Ingredients

Makes 30ml (1fl oz)
Olive oil 2 tbsp
Lavender essential oil 1 drop
Palmarosa essential oil 1 drop
Patchouli essential oil 1 drop

How to **make**

1 Combine all the ingredients together in a bowl. Transfer to a sterilized dark glass bottle and seal with a cap or dropper.

2 Gently massage into your baby's scalp. Leave the oil overnight, then use a soft-bristled baby brush to gently remove loose flakes in the morning before washing with a baby shampoo. Don't be tempted to pick at or remove flakes that aren't already lose as this could damage skin and lead to infection.

3 Store the oil in a cool, dark place. Keeps for up to 3 months.

Lavender shampoo

Gently washing your baby's hair and scalp with a mild shampoo can help prevent a build-up of scales. In addition to its skin-healing properties, lavender is a gentle oil to use on your baby's scalp.

Ingredients

Makes 2 applications
Unscented baby shampoo 1 tbsp
Lavender essential oil 2 drops

How to **make**

1 Mix 2 drops of lavender essential oil in an unfragranced shampoo.

2 Gently wash your baby's hair, taking care not to remove flakes that aren't already loose. Rinse with just warm water.

Dandruff

The body continually sheds dead skin cells as new cells are formed.

In most cases, this is a gradual process that goes unnoticed. However, if the process speeds up, it can produce a buildup of dead skin cells that appear prominent and feel unsightly. Dandruff is a common skin condition that causes dry white or grey flakes of dead skin to appear on the scalp or attached to hair. The scalp may feel dry and itchy. It's not always clear why this happens, but possible causes include seborrhoeic dermatitis, which is a common skin condition that causes oily skin. Certain factors can make dandruff worse, for example, an overuse of hair products, emotional stress, and washing hair too much or too little. The following treatments can help to condition the scalp.

Invigorating scalp massage

The stimulating action of a scalp massage can be used with essential oils to create an effective dandruff treatment. Thyme essential oil has an anti-fungal action that is useful for treating conditions such as dandruff, while tea tree helps to balance oils and keep the scalp healthy.

Ingredients

Makes 2 applications
Coconut oil solid 1 tbsp
Tea tree essential oil 3 drops
Lavender essential oil 2 drops
Thyme essential oil 2 drops

How to **make**

1 Melt the coconut oil solid in a bain marie, then add the essential oils and pour the blend into a sterilized glass jar. Massage half the oil blend into the scalp. Do this before bed, then cover the pillow with a towel to avoid the oil blend staining the pillowcase.

2 Leave the oil on overnight and then rinse it out in the morning, applying shampoo before wetting and rinsing the hair.

Peppermint hair rinse

Combining essential oils with dried herbs creates a natural hair tonic that can add shine and help to tone and balance oils on the scalp and control flaky dandruff. Adding soothing peppermint to stimulating rosemary can help to condition the scalp and combat dandruff.

Ingredients

Makes 45ml (1½fl oz)
Dried peppermint 1 tbsp
Dried rosemary herb 1 tbsp
Cider vinegar 1 tbsp
Peppermint essential oil 2 drops
Rosemary essential oil 1 drop

How to **make**

1 To make the infusion, place the dried herbs in a teapot and add 200ml (7fl oz) boiling water. Leave to infuse for around 10 minutes then strain the water.

2 Add the essential oils to the cider vinegar, then to the herbal infusion.

3 Use the infusion as a final hair rinse after shampooing. Finish with a final rinse of warm water only.

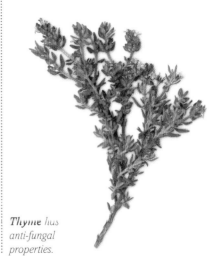

Thyme has anti-fungal properties.

Allergic reactions

Our immune system is designed to **protect** the body against harmful foreign substances. Sometimes, however, the body develops a **sensitivity** to a substance that doesn't pose a threat and reacts as though it is harmful, releasing the substance histamine, which triggers an allergic reaction. Essential oils can help to **calm** allergic responses and **soothe** symptoms.

Allergies and hay fever

An allergy is the body's reaction to a particular food or substance, known as an allergen. Allergic reactions are most common in children. The severity of a reaction can vary. Most are mild, but occasionally a severe reaction, called anaphylaxis, or anaphylactic shock, can occur, which is a medical emergency and requires urgent treatment. Allergic reactions can usually be kept under control with careful management. Common allergens include dust mites, medication, food such as nuts, shellfish, fruit, and cows' milk, and animal fur.

Hay fever is a common allergic reaction to pollen in the warmer months. Many types of pollen are released by plants at different times of the year, causing symptoms such as sneezing, a runny nose, and itchy eyes. Remedies with calming oils can help control symptoms.

Clearing eucalyptus inhalation

Essential oils can help open the airways. Here, the sharp aroma of eucalyptus blends with ravensara for an effective decongestant. The addition of calming lavender helps to quell the stress and anxiety caused by allergic reactions.

Ingredients

Makes 1 inhalation
Eucalyptus radiata essential oil 5 drops
Lavender essential oil 3 drops
Ravensara essential oil 2 drops

How to **make**

1 Add the essential oils to a bowl of hot water. Cover your head with a towel, make a tent over the bowl of hot water, and then lean forwards over the bowl. For children or asthma sufferers, don't cover the head with a towel.

2 Inhale the steam for 5 minutes, taking a break if needed.

Chamomile nose balm

Essential oils provide a simple yet effective way to reduce hay fever and allergy symptoms. Using calming oils, such as chamomile, in a balm can trap pollen and soothe irritated skin.

Ingredients

Makes 20 to 30 applications
Beeswax 1 tbsp
Sunflower oil 1 tbsp
German chamomile essential oil 1 drop
Lavender essential oil 1 drop
Peppermint essential oil 1 drop

How to **make**

1 Gently melt the wax and sunflower oil in a bain marie.

2 Add the essential oils and mix together. Pour into a sterilized jar and leave to cool, then seal with a lid.

3 Apply the balm around the nose as required to soothe irritated skin.

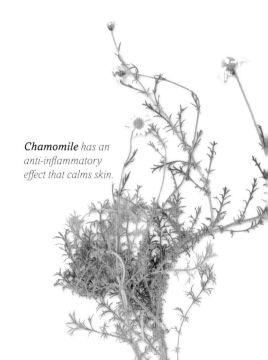

Chamomile has an anti-inflammatory effect that calms skin.

Mind and wellbeing

Stress is a common modern-day malady and it can have profound effects on mental health. Addressing over-hectic lifestyles can help to **combat stress**, and essential oils can be a great support here as their numerous therapeutic benefits work **holistically** to **soothe** and calm emotions, ease anxiety and tension, and **balance moods**, creating an enhanced sense of wellbeing.

Anxiety

We all experience anxiety at some point in life. The feeling of unease or worry that can be mild or severe is a normal response to the stresses of life. For example, you may feel worried about an exam, or anxious about a medical test or an interview. Feeling anxious at stressful times is normal, but if it becomes hard to control worries, and feelings of anxiety become constant, talk to your doctor. Using oils in a diffuser creates a reassuring and calm environment.

Lemon balm diffusion

There are a number of relaxing oils for reducing anxiety that can be used in a massage, in the bath, or diffused into a room to create a peaceful environment.

Ingredients

Makes 1 diffusion
Lemon balm essential oil 5 drops
Lemon essential oil 3 drops
Cypress essential oil 3 drops
Bergamot essential oil 2 drops

How to **make**

1 Add the essential oil blend to a diffuser, vaporizer or oil burner.

2 Gently fragrance your chosen environment.

Depression

Difficult events and experiences can leave us feeling in low spirits. If this low feeling persists we can develop depression.

Some common causes of depression include relationship problems, bereavement, sleep problems (which may arise from stress and other concerns), stress at work, bullying, and chronic illness and pain. Sometimes it's possible to feel down without there being an obvious reason. Depression can also come on at specific points in life or at specific times, for example after the birth of a child or during the winter months.

A low mood that lasts for two weeks or more can be a sign of depression. Other symptoms of depression include: not getting any enjoyment out of life, feeling hopeless, feeling tired or lacking energy, not being able to concentrate on everyday tasks such as reading the paper or watching television, comfort eating or losing one's appetite, sleeping more than usual or being unable to sleep, having suicidal thoughts or thoughts about harming yourself. It's always important to talk to your doctor about how you are feeling if you are experiencing any of the above symptoms and a low mood persists for an extended period of time.

Therapeutic essential oils can be very beneficial for helping to lift feelings of depression and bring a feeling of calm that can release anxiety and tension.

Calming diffusion

Essential oils can be wonderful remedies for providing emotional support. In this diffusion, calming frankincense helps to lift the spirits and is especially helpful when you are feeling tired or overwhelmed, while mandarin soothes frayed nerves, promoting relaxation, and uplifting neroli helps to balance emotions and is effective for relieving stress.

Ingredients

Makes 1 diffusion
Frankincense essential oil 5 drops
Neroli essential oil 3 drops
Mandarin essential oil 2 drops

How to **make**

1 Add the essential oil blend to a diffuser, vaporizer or oil burner.

2 Gently fragrance your chosen environment.

Grief and shock

Times of emotional crisis and upset often involve some kind of loss or bereavement. This may be the loss of a loved one, or the end of a marriage or important relationship. Most people grieve when they lose something or someone important to them. Grieving can feel unbearable at times, but it's a necessary process to work through. There are many different reactions to loss, and no one right reaction, but grief usually does consist of a few key emotions: these include anxiety and helplessness, and anger and sadness. Eventually, you adjust to a loss and though your feelings can remain as intense, they tend to become less frequent. Essential oils can be especially helpful at times of loss or trauma, helping to lift spirits and ground emotions.

Neroli "rescue" remedy

Neroli essential oil is considered to be the "rescue remedy" of essential oils and is particularly helpful during times of grief and shock. Here, its effects are supported by uplifting bergamot and calming petitgrain essential oils. Disperse this blend of oils in your environment to help calm emotions and ease feelings of anxiety.

Ingredients

Makes 1 diffusion
Neroli essential oil 5 drops
Petitgrain essential oil 3 drops
Bergamot essential oil 2 drops

How to **make**

1 Add the essential oil blend to a diffuser, vaporizer or oil burner.

2 Gently fragrance your chosen environment.

Soothing rose and geranium massage

Essential oils with uplifting and euphoric properties are very useful for helping to deal with grief. Geranium is uplifting and calming at the same time, which makes it useful for warding off the feelings of depression that often accompany grief. Frankincense essential oil also helps to lift the spirits, and the calming aroma of rose promotes relaxation and helps to reduce feelings of anxiety and releases tension, helping to create a sense of wellbeing that can punctuate the grief.

Ingredients

Makes 2 tbsp of massage oil
Almond oil 2 tbsp
Frankincense essential oil 4 drops
Rose absolute or essential oil 3 drops
Geranium essential oil 1 drop

How to **make**

1 Combine all the ingredients together in a bowl. Transfer to a sterilized dark glass bottle and seal with a cap or dropper.

2 Massage into the skin (avoiding the face). Allow the oil to absorb into the skin before you get dressed. Store the remaining oil in a cool, dark place. Keeps for up to 3 months.

Uplifting jasmine bath

This combination of oils provides a revitalizing bath soak that can create a feeling of wellbeing. Jasmine essential oil or absolute helps to increase optimism, combating the feelings of listlessness, while sandalwood promotes restful sleep and helps to restore vitality.

Ingredients

Makes 1 tbsp
Almond oil or full-fat milk 1 tbsp
Sandalwood essential oil 4 drops
Jasmine absolute or essential oil 4 drops
Grapefruit essential oil 2 drops

How to **make**

1 Combine all the ingredients together in a bowl.

2 Disperse the blend immediately in the bath and enjoy a reviving and soothing soak.

Stress and insomnia

Stress is one of the major health problems in the Western world and is responsible for many

of our illnesses. It has numerous causes and can affect us in a number of different ways, both mentally and physically. The body's natural response to stress is controlled by the autonomic nervous system and involves the release of the hormones adrenaline and cortisol, which also control the "fight or flight" mechanism – the body's inbuilt reaction to dangerous or threatening situations. While a certain amount of stress is good for us, helping to keep us motivated and interested in tasks, if stress starts to impact on our moods, digestion, and sleep, it becomes more of an issue. Try these relaxing and soothing remedies to help yourself wind down and let go of tension.

De-stressing clary sage massage

Using therapeutic essential oils in a massage blend is an excellent way to help the body to manage chronic stress, promote relaxation, and improve the quality of sleep if stress is causing insomnia. You can also enjoy this oil blend in a soothing bedtime bath by adding the essential oils to 1 tablespoon of either base oil or full-fat milk, and dispersing immediately in the bath, then enjoy a relaxing pre-bedtime soak.

Ingredients

Makes 2 tbsp
Almond oil 2 tbsp
Clary sage essential oil 5 drops
Frankincense essential oil 5 drops
Geranium essential oil 5 drops

How to **make**

1 Combine all the ingredients together in a bowl. Transfer to a sterilized dark glass bottle and seal with a cap or dropper.

2 Massage into the skin (avoiding the face). Allow the oil to absorb into the skin before you get dressed. Store the remaining oil in a cool, dark place. Keeps for up to 3 months.

Litsea and bergamot calming diffusion

Litsea essential oil is a useful stress buster. Its naturally soothing properties calm the rapid heartbeat that can accompany stress and panic, helping you to think more rationally. Bergamot is grounding and helps to balance the mind. The addition of uplifting orange adds to the calming effect of this blend.

Ingredients

Makes 1 diffusion
Litsea essential oil 6 drops
Orange essential oil 4 drops
Bergamot essential oil 4 drops

How to **make**

1 Add the essential oil blend to a diffuser, vaporizer or oil burner.

2 Gently fragrance your chosen environment.

Ylang ylang bedtime spray

If stress and anxiety keep you awake at night, or you find it difficult to switch off at bedtime and find that you wake in the morning feeling groggy, try this wonderfully relaxing pillow spray. Calming chamomile and rose essential oils are joined by the uplifting, sweetly scented ylang ylang, which helps to calm breathing, and grounding vetiver, which has a profoundly calming effect when you feel overwhelmed by stress.

Ingredients

Makes 30ml (1fl oz)
Ylang ylang essential oil 6 drops
Rose essential oil 6 drops
Vetiver essential oil 2 drops
Roman chamomile essential oil 1 drop

How to **make**

1 Mix the essential oils with 2 tablespoons cold water and pour into a sterilized bottle with an atomizer.

2 Spritz your room before bedtime. Shake before use, and avoid spraying directly onto fabric.

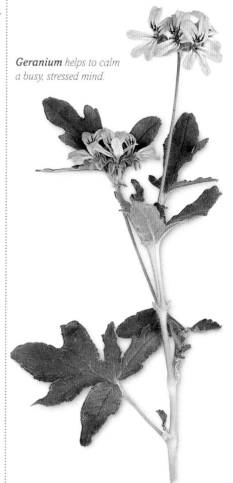

Geranium helps to calm a busy, stressed mind.

Women's health

Women's hormones go through a number of changes throughout life, causing physical and **emotional** symptoms, many of which can be helped by essential oils. Premenstrual fluid retention can be alleviated using oils and massage, and premenstrual tension can be **soothed** with **calming oils.** Uplifting oils can alleviate depression after birth and during the menopause.

Premenstrual symptoms

Many women experience a mix of emotional and physical symptoms in the run up to menstruation.

For some women, these symptoms are mild and occur for just a couple of days before menstruation begins. For others, symptoms can be wider ranging, more pronounced, and can start as early as two weeks before the onset of menstruation.

Physical premenstrual symptoms include fluid retention and bloating, fatigue, breast tenderness, lower back ache, and abdominal discomfort. Emotional symptoms include general anxiety, irritability, stress, and a low mood, or unpredictable mood swings. Therapeutic essential oils are a great help for premenstrual complaints as their holistic nature helps to treat the whole range of symptoms, relieving physical complaints and providing emotional support by calming and balancing emotions.

Juniper compress for fluid retention

Essential oils with a mild diuretic action, such as juniper, geranium, and fennel, are effective for flushing out toxins and reducing the uncomfortable fluid retention and puffiness commonly experienced before menstruation. As well as their physical benefits, the oils relieve emotional premenstrual symptoms, too. Juniper helps to revive flagging spirits and calms nervous tension, and geranium balances the emotions, which can ward off mood swings. A hot or cold compress using this essential oil blend makes a soothing and effective premenstrual remedy. Avoid this blend in pregnancy.

Ingredients

Makes 1 compress
Almond oil 1 tsp
Calendula macerated oil 2 tsp
Wheatgerm oil 1 tsp
Juniper essential oil 5 drops
Fennel essential oil 5 drops
Geranium essential oil 5 drops

How to **make**

1 Fill a bowl with hot or cold water, whichever is your preference. Add the oil blend.

2 Soak a flannel in the bowl, then remove the flannel and squeeze out the excess water.

3 If the flannel is hot, place a towel or piece of cling film over it to insulate it, if you wish. Place the compress on the area requiring treatment. Leave the flannel in place while it reaches body temperature. Repeat 3 times.

Pre-menstrual rose and geranium bath

Pre-menstrual tension (PMT) can be stressful and tiring as hormonal changes lead to sudden mood swings, or bring on a general low mood, and feelings of tension and anxiety can feel overwhelming. Try this soothing and grounding essential oil bath soak for a pre-menstrual stress-reducing tonic that will leave you feeling more grounded, calm, and uplifted.

Ingredients

Makes 1 tbsp
Base oil or full-fat milk 1 tbsp
Rose essential oil 5 drops
Clary sage essential oil 2 drops
Geranium essential oil 2 drops

How to **make**

1 Combine all the ingredients together in a bowl.

2 Disperse the oil blend immediately in a hot bath, and then enjoy a reviving and uplifting soak that can leave you feeling revived.

Pregnancy

Many essential oils aren't advised in pregnancy (see Safe usage in the A–Z for each oil), but some are safe and help with relaxation and some pregnancy symptoms. For example, juniper, mandarin, rose, rosemary, marjoram, and neroli are popular pregnancy oils. See page 195 for oils that are safe in pregnancy.

Skin-nourishing pregnancy massage

Enjoy a backache-relieving massage or a calming facial massage. Stick to 1 per cent dilutions as your sense of smell is heightened in pregnancy. The massage blend below nourishes skin and improves elasticity. Used daily from the fifth month of pregnancy, it can help to prevent stretch marks. It is best not to use essential oils until you are past the first trimester (unless you have had advice from a qualified aromatherapy practitioner).

Ingredients

Makes 30ml (1fl oz)
Almond oil 1 tbsp
Wheatgerm oil 1 tbsp
Mandarin essential oil 2 drops
Lavender essential oil 2 drops
Neroli essential oil 2 drops

How to **make**

1 Combine the ingredients in a bowl. Transfer to a sterilized dark glass bottle. Seal with a cap or dropper.

2 Gently massage the skin. Allow the oil to absorb into the skin before you get dressed. Store the remaining oil in a cool, dark place. Keeps for up to 3 months.

Postnatal and menopause

Hormonal swings after birth can affect mood, leading to the baby blues, and sometimes longer-lasting postnatal depression. Similarly, hormonal changes in the menopause can affect mood, causing irritability and depression. Menopause also has a range of physical symptoms, one of the best-known being hot flushes, characterized by a sudden feeling of heat sweeping over the body. Calming and relaxing essential oils can help to ease symptoms and lift the spirits.

Soothing blend for hot flushes and irritability

This cooling blend of oils is ideal for hot flushes and general irritability. Bergamot is particularly helpful when the body is overheated. Roman chamomile calms and soothes, while rose and geranium enhance wellbeing.

Ingredients

Makes 90ml (3fl oz)
Bergamot essential oil 5 drops
Rose absolute oil 5 drops
Geranium essential oil 2 drops
Roman chamomile essential oil 2 drops

How to **make**

1 Add the oils to 90ml (3fl oz) water. Transfer to an atomizer bottle.

2 Spritz the face to cool hot flushes, or spray a room to create a calming environment. Alternatively, add the blend to a diffuser and gently fragrance your chosen environment.

Hormone-balancing fennel massage

Cooling fennel is blended with soothing rose and geranium oils here to create a gentle balancing and grounding blend. Avoid this blend in pregnancy.

Ingredients

Makes 2 tbsp
Almond oil 2 tbsp
Fennel essential oil 3 drops
Rose absolute oil 5 drops
Geranium essential oil 5 drops

How to **make**

1 Combine all the ingredients together in a bowl. Transfer to a sterilized glass dark bottle and seal with a cap or dropper.

2 Gently massage the body (avoid the face). Allow the oil to absorb into the skin before getting dressed. Store the remaining oil in a cool, dark place. Keeps for up to 3 months.

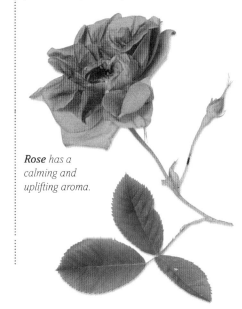

Rose has a calming and uplifting aroma.

Men's health

As with women, men can encounter specific health issues. Prostate health is important for men, and the effects of stress can feature prominently. Essential oils have clear benefits for these areas. Remedies that work **holistically** on **body** and **mind** help to counter the negative effects of stress, and antiseptic and diuretic oils target prostate problems **alongside medical treatments**.

Heart health and stress

Cardiovascular disease is one of the leading causes of death for men in the United States and is a growing health concern worldwide. General heart health can be improved by exercising regularly, eating a healthy, balanced diet, giving up smoking, and finding ways to reduce and manage everyday stress. See pages 318–19 for other remedies for circulation. Essential oils have numerous properties that can help with problems that are associated with the cardiovascular system, such as high blood pressure and sluggish circulation.

Bergamot and neroli bath oil blend

This bath oil remedy can also be used as a massage blend, added to a shower gel, or the essential oils can be added to a diffuser. Here, relaxing essential oils are used in a warm bath to help release tension in the body and combat the effects of stress and anxiety.

Ingredients

Makes 15ml (½fl oz)
Almond oil 1 tbsp
Bergamot essential oil 5 drops
Neroli essential oil 2 drops
Sandalwood essential oil 5 drops

How to **make**

1 Combine all the ingredients together in a bowl.

2 Disperse the oil blend immediately in the bath and enjoy a relaxing soak.

Prostate problems

Problems with the prostate are increasingly common in older men. The prostate gland can become enlarged, which can sometimes be due to bacterial infection. Anti-inflammatory and antiseptic essential oils can help to calm swelling and kill off bacteria. It's also important that men get the prostate checked regularly so that changes in size are spotted and any necessary treatment given.

Prostate massage

Antiseptic and anti-inflammatory frankincense blends well with myrrh and anti-bacterial rosemary. Massage around the genital area regularly to stimulate circulation and improve prostate health.

Ingredients

Makes 15ml (½fl oz)
Almond oil 1 tbsp
Rosemary essential oil 1 drop
Frankincense essential oil 1 drop
Myrrh essential oil 1 drop

How to **make**

1 Combine all the ingredients together in a bowl. Transfer to a sterilized dark glass bottle and seal with a cap or dropper.

2 Gently massage into the area around and below the genitals. Allow the oil to absorb into the skin before getting dressed. Store the remaining oil in a cool, dark place. Keeps for up to 3 months.

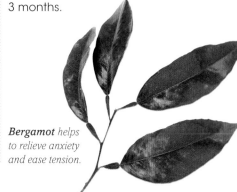

Bergamot helps to relieve anxiety and ease tension.

First aid

Essential oils are a valuable addition to a home first-aid kit. Alongside the bandages and plasters, oils act as antiseptics for cuts and wounds and can **soothe** and **calm** irritated skin, bites and stings, and minor burns and scalds. Oils such as tea tree can be applied neat to protect wounds from infection, while **cooling** and **warming oils** can counter the effects of weather.

Blisters

Blisters on the skin often occur after an injury, burning, scalding, repetitive rubbing or an insect sting. They can be painful and also very annoying. A blister develops when there is an accumulation of fluid underneath the skin. When the blister bursts, the revealed tissue beneath may be sore and become infected.

Tea tree and lavender ointment

Regular application of lavender essential oil directly onto the affected area can help reduce swelling and prevent infection and ease pain.

Ingredients

Makes 1 application
Tea tree essential oil 1 drop
Lavender essential oil 1 drop

How to **make**

1 Apply the essential oils directly to the blister with a cotton bud.

2 Cover the blister carefully with a plaster to reduce the chance of an infection.

Heat exhaustion and fever

Heat exhaustion is when too much heat or sunlight causes lethargy, dizziness, nausea, vomiting, and a headache. A person with heat exhaustion should be moved to a cool place and given water.

Fever is the body's defence against infections. Seek medical help if a temperature rises quickly.

Cooling compress

Cool the body with this compress.

Ingredients

Makes 1 compress
Witch hazel 1 tbsp
Peppermint essential oil 2 drops
Lavender essential oil 3 drops

How to **make**

1 Fill a bowl with cold water. Add the essential oils to the witch hazel and then to the water.

2 Soak a flannel in the bowl, remove and wring out.

3 Place the compress on the skin. Leave in place while it reaches body temperature. Repeat 3 times.

Insect bites and stings

The severity of bites and stings depends on the type of insect and a person's sensitivity. A serious allergic reaction will require immediate medical help.

Lavender compress

This soothing compress reduces itching.

Ingredients

Makes 1 compress
Witch hazel 1 tbsp
Lavender essential oil 3 drops
Roman chamomile essential oil 1 drop

How to **make**

1 Fill a bowl with cold water. Add the essential oils to the witch hazel and then to the water.

2 Soak a flannel in the bowl, remove and wring out.

3 Place the flannel on the skin. Leave it in place while it reaches body temperature. Repeat 3 times.

Treatment reference charts

Essential oils are versatile and the choice can be overwhelming, which can make it hard to decide which oils have the right properties for your specific needs. The quick reference charts below are designed to help you rapidly pinpoint the essential oils particularly suited to your requirements. The chart on pages 340-342 lists essential oils for common complaints, while the charts on page 343 recommend essential oils for mind and wellbeing and essential oils for cosmetic use.

Common **complaints**

Everyday common complaints include chronic conditions that require long-term management, such as arthritis, depression, and stress; occasional problems, such as headaches or diarrhoea; one-off first-aid situations; skin complaints, such as eczema, athlete's foot, and dandruff; and menstrual and menopausal complaints. This chart helps you to identify at a glance which essential oils are especially recommended to help with specific concerns. Always consult your doctor about symptoms and use essential oils as complementary treatments alongside medications when necessary. For information on each essential oil, check the A–Z listings on pages 196–293.

HEALING OILS

Certain essential oils have specific properties that make them ideal for treating a particular complaint. The remedies in this chapter show you how to use oils in massage, compresses, inhalations, and ointments to treat a range of conditions.

Common complaint	Recommended essential oils
Allergies	Yarrow, Helichrysum, Lavender, Chamomile
Appetite loss	Buchu, Galangal, Dill, Tarragon, Cinnamon, Lemon, Lemongrass, Fennel, Wintergreen, Litsea, Peppermint, Nutmeg, Ginger
Arthritis	Yarrow, Lemon verbena, Mugwort, Birch leaf, Frankincense, Cedarwood, Cypress, Wintergreen, Helichrysum, Star anise, Juniper, Lavender, Nutmeg, Marjoram, Parsley, Black pepper, Benzoin, Plai, Ginger
Asthma	Frankincense, Caraway, Lemon, Eucalyptus, Lavender, Roman chamomile, Niaouli, Lemon balm, Peppermint, Myrtle, Sandalwood, Clove
Athlete's foot	Galangal, Cedarwood, Lemongrass, Palmarosa, Eucalyptus, Wintergreen, Star anise, Lavender, Manuka, Tea tree, Cajuput, Oregano, Geranium, Patchouli, Summer savory, Tagetes, Thyme
Backache and neck pain	Tarragon, Coriander, Camphor, Grapefruit, Bay laurel, Lavender, Niaouli, Marjoram, Geranium, Allspice, Black pepper, Rosemary, Ginger
Bites and stings	Lime, Lavender, Manuka, Roman chamomile, Lemon balm, Peppermint, Allspice, Patchouli, Summer savory
Blisters	Lavender, Tea tree
Body odour	Galangal, Tarragon, Petitgrain, Lemon, Grapefruit, Coriander, Cypress, Lemongrass, Palmarosa, Cardamom, Star anise, Manuka, Litsea, Pine, Sage, Vetiver

Common complaint	Recommended essential oils
Bruising	Yarrow, Lavender
Constipation	Orange, Fennel, Marjoram, Peppermint, Pine, Black Pepper, Rosemary
Coughs and colds	Frankincense, Cedarwood, Lemon, Cypress, Eucalyptus, Fennel, Helichrysum, Lavender, Tea tree, Peppermint, Marjoram, Pine, Ravintsara, Rosemary, Clary sage, Thyme
Cradle cap	Palmarosa, Lavender, Patchouli
Dandruff	Birch, Cedarwood, Lime, Lemon, Wintergreen, Juniper, Bay laurel, Lavender, Tea tree, Peppermint, Geranium, Rosemary, Sage, Thyme
Depression	Frankincense, Ylang ylang, Cedarwood, Cinnamon, Neroli, Bergamot, Mandarin, Orange, Lemongrass, Helichrysum, Jasmine, Litsea, Basil, Geranium, Tuberose, Ravintsara, Clary sage, Benzoin
Diarrhoea	Neroli, Mandarin, Cypress, Eucalyptus, Fennel, Chamomile, Peppermint, Black pepper, Ginger
Eczema and psoriasis	Yarrow, Frankincense, Cedarwood, Cistus, Cumin, Helichrysum, Juniper, Lavender, German chamomile, Lemon balm, Geranium, Sandalwood, Benzoin, Fenugreek
Fluid retention	Yarrow, Buchu, Dill, Cedarwood, Cistus, Lime, Lemon, Grapefruit, Mandarin, Orange, Cypress, Carrot seed, Juniper, Geranium, Parsley seed, Rosemary
Grief	Frankincense, Cistus, Neroli, Petitgrain, Bergamot, Geranium, Rose
Headaches and migraines	Rosewood, Grapefruit, Coriander, Lemongrass, Eucalyptus, Bay laurel, Lavender, Lemon balm, Peppermint, Marjoram, Rosemary, Ginger
Heat exhaustion and fever	Lime, Bergamot, Lavender, Lemon balm, Peppermint, Vetiver
High blood pressure	Ylang ylang, Cumin, Lavender, Marjoram, Clary sage, Valerian
Hot flushes	Bergamot, Roman chamomile, Geranium, Rose, Clary sage

Essential oils make useful additions to your home remedy cabinet.

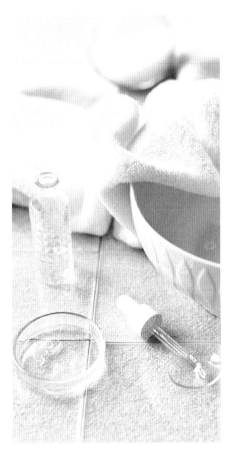

Using oils therapeutically *in steam inhalations can be an excellent way to relieve congestion.*

Common complaint	Recommended essential oils
Insomnia	Yarrow, Dill, Neroli, Petitgrain, Bergamot, Lemon, Orange, Star anise, Bay laurel, Lavender, Roman chamomile, Nutmeg, Myrtle, Marjoram, Allspice, Tuberose, Sandalwood, Valerian, Vetiver
Mouth and gum care	Cistus, Myrrh, Cardamom, Fennel, Tea tree, Peppermint, Nutmeg, Clove
Muscular aches and pains	Eucalyptus, Lavender, Peppermint, Nutmeg, Rosemary, Clove, Thyme, Ginger
Nausea and sickness	Buchu, Lemon verbena, Galangal, Dill, Mandarin, Cardamom, Litsea, Roman chamomile, Lemon balm, Peppermint, Nutmeg, Parsley seed, Allspice, Black pepper, Rose, Clary sage, Fenugreek, Ginger
Pre-menstrual tension	Fennel, Juniper, Marjoram, Geranium, Rose, Clary sage
Prostate health	Frankincense, Myrrh, Rosemary
Reflux and indigestion	Dill, Mandarin, Coriander, Cardamom, Fennel, Chamomile, Peppermint, Basil, Parsley, Ginger
Sprains and strains	Lemongrass, Marjoram, Black pepper, Rosemary, Thyme, Ginger
Stress and anxiety	Frankincense, Ylang ylang, Cedarwood, Neroli, Petitgrain, Bergamot, Lemon, Mandarin, Orange, Jasmine, Lavender, Litsea, Chamomile, Lemon balm, Basil, Marjoram, Geranium, Patchouli, Rose, Rosemary, Clary sage, Sandalwood, Vetiver
Sunburn	Bergamot, German chamomile, Lavender, Tea tree
Urinary tract infections	Lavender, German chamomile, Peppermint
Varicose veins/ haemorrhoids	Lemon, Cypress, Helichrysum, Juniper, Geranium

Each essential oil has a range of therapeutic properties.

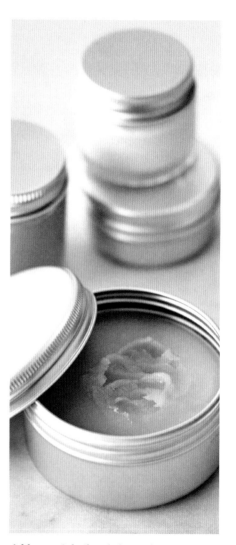

Add essential oils *to balms and creams to create healing remedies and nourishing cosmetic products.*

Mind and **wellbeing**

An important and key element of aromatherapy is its ability to treat holistically, looking beyond isolated symptoms and treating both body and mind. For example, when oils are used to promote relaxation or to energize, they can also help the body to deal with other specific complaints. The chart, right, suggests key oils for mental and physical wellbeing.

Mind and wellbeing	Recommended essential oils
Calming and soothing	Ylang ylang, Cypress, Palmarosa, Helichrysum, Lavender, Chamomile, Patchouli, Rose, Clary sage, Sandalwood
Concentration and focus	Cardamom, Peppermint, Basil, Thyme
Energizing	Lemongrass, Juniper, Pine, Rosemary, Clove, Thyme
Relaxation	Ylang ylang, Neroli, Orange, Lavender, Rose, Sandalwood, Vetiver
Stimulating and invigorating	Citronella, Basil, Black pepper, Rosemary, Ginger
Uplifting	Lime, Neroli, Petitgrain, Bergamot, Lemon, Grapefruit, Orange, Lemongrass, Palmarosa, Litsea, Lemon balm, Peppermint, Geranium, Rose
Warming	Cinnamon, Nutmeg, Marjoram, Black pepper, Clove

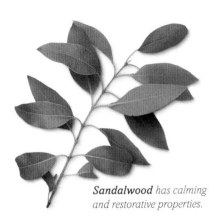

Sandalwood *has calming and restorative properties.*

Cosmetic **treatments**

Essential oils can play a key role in cosmetics, where their properties prove extremely useful for balancing and enhancing skin. The chart, right, helps you to choose oils and tailor blends to suit your particular skin type. When using oils cosmetically, ensure you first dilute them in a base oil or combine them with a cream or lotion base. The recipes in chapter five show you how to create cosmetic products using essential oils.

Skin conditions	Recommended essential oils
Dry and mature skin	Frankincense, Ylang ylang, Neroli, Palmarosa, Jasmine, Lavender, Chamomile, Patchouli, Rose, Sandalwood
Dry/oily hair	Cedarwood, Grapefruit, Tea tree, Rosemary
Oily and acne-prone skin	Ylang ylang, Petitgrain, Bergamot, Lime, Neroli, Lemon, Mandarin, Cypress, Palmarosa, Juniper, Bay laurel, Lavender, Tea tree, Niaouli, Geranium, Rose, Rosemary, Clary sage, Sandalwood
Scars/stretch marks	Frankincense, Neroli, Mandarin, Palmarosa, Jasmine, Lavender, Patchouli, Sandalwood, Vetiver, Plai
Sensitive skin	Neroli, Helichrysum, Lavender, Chamomile, Sandalwood

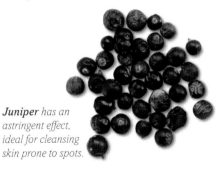

Juniper *has an astringent effect, ideal for cleansing skin prone to spots.*

Blending essential oils

The **art of blending** oils successfully to create **pleasing** and uplifting scents comes with practice. The fragrance families on pages 346–47 will help you understand which scents work especially well together. Below are a few practical **guidelines** to help you get started. Enjoy **experimenting** with scent combinations and discovering which aromas appeal to you. Over time, your confidence will grow and you will develop an **instinct** for blending.

How oils work **together**

Each essential oil is made up of multiple components, all of which are responsible for the different attributes and properties of the oil. The beauty of essential oils is that a fragrance is not just one individual note, but is composed of a complex harmony of notes (see box, right). You can work with these different notes to create favourite blends, adding citrus notes by blending with lemon, grapefruit, or lime, for example; or enhancing a blend with spicy notes by adding cardamom or black pepper.

The art of creating a beautiful blend of oils often comes down to practice, but there are some tips you can use to make life easier. And while you won't want to waste oils, a little trial and error can help you to understand how they work together and to gain confidence blending, so don't be afraid to make a few mistakes.

Blending guidelines Start off by creating very simple blends. As you work with the essential oils and become more familiar with them, you will notice that some are stronger smelling and more pervasive than others. These oils will dominate the ones that have a more subtle smell, so do bear this in mind and blend carefully, drop by drop, while you are practising and gaining confidence.

● **Always dilute essential oils** before applying to the skin (see the blending table on page 195 for guidelines of quantities of essential oil to base oil).

Aromatherapists use the following guidelines: 1 per cent dilution in a base oil for a product for sensitive skin, for a facial oil, for children, the elderly or for those with a weak immune system; 2.5 per cent dilution in a base oil for a product for the body of a healthy adult; and 5 per cent dilution for a local or topical application, for example for a compress.

● **Aim to use four to seven oils** per blend and avoid adding more than seven oils. When you start blending, you might prefer to blend just two or three oils at once, and these simple blends can be effective. As you gain confidence and discover scent combinations you like, you can begin to add a few more oils.

● **If you make a mistake** while blending oils, perhaps adding an oil whose smell you aren't keen on, it is hard to rectify the mistake. In this case, it's best to abandon the blend and start again.

● **Blend oils** in a small beaker or cup. If you need to store a blend, transfer it to a sterilized dark glass bottle and label the bottle with the date and the ingredients of the blend.

Top, middle, and base notes

Fragrances are built using "accords", which means that individual scents, or notes, are blended to create a new, unified aroma. Each fragrance is made up of top, middle, and base notes, which are combined to give structure to the blend and to create appealing, balanced, long-lasting fragrances.

● *Top notes* are light and refreshing and give the first impression.

● *Middle notes* are the heart of the fragrance and include most of the herbaceous scents, such as geranium.

● *Base notes* are rich aromas, such as sandalwood and ylang ylang, which give a scent body and longevity.

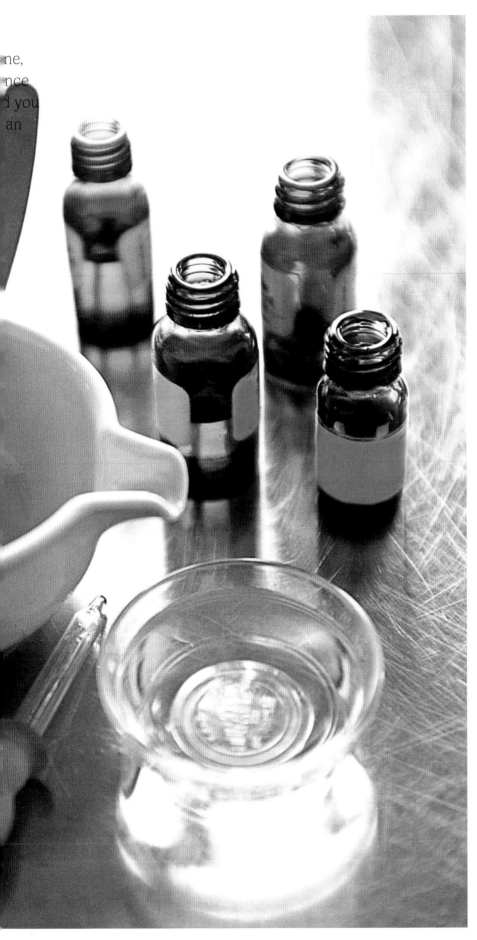

ne,
nce
d you
an

BLEND
VARIATION
Throughout the recipes, blend
variations are suggested to
encourage you to experiment
with oils and find your
favourite combinations.

Mix small
quantities of
oil to start with
as you learn the
art of blending.

Perfect blends

Essential oils can be categorized into **fragrance "families"**, which can guide your blending choices. Typically, the **aromas** each of us most enjoy belong to just one or two families. Here, families are arranged in a circle. While there are no rules, scents tend to marry well with those in their own family, and also with **neighbouring families**.

Floral oils

Florals are full-bodied scents such as rose that form the heart of an aroma. They can be used alone, or blended for more complex scents. Add citrus oils to lighten heady florals; spicy oils for a warm scent; or herbaceous oils for a cool aroma.

Essential oils
- Rosewood • Violet • Geranium
- Neroli • Rose • Ylang ylang
- Jasmine • Lavender
- Tagetes • Helichrysum
- Palmarosa • Mimosa

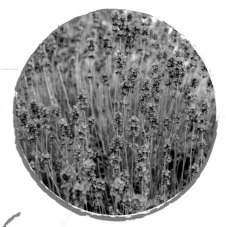

Floral lavender

Herbaceous oils

Herbaceous oils, such as basil, parsley, and chamomile, have a natural, elegant "green" scent and often form the "middle" note (p.344) of an aroma. Their clear scent can temper sweeter floral oils, and they can soften sharper citrus ones.

Essential oils
- Basil • Clary sage • Oregano • Parsley • Tarragon • Thyme • Yarrow • Dill
- Mugwort • Caraway • Carrot seed
- Chamomile • Fennel • Marjoram
- Myrtle • Summer savory • Manuka

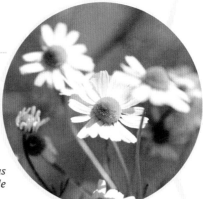

Herbaceous chamomile

THE FRAGRANCE WHEEL

In 1983, Michael Edwards, a fragrance industry consultant, devised a fragrance "wheel". He divided scents into floral, oriental, woody, and fresh, and most groupings are based on these classifications.

Essential oil families can be blended to create more complex aromas.

Citrus oils

Zingy and vibrant, the citrus family includes citrus oils, as well as oils such as fragonia that have scents reminiscent of citrus. These oils add tartness to floral and herbaceous oils, and make a crisp scent when blended with medicinal oils.

Essential oils
- Bergamot • Lemon • Grapefruit
- Mandarin • Orange • Lemon verbena • Lemongrass • Lemon balm • Lime • Buchu • Fragonia
- Petitgrain • Citronella • Litsea

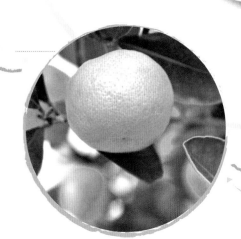

Citrus orange

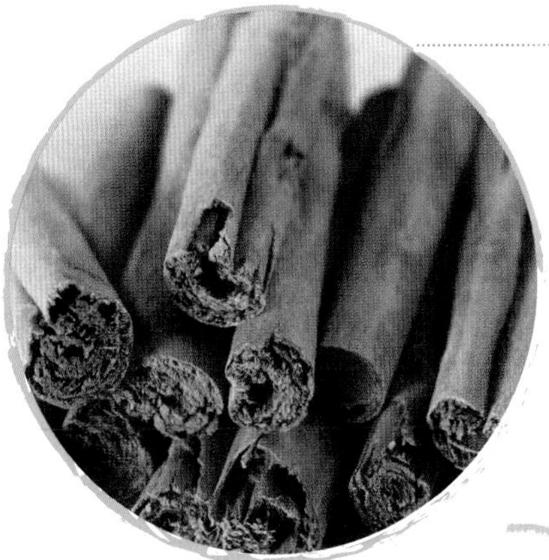

Spicy oils

This exotic family of scents is made up of warm, sensual, spicy, and velvety aromas. Oils such as cinnamon can form the central note in a scent, and rich oils such as vanilla create a "base" note (p.344), giving longevity to a scent. Try marrying spicy oriental oils with woody ones, such as sandalwood, to create blends that are earthy and deep. Oriental oils also blend naturally with many floral scents, such as ylang ylang, jasmine, and lavender, where the floral note tempers the oriental one to prevent it overpowering.

Essential oils
- Vanilla • Cinnamon • Nutmeg • Cardamom • Clove • Juniper
- Coriander • Black pepper • Cumin • Galangal • Litsea • Fenugreek
- Ginger • Star anise • Tuberose • Allspice • Cistus

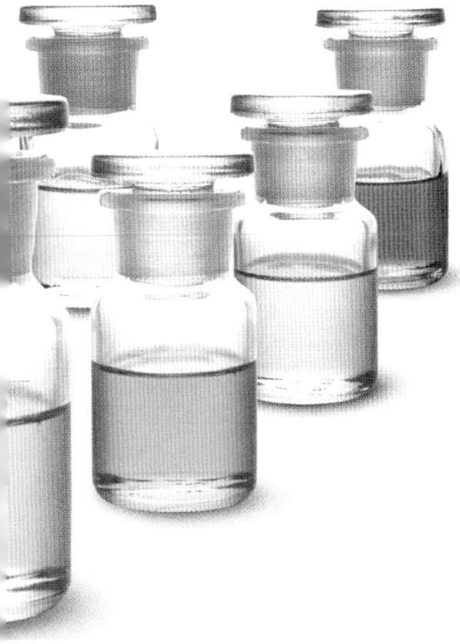

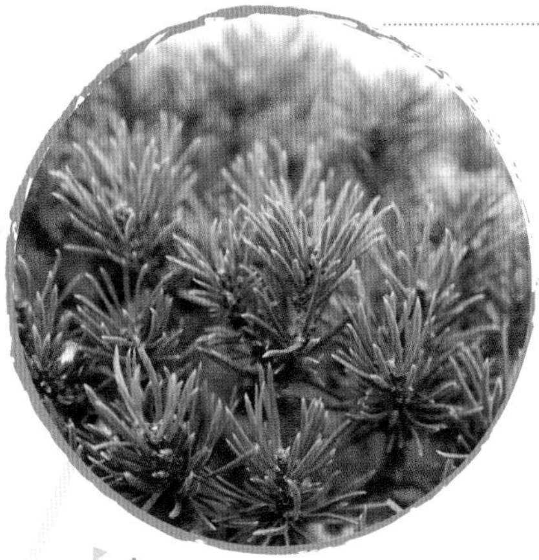

Spicy cinnamon

Woody oils

Earthy, mossy, musky, and dense, these complex scents contain many dominant aromas. Woody scents tend to be deeply grounding and are often sensual, as with sandalwood; and oils such as cedarwood and myrrh accentuate oriental aromas. Adding zesty citrus notes to woody oils creates a lively, fresher scent, while mixing woody oils with medicinal ones, such as eucalyptus, creates cool, resinous, minty aromas that offset the deep woody tones.

Essential oils
- Frankincense • Cypress • Pine • Myrrh
- Patchouli • Sandalwood • Cedarwood
- Angelica • Elemi • Benzoin • Valerian • Vetiver

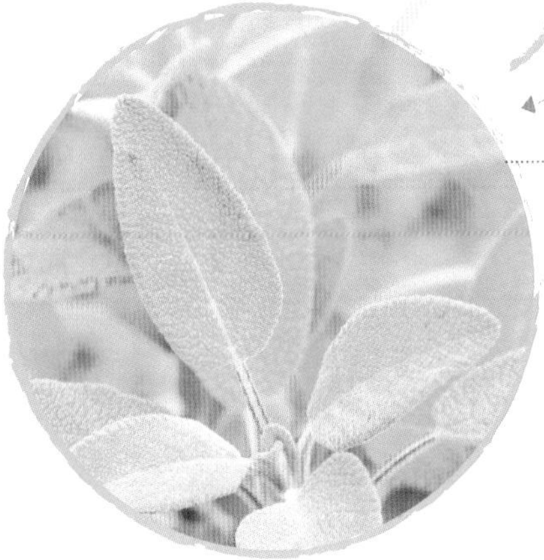

Woody pine

Medicinal oils

Crisp and clean, these, often lighter, scents produce a refreshing "top" note (see p164) to complement heavier woody aromas. Try also blending with woody or herbaceous oils to create a layered scent.

Essential oils
- Camphor • Sage • Wintergreen • Birch • Tea tree • Cajuput • Niaouli
- Ravintsara • Rosemary • Bay laurel • Peppermint • Eucalyptus • Plai

Medicinal sage

Additional ingredients

Essential oils can be combined with various ingredients to make a **range** of bath and body products and treatments. For **basic blends**, the oils on pages 296–309 make the ideal base for essential oils. In the following recipes, additional ingredients are used, such as **waxes**, floral waters, mineral salts, and citric acid to create **creams**, lotions, balms, scents, and infusions.

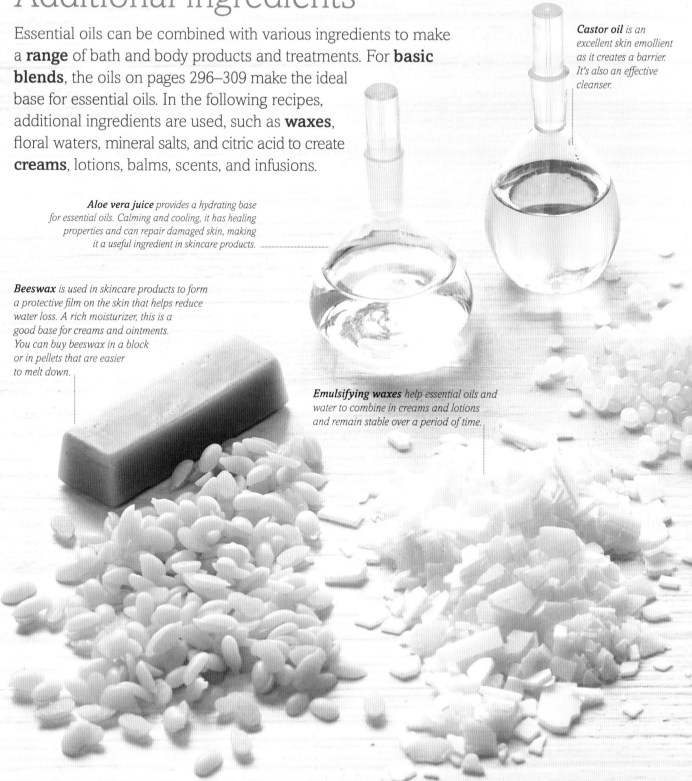

Castor oil is an excellent skin emollient as it creates a barrier. It's also an effective cleanser.

Aloe vera juice provides a hydrating base for essential oils. Calming and cooling, it has healing properties and can repair damaged skin, making it a useful ingredient in skincare products.

Beeswax is used in skincare products to form a protective film on the skin that helps reduce water loss. A rich moisturizer, this is a good base for creams and ointments. You can buy beeswax in a block or in pellets that are easier to melt down.

Emulsifying waxes help essential oils and water to combine in creams and lotions and remain stable over a period of time.

Rose floral water is a by-product of the steam-distillation of the essential oil. Beautifully fragrant, it can be used on its own as a toner or added to recipes. Floral waters share some of the oil's properties, but are less concentrated.

Kaolin powder can be added to skin products to work as an exfoliator, helping to remove dead skin cells and cleanse skin.

Sodium bicarbonate helps reduce inflammation and is cleansing. It soothes and softens the skin and promotes the release of toxins.

Candle wax can be made from beeswax, vegetable wax, or paraffin wax.

Glycerine is a colourless and odourless humectant, or moisturizer, that hydrates skin. It is a useful ingredient in cosmetics, and especially helpful in dry-skin treatments.

Citric acid is a naturally occurring fruit acid that cleanses the skin and helps to even skin tone.

Mineral salts are rich in detoxifying minerals that help to stimulate the lymphatic system, and magnesium, which helps reduce fatigue and soothes muscles after exercising.

Aromatherapy blends

Using fragrant blends of essential oils in the way that best suits your lifestyle is a great way to enhance general wellbeing and health. Essential oils have wonderful properties that are calming, balancing, anxiety-reducing, uplifting, cleansing, and stimulating, all of which will help you to relax, unwind, and release stress, as well as provide an overall boost to your body.

MASSAGE OIL

BATH OIL

DIFFUSER

Blend for relaxation

Allowing ourselves time to relax is key to wellbeing. Lavender essential oil is well known for **aiding relaxation** and blends well with **calming** rose oil. Vetiver oil has a woody, earthy, slightly bitter fragrance with relaxing and **sedative properties**, making it ideal for use before bedtime.

Ingredients

Makes 30ml (1fl oz)
Almond oil 2 tbsp
Lavender essential oil 5 drops
Rose essential oil 3 drops
Vetiver essential oil 2 drops

How to **make**

For a massage oil, combine all the ingredients in a bowl, then transfer the blend to a sterilized dark glass bottle and seal with a cap or dropper, ready for use. Store the blend in a cool, dark place. It will keep for up to 3 months.

How to **use**

As a massage oil Massage into the skin on the body (avoiding your face). Allow the oil to absorb into the skin before you get dressed.

In the bath For a relaxing bedtime wind-down soak, mix the essential oils with just 1 tablespoon of the almond oil, or alternatively mix the essential oils with 1 tablespoon full-fat milk, then add to a warm bath.

In a diffuser Add the essential oils on their own to a diffuser, vaporizer or oil burner and gently fragrance your chosen environment as you relax and unwind.

Safe usage *Take care not to slip when getting into and out of the bath.*

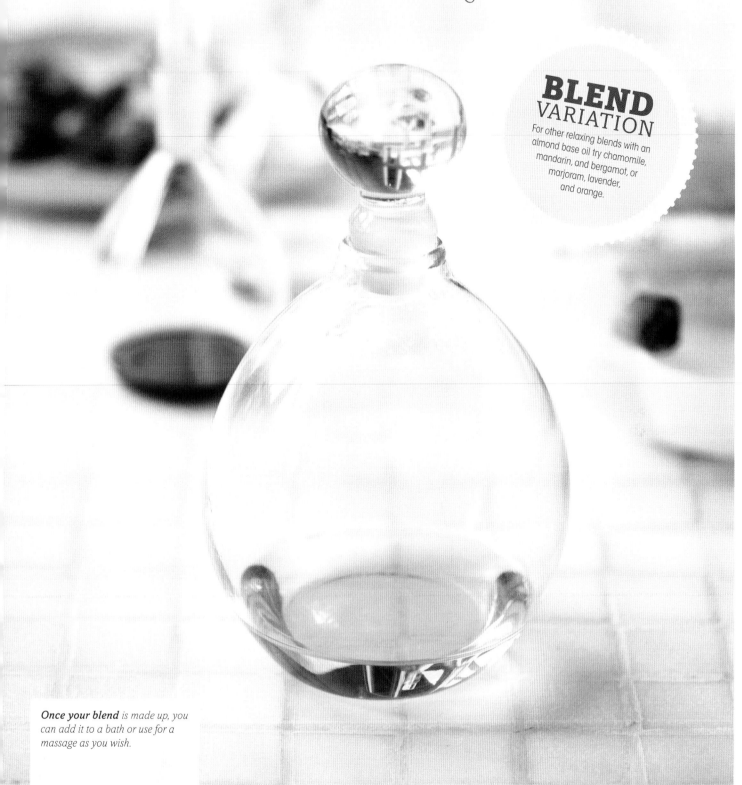

Unwind and relax with a soothing aromatic blend.

BLEND VARIATION

For other relaxing blends with an almond base oil try chamomile, mandarin, and bergamot, or marjoram, lavender, and orange.

Once your blend *is made up, you can add it to a bath or use for a massage as you wish.*

SHOWER

Uplifting blend

This trio of **reviving** oils can lift spirits and boost flagging energy. Zesty, **energizing** grapefruit stimulates body and mind and geranium helps to balance emotions by being both **calming** and **uplifting**. Jasmine completes the blend perfectly, its heady aroma increasing feelings of wellbeing.

Ingredients

Makes 30ml (1fl oz)

Unscented shower gel 2 tbsp

Grapefruit essential oil 4 drops

Jasmine absolute or essential oil 4 drops

Geranium essential oil 1 drop

How to **make**

Mix the essential oil drops with the unscented shower gel.

How to **use**

In the shower Use this uplifting blend first thing in the morning for an energizing shower that will help you start the day on a positive note.

MASSAGE OIL   DIFFUSER

Soothing blend

Calming aromatherapy provides a natural and easy way to deal with the symptoms of stress and feelings of anxiety. **Uplifting** floral essential oils, such as neroli, can be blended with other mood-boosting oils, such as frankincense, to create a wonderfully **soothing** massage or diffusion.

Ingredients

Makes 30ml (1fl oz)

Almond oil 2 tbsp

Frankincense essential oil 3 drops

Neroli essential oil 3 drops

Orange essential oil 2 drops

How to **make**

For a massage oil, combine all the ingredients in a bowl, then transfer the blend to a sterilized dark glass bottle and seal with a cap or dropper, ready for use. Store in a cool, dark place. It will keep for up to 3 months.

How to **use**

As a massage oil Massage into the skin on the body (avoiding your face). Allow the oil to absorb into the skin before you get dressed.

In a diffuser Add the essential oils on their own to a diffuser, vaporizer or oil burner to create a calming and tranquil environment.

BLEND
VARIATION
For an alternative uplifting blend combination, try combining sandalwood, rose, and cypress essential oils.

Enjoy the therapeutic benefits of essential oils by dispersing in a diffuser or vaporizer.

MASSAGE OIL

DIFFUSER

BATH OIL

Calming blend

The aromatherapeutic properties of certain oils work on both mind and body, helping to **calm** and **balance** the emotions and soothe skin. Rose essential oil helps to calm skin, reducing redness and inflammation, while geranium oil can balance oily skin and calm unsettled **emotions**. Light, versatile, and gentle on the skin, almond base oil makes an ideal carrier for this blend.

Ingredients

Makes 30ml (1fl oz)

Almond oil 2 tbsp

Rose absolute or essential oil 7 drops

Geranium essential oil 7 drops

How to **make**

For a massage oil, combine all the ingredients in a bowl, then transfer the blend to a sterilized dark glass bottle and seal with a cap or dropper, ready for use. Store in a cool, dark place. It will keep for up to 3 months.

How to **use**

As a massage oil Massage into the skin on the body (avoiding your face). Allow the oil to absorb into the skin before you get dressed. For a calming facial oil, blend 2 tablespoons almond or calendula oil with 1 drop each of rose and lavender essential oils.

In a diffuser Add the essentials oils on their own to a diffuser, vaporizer or oil burner and gently fragrance your environment with this soothing blend.

In the bath Mix the essential oils with just 1 tablespoon of the almond oil, or alternatively mix the oils with 1 tablespoon full-fat milk or a bath oil base, then add to a warm bath.

Safe usage If using the oils in a bath, take care not to slip when getting into and out of the bath.

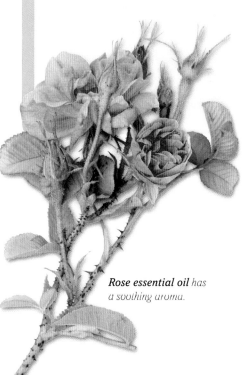

Rose essential oil has a soothing aroma.

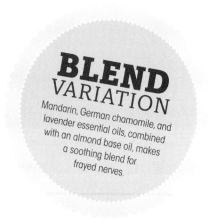

BLEND
VARIATION
Mandarin, German chamomile, and lavender essential oils, combined with an almond base oil, makes a soothing blend for frayed nerves.

FRAGRANCE

Blend for focus

Essential oils have long been used to facilitate meditation as they help to deepen and slow breathing, as well as **balance** and **centre energy**. Rosemary essential oil has a **stimulating** effect on the central nervous system so is useful for improving poor concentration. Clove and peppermint essential oils help to keep sleepiness at bay, so they are an ideal combination for maintaining focus.

Ingredients

Makes 30ml (1fl oz)
Sunflower oil 2 tbsp
Rosemary essential oil 6 drops
Clove essential oil 2 drops
Peppermint essential oil 2 drops

How to **make**

Combine the ingredients in a bowl, then transfer to a sterilized dark glass bottle and seal with a cap or dropper, ready for use. Store in a cool, dark place. It will keep for up to 3 months.

How to **use**

On the skin Dab the fragranced blend onto the pulse points on the wrists and temples. Use a bottle with a roller ball for easy application.

This centring group of oils helps to enhance concentration.

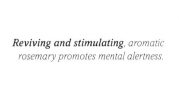

Reviving and stimulating, aromatic rosemary promotes mental alertness.

MASSAGE OIL

STEAM
INHALATION

DIFFUSER

Purifying and cleansing blend

Enjoy a **detox** massage or **cleanse** your environment by using essential oils with key **purifying** properties. You can also deep-cleanse skin by adding the oils to an unscented facial wash or oil blend, or to a steam inhalation to open pores. Juniper has stimulating and astringent properties, frankincense tones skin and helps to close pores, and lemon's citrussy scent refreshes, eliminating unwelcome odours.

Ingredients

Makes 30ml (1fl oz)
Jojoba oil 2 tbsp
Juniper essential oil 8 drops
Frankincense essential oil 4 drops
Lemon essential oil 2 drops

How to **make**

For a massage oil, combine all the ingredients in a bowl, then transfer the blend to a sterilized dark glass bottle and seal with a cap or dropper, ready for use. Store the blend in a cool, dark place. It will keep for up to 3 months.

How to **use**

As a massage oil Massage into the skin on the body (avoiding your face). Allow to the oil to absorb into the skin before you get dressed.

In an inhalation Add the essential oils on their own to hot water, cover your head with a towel, and allow the steam to act on your skin for 5 minutes. Wash skin with cool water and pat it dry with a clean towel.

In a diffuser Add the essential oils on their own to a diffuser, vaporizer or oil burner and diffuse in a sick room or your chosen room to cleanse and freshen the air.

Gently astringent and toning, this blend of essential oils has a potent cleansing action.

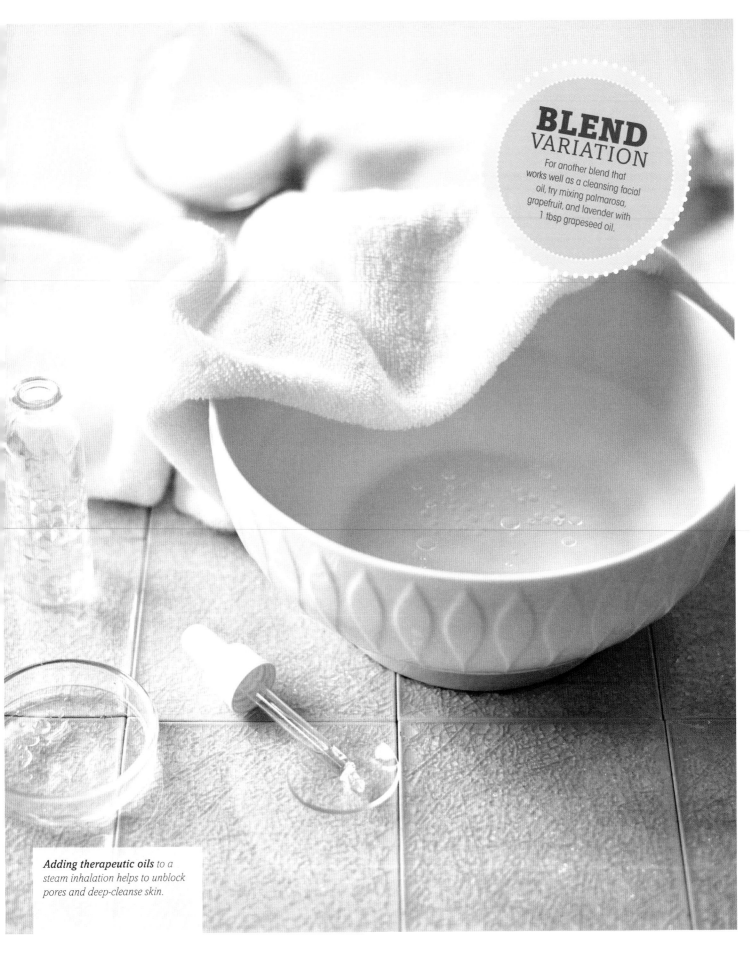

BLEND
VARIATION

For another blend that
works well as a cleansing facial
oil, try mixing palmarosa,
grapefruit, and lavender with
1 tbsp grapeseed oil.

Adding therapeutic oils to a
steam inhalation helps to unblock
pores and deep-cleanse skin.

MASSAGE OIL

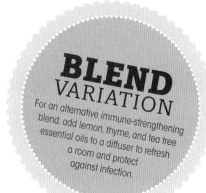

BLEND
VARIATION

For an alternative immune-strengthening blend, add lemon, thyme, and tea tree essential oils to a diffuser to refresh a room and protect against infection.

Immune-boosting blend

Immunity is the final line of **defence** against disease. Poor nutrition, lack of exercise, stress, and other lifestyle issues all place extra strain on the body's ability to function well, which can lead to an accumulation of toxins that can cause disease. Niaouli, lavender, and rosemary essential oils help **support** a compromised immune system and are strongly **antimicrobial**, helping the body to fight off infection.

Ingredients

Makes 30ml (1fl oz)

Grapeseed oil 2 tbsp

Lavender essential oil 2 drops

Niaouli essential oil 2 drops

Rosemary essential oil 2 drops

How to **make**

Combine all the ingredients in a bowl, then transfer the blend to a sterilized dark glass bottle and seal with a cap or dropper, ready for use. Store the blend in a cool, dark place. It will keep for up to 3 months.

How to **use**

As a massage oil Massage into the skin on the body (avoiding the face). Allow to the oil to absorb into the skin before you get dressed.

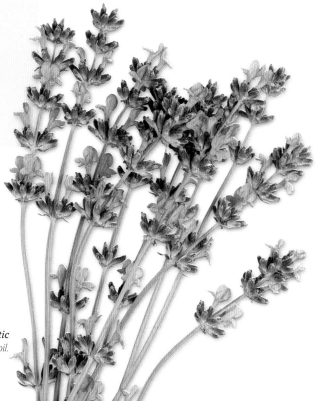

Harness the antiseptic properties of lavender essential oil.

MASSAGE OIL

BATH OIL

Regenerating blend

Essential oils can be used to encourage **skin-cell regeneration**, which is useful in the case of cuts, burns, scars, and stretch marks. Myrrh essential oil is ideal for slow-to-heal wounds and weepy eczema, while **anti-inflammatory** helichrysum can help speed up the **wound-healing** process, and frankincense encourages the growth of new cells – all of which help with skin healing and regeneration.

Ingredients

Makes 30ml (1fl oz)

Rosehip seed oil 1 tbsp

Calendula macerated oil 1 tbsp

Frankincense essential oil 6 drops

Helichrysum essential oil 4 drops

Myrrh essential oil 2 drops

How to **make**

For a massage oil, combine all the ingredients in a bowl. Transfer to a sterilized dark glass bottle and seal with a cap or dropper. Store in a cool, dark place. Keeps for up to 3 months.

How to **use**

As a massage oil Massage into the skin on the body (avoiding the face). Allow the oil to absorb into the skin before you get dressed.

In the bath Mix the essential oils with 1 tablespoon combined rosehip and calendula oil or 1 tablespoon full-fat milk. Disperse in a warm bath.

Safe usage Do not use the blend on broken skin. Take care not to slip when getting in and out of the bath.

This healing blend of essential oils has a generally rejuvenating effect on the skin.

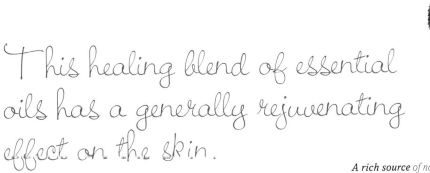

A rich source of nourishing fatty acids, rosehip is ideal for skin healing.

MASSAGE OIL   BATH OIL

Stimulating blend

Essential oils can be used to **stimulate** the appetite, digestive system, circulation, and lungs. This dynamic blend is ideal if you're feeling generally below par: ginger **calms** the digestive system and restores appetite; black pepper stimulates circulation; and tea tree helps **boost immunity**.

Ingredients

Makes 30ml (1fl oz)
Almond oil 2 tbsp
Ginger essential oil 6 drops
Black pepper essential oil 4 drops
Tea tree essential oil 4 drops

How to **make**

For a massage oil, combine all the ingredients in a bowl, then transfer the blend to a sterilized dark glass bottle and seal with a cap or dropper, ready for use. Store the blend in a cool, dark place. It will keep for up to 3 months.

How to **use**

As a massage oil Massage into the skin (avoiding the face). Allow the blend to absorb into the skin before you get dressed.

In the bath Mix the essential oils with just 1 tablespoon almond oil or, if you wish, 1 tablespoon full-fat milk. You can also enjoy a stimulating shower by mixing the essential oils with a fragrance-free shower gel.

Safe usage Take care not to slip when getting in and out of the bath.

DIFFUSER

Refreshing blend

If you feel sluggish and overcome by nervous exhaustion, this **energizing** blend could be the perfect pick-me-up. Pine oil has a **refreshing** effect, stimulating the nervous system and, along with eucalyptus, **enhancing concentration**, and peppermint is **reviving** and uplifting.

Ingredients

Makes 1 diffusion
Pine essential oil 2 drops
Peppermint essential oil 2 drops
Eucalyptus essential oil 1 drop

How to **make**

Add the essential oils to a diffuser, vaporizer or oil burner, according to the manufacturer's instructions.

How to **use**

In a diffuser Allow the oil blend to disperse and gently fragrance your chosen environment.

Safe usage Peppermint oil may be irritating to the skin. Don't use in concentrations above 2 per cent, and avoid near babies and young children.

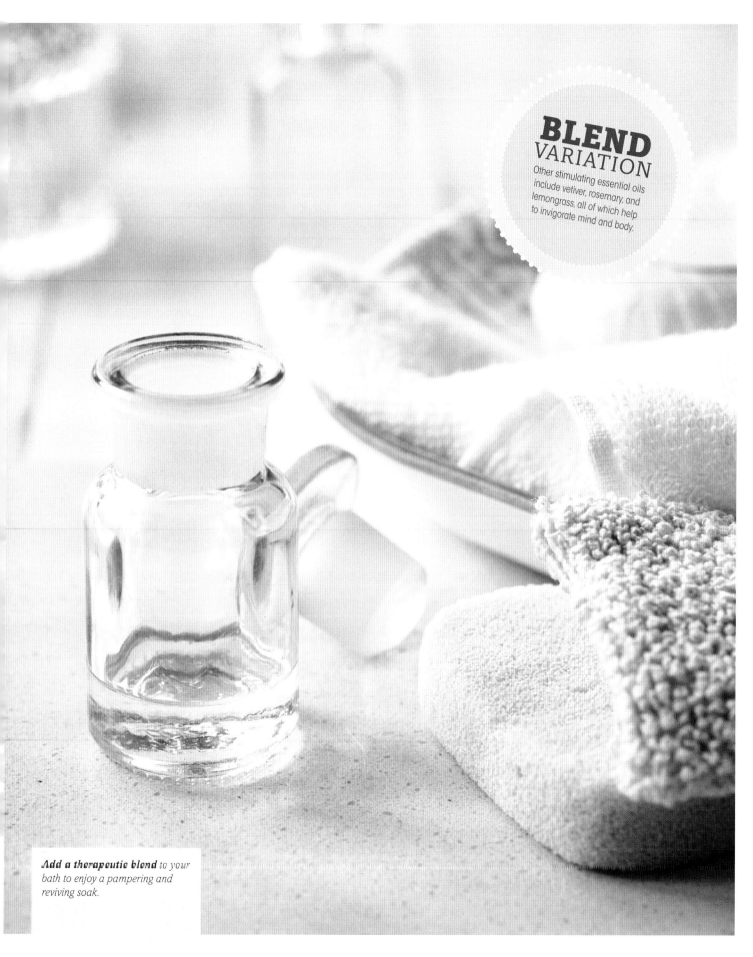

BLEND
VARIATION

Other stimulating essential oils include vetiver, rosemary, and lemongrass, all of which help to invigorate mind and body.

Add a therapeutic blend to your bath to enjoy a pampering and reviving soak.

Healing
Outside and In

Unlock the power of herbs to nurture and heal **inside** and **outside**. These simple recipes use **all-natural ingredients** to create restorative drinks, tinctures, and syrups and pampering products to help **revive body** and mind.

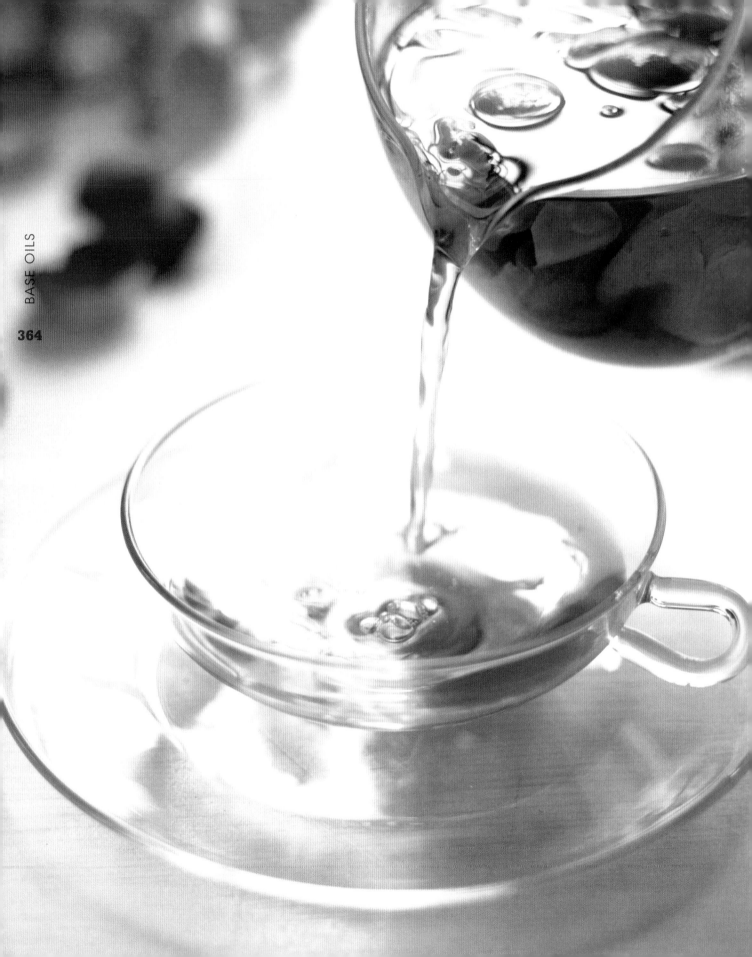

MAKING TEAS

The recipes for the tea blends provided here allow you to explore the wonderful flavours of plants, with subtle nurturing and healing qualities in a single cup. All the plants mentioned here can be used either fresh or dry – and may inspire you to grow your own healing teas in your garden.

Lemon balm and rose tea

 ENHANCES MOOD

Makes 2–3 servings

This herbal tea contains a fusion of empowering yet relaxing lemon balm and mood-enhancing, sensual rose petals to make the ultimate summer refreshment. It can be enjoyed hot or cold, and is best drunk slightly bitter. For the best results, pick fresh lemon balm leaves and fresh perfumed rose petals from the damask rose (*Rosa* x *damascena*) or French rose (*Rosa gallica*).

INGREDIENTS

16 leaves of fresh lemon balm (the soft flowering tops can also be used), or 1 tbsp dried lemon balm

2 rose heads with petals removed, or 2 tbsp dried rose petals

METHOD

1 Put the fresh lemon balm leaves and rose petals in a large teapot. If using dried lemon balm and rose petals, spoon them into the teapot instead.

2 Boil 500ml (16fl oz) of water, allow to cool for 5 minutes, then pour it into the teapot. Allow to infuse for 5 minutes and then serve. More water can be added later if needed to re-infuse the leaves and rose petals.

Jasmine and lemongrass tea

 ALLEVIATES ANXIETY   **REVIVES PASSION**   **REVIVES PASSION**

Makes 2 servings

This tea, known for being an oriental love potion, is great to serve with oriental foods. Both jasmine flowers and lemongrass help to relax the mind, alleviate anxiety, improve communication, and revive passion. For the best flavour, buy fresh lemongrass from your local oriental greengrocer or a supermarket.

INGREDIENTS
1 stem lemongrass, chopped
1 tbsp jasmine flowers
a dash of lime juice

METHOD
1 Place the chopped lemongrass in a teapot and add the jasmine flowers.
2 Dilute 200ml (7fl oz) of boiled water with 100ml (3½fl oz) of cold water so that the temperature of the hot water is approximately 70°C (158°F).
3 Pour the water into the teapot, allow the aroma to develop, and serve. In hot weather this tea can be served chilled.

Goji berry and damiana tea

 ENHANCES SEXUAL EXPRESSION   **ENHANCES SEXUAL EXPRESSION**

Makes 2 servings

Damiana has a distinctive fragrance and flavour. It lifts depression, relieves anxiety, alleviates fatigue, and enhances reproductive energy. Goji berries also improve fertility, strengthen the heart, improve disease resistance, and alleviate menopausal symptoms. Liquorice is a tonic that is restorative to the adrenal glands and alleviates fatigue.

INGREDIENTS
1 tbsp goji berries, fresh or dried
1 tsp damiana (*Turnera diffusa*)
½ tsp liquorice root powder

METHOD
Place all the ingredients in a teapot, cover with 300ml (10fl oz) of boiling water, allow to stand for 10–15 minutes, then serve. The infusion can also be left to cool and served as a cold drink.

NOTE: This tea is not suitable for use during pregnancy.

Rosehip and bilberry tea

 REJUVENATES

Makes 2 servings

Rosehip helps to maintain healthy collagen in the skin, bilberries enhance blood perfusion to give skin a rosy, plumped complexion, and bilberries and goji berries are anti-inflammatory. These fruits are also known to be powerful antioxidants, while orange rind harmonizes the digestive system and helps to improve the absorption of nutrients. This tea is also delicious served cold.

INGREDIENTS
1 tbsp rosehip shells, fresh or dried
1 tbsp bilberries, fresh or dried
1 tsp orange rind
1 tsp goji berries, fresh or dried

METHOD
Place all ingredients in a teapot and cover with 300ml (10fl oz) of boiling water. Allow to infuse for 10–15 minutes, strain, and serve. (After straining, all the ingredients can be added to breakfast porridge and eaten.)

Chrysanthemum and elderflower tea

 PROTECTS AGAINST HAY
FEVER, COLDS, AND FLU

Makes 2 servings

This is a good tea to drink to alleviate symptoms of hay fever or to ward off colds or flu. All the ingredients reduce sweating, defend the body from pathogenic influences, have anti-allergic activity, and calm allergic reactions – especially to pollen and dust. Chrysanthemum also cools the body, neutralizes toxins, improves and brightens the eyes, and protects against liver damage.

INGREDIENTS
½ tbsp chrysanthemum flowers
  (*Chrysanthemum morifolium*)
½ tbsp elderflowers
½ tbsp peppermint
½ tbsp nettle leaves

METHOD
Place all the ingredients in a teapot, cover with 300ml (10fl oz) of boiling water, allow to infuse, and serve. Drink 3–4 cups a day during the hay fever season.

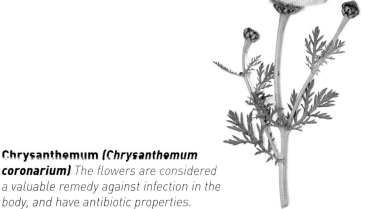

Chrysanthemum (*Chrysanthemum coronarium*) *The flowers are considered a valuable remedy against infection in the body, and have antibiotic properties.*

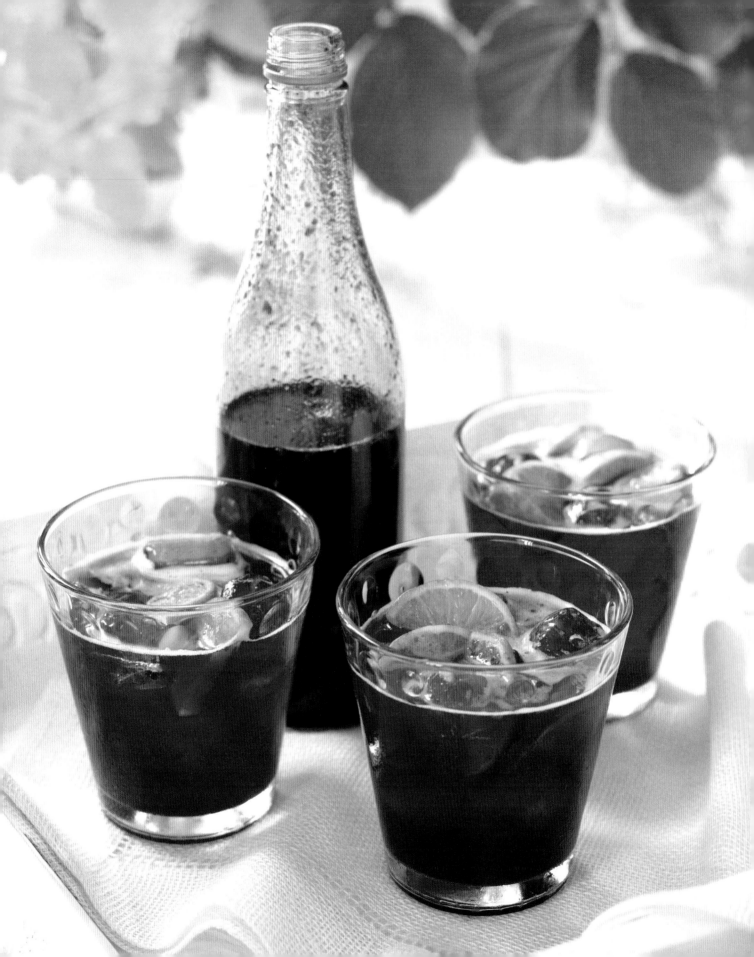

MAKING CORDIALS AND SYRUPS

Fruit cordials and syrups help to increase energy levels and nourish the body. The natural benefits of the plants in these cordial and syrup recipes are aided by sugar and honey, which help to alleviate dry coughs, sore throats, and general irritations of the respiratory system.

Blackberry and lime cordial

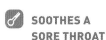 SOOTHES A
SORE THROAT

REJUVENATES

INGREDIENTS
1kg (2¼lb) fresh blackberries
juice of 4 limes
350g (12oz) caster sugar

Makes 500ml (16fl oz)

Blackberries are packed with antioxidants and are used in many recipes as a traditional remedy for colds and sore throats. This cordial also benefits from the antiseptic and refreshing taste of limes, which help to detoxify and cool the body.

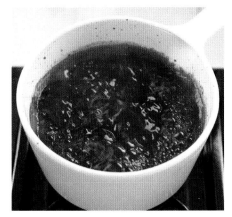

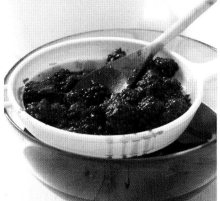

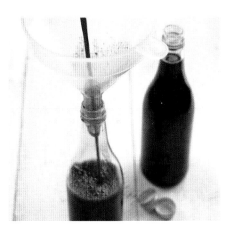

1 *Over a low heat, simmer the blackberries and lime juice in 600ml (1 pint) of water in a saucepan for approximately 15 minutes.*

2 *Leave to cool for 10 minutes or so, then push the mixture through a sieve and discard the pulp and pips. Pour the strained juice into a clean saucepan, and add the sugar. Stir over a low heat until the sugar has dissolved, and then simmer for about 5 minutes until the mixture is syrupy.*

3 *Pour into sterilized bottles, (p.370) seal, refrigerate, and use within a few days. Dilute to taste with fizzy or still mineral water and fresh mint or lime slices to make a refreshing drink.*

Rose petal syrup

 RELAXES　　　 **RELIEVES PERIOD PAIN**

Makes approximately 500ml (16fl oz)

This fragrant syrup can be served as a sweetener for herbal infusions, poured over pancakes and ice cream, or as a cordial diluted with water. The dark-coloured, perfumed rose petals of the damask rose (*Rosa* x *damascena*) or French rose (*Rosa gallica*) are best for this recipe. Keeping the temperature low is the key to making a successful syrup.

INGREDIENTS

225g (8oz) granulated sugar
juice of 1 lemon, strained
juice of 1 orange, strained
100g (3½oz) dried rose petals or
　10 fresh rose heads

METHOD

1 Dissolve the sugar in 300ml (10fl oz) of water in a small saucepan over a low heat, and do not allow it to boil, as this will make the mixture cloudy. Add the strained lemon and orange juices, turn the heat down and simmer over a low heat for 5 minutes.

2 Over the next 15 minutes, add the rose petals, a tablespoon at a time, and stir thoroughly before adding more. Remove from the heat, allow to cool, and strain. Pour into a sterilized glass bottle, seal, and label. Keep refrigerated and use within 6 weeks.

NOTE: To sterilize a glass jar or bottle, wash it and its lid in hot water, drain upside down, and put into a cool oven (140°C/275°F) for 15 minutes.

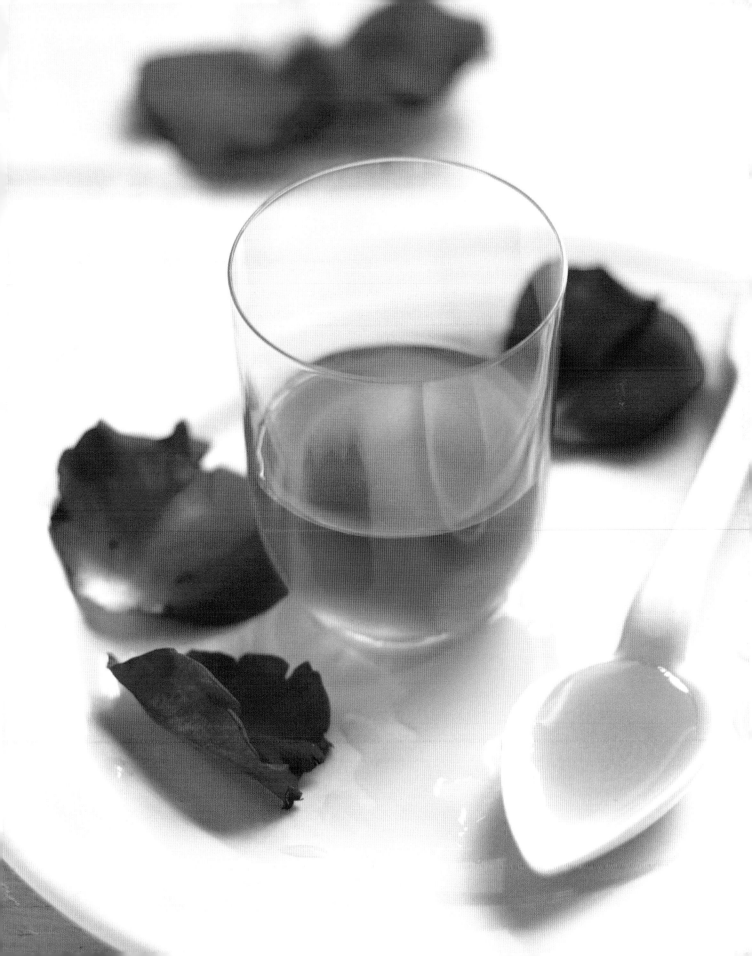

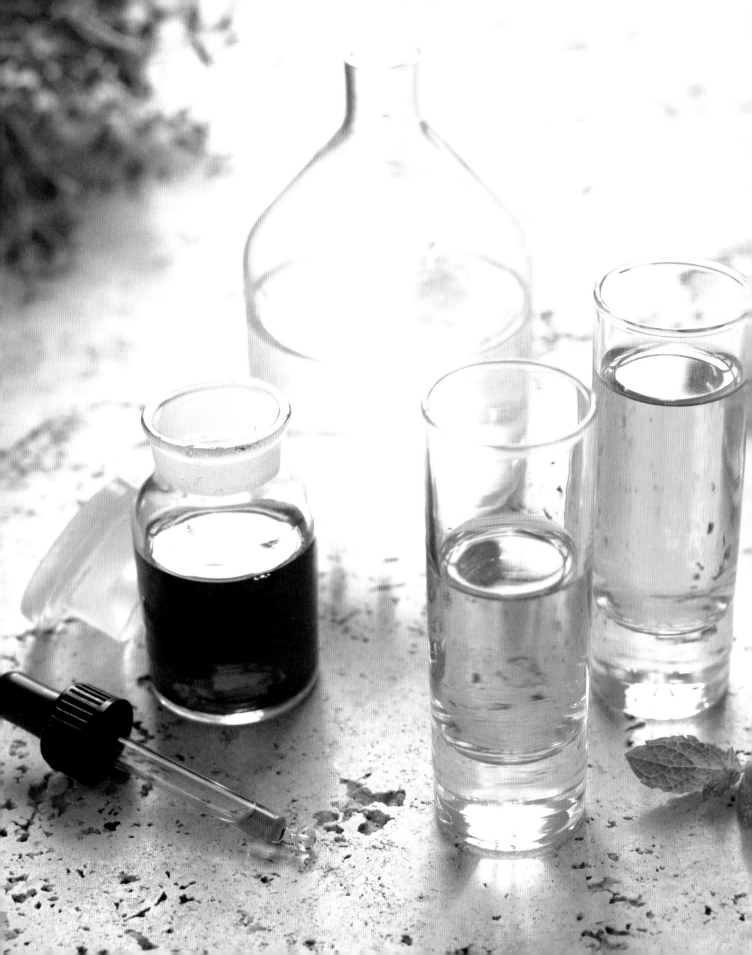

HOW TO MAKE TINCTURES

Tinctures are concentrated, alcohol-based extracts of plant materials, and are much more portable and long-lasting than herbal teas. These recipes enable you to produce simple extracts and further explore the benefits of medicinal herbs.

Peppermint and thyme tincture

 CALMS A NERVOUS GUT

INGREDIENTS
25g (scant 1oz) peppermint
15g (½oz) thyme
25g (scant 1oz) chamomile
20g (¾oz) yarrow
15g (½oz) liquorice root
500ml (16fl oz) good-quality vodka

Makes approx 500ml (16fl oz)

This tincture tastes good enough to serve as an aperitif. It aids digestion and benefits the activity of the large intestine, and helps to expel wind and soothe a nervous stomach. Use within 6 months.

NOTE: This tincture is not suitable for use during pregnancy.

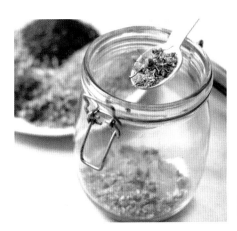

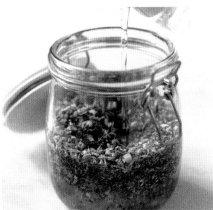

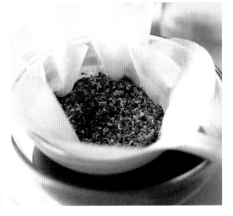

1 *Place all the ingredients* *except the vodka in a large jar.*

2 *Cover with the vodka,* *stir, and make sure all the ingredients are well immersed. Seal the jar tightly and place it in a dark cupboard. Give the jar a few good shakes every day for 3 weeks.*

3 *Open the jar* *and strain the ingredients through a muslin-lined sieve into a shallow bowl. Discard the ingredients in the muslin and pour the liquid into an amber glass bottle. Label the tincture bottle with the names of all the ingredients and the date. Take 1 teaspoon in a glass of warm or cold water and sip before or after meals.*

Elderberry and liquorice tincture

 **ACTS AS A
WINTERTIME TONIC**

Makes 300–350ml (10–12fl oz)

In autumn, winter, and early spring, most of us require something to nurture our immunity, defend us from external pathogenic influences (rampant cold and flu viruses), stimulate our blood, warm our body, and keep our strength up. These plants are known to do just that. This blend may also be taken to shorten the duration of a cold or flu.

INGREDIENTS

25g (scant 1oz) elderberries
25g (scant 1oz) echinacea root
10g (¼oz) liquorice root
10g (¼oz) fresh ginger root, grated
10g (¼oz) cinnamon stick, broken into small pieces
20g (¾oz) peppermint
400ml (14fl oz) good-quality vodka

METHOD

1 Ensure that all the dried ingredients are finely chopped, but not powdered.

2 Place all the ingredients except the vodka into a large glass jar with a secure-fitting lid. Pour in the vodka, close the lid tightly, and shake a few times.

3 Label the jar with all the ingredients and the date. Place the jar in a dark cupboard and shake it at least once every day for 3 weeks.

4 Strain the contents of the jar through a muslin bag into a measuring jug and pour the tincture into an appropriately sized (350–400ml/12–14fl oz) sterilized amber glass bottle (p.370) Seal the bottle.

5 Label with all the ingredients and the original starting date. Start by taking a few drops each day and build up to 1 teaspoon 2–3 times a day. Use within 6 months.

NOTE: This tincture is not suitable for use during pregnancy.

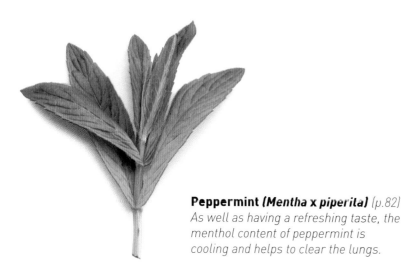

Peppermint (Mentha x piperita) *(p.82)*
As well as having a refreshing taste, the menthol content of peppermint is cooling and helps to clear the lungs.

Lime flower and hawthorn berry tincture

 RELIEVES SYMPTOMS OF STRESS   **ACTS AS A HEART TONIC**

Makes 300–350ml (10–12fl oz)

This heart tonic is good for relieving nervous palpitations and discomfort due to stress and anxiety. Hawthorn berries and lemon balm have heart-strengthening and nourishing qualities, while lime flowers and lemon balm relax the mind and improve sleep patterns. Yarrow and cramp bark relax the blood vessels, enabling a better supply of blood to the heart, and also lower blood pressure.

INGREDIENTS
20g (¾oz) lime flowers
20g (¾oz) hawthorn berries
20g (¾oz) yarrow
20g (¾oz) lemon balm
20g (¾oz) crampbark
400ml (14fl oz) good-quality vodka

METHOD
1 Ensure that all the dried ingredients are finely chopped, but not powdered.
2 Place all the ingredients except the vodka into a large glass jar with a secure-fitting lid. Pour in the vodka, close the lid tightly, and shake a few times.
3 Label the jar with all the ingredients and the date. Place the jar in a dark cupboard and shake it at least once every day for 3 weeks.
4 Strain the contents of the jar through a muslin bag into a measuring jug and pour the tincture into an appropriately sized (350–400ml/12–14fl oz) sterilized amber glass bottle (p.370). Seal the bottle.
5 Label with all the ingredients and the original starting date. Start by taking a few drops each day and build up to 1 teaspoon 2–3 times a day. Use within 6 months.

NOTE: This tincture is not suitable for use during pregnancy or if taking prescribed medication.

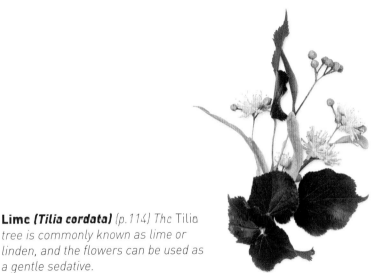

Lime (Tilia cordata) *(p.114) The Tilia tree is commonly known as lime or linden, and the flowers can be used as a gentle sedative.*

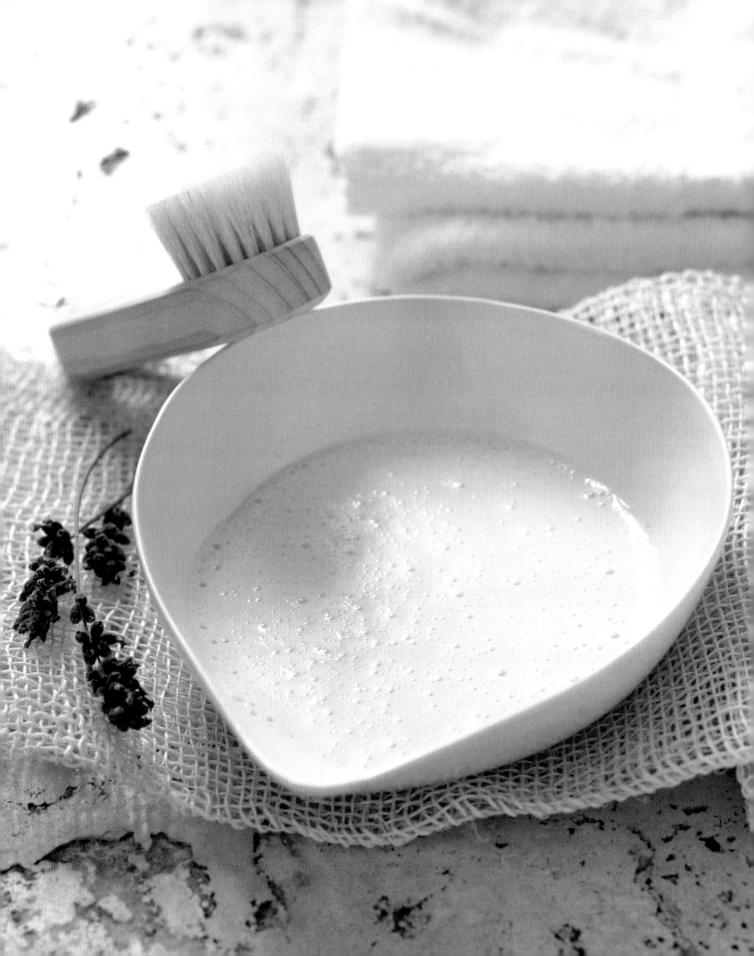

MAKING CLEANSERS

A cleansing routine is essential to support and maintain healthy skin, especially if you live or work in an urban environment with higher levels of pollution. If you have very sensitive skin, test any skin product on a small area of skin first to check that it does not provoke a reaction.

Soothing lavender cleanser

 CLEANSES SKIN

Makes 60ml (2fl oz)

This is a simple cleanser for sensitive or dry skin. Oats have long been used for their skin-soothing properties, as they are rich in natural polysaccharides that become glutinous in water to create a nurturing wash for delicate skin. Almond oil also soothes and enriches skin, helping to prevent moisture loss, while lavender soothes the skin and adds a gentle fragrance.

INGREDIENTS
25g (scant 1oz) organic oats
a little mineral water
1 egg yolk
3½ tbsp almond oil
5 drops lavender essential oil

METHOD
1 Put the oats in a bowl, pour on enough mineral water to cover, and leave to soak for at least 1 hour.
2 Whisk the egg yolk in a blender or food processor, adding a drop of almond oil at a time. The mixture should be a thick emulsion when all the oil has been added. Add the lavender essential oil, adding a drop at a time so it blends in well.
3 Strain the oats, squeezing all the liquid (oatmilk) into a bowl. Reserve the oatmilk, but discard the oats. Add the oatmilk slowly to the egg mixture, stirring or blending it in gently so that it thins to the consistency of a lotion.
4 Store in a sterilized glass bottle (p.370) with a tight-fitting lid. Refrigerate and use within 3 days.

Rose clay mask

 CONDITIONS SKIN

Makes enough for 1–2 treatments

This nourishing mask purifies and smoothes the skin. Rose, used for its cooling and balancing properties, is combined with aloe vera – an extremely soothing plant extract that is rich in vitamins, amino acids, enzymes, and proteins, and has excellent moisturizing properties. Store in a sterilized dark glass jar (p.370) with a tight-fitting lid and use within 2 months

INGREDIENTS
2 tbsp aloe vera juice
1 tsp rose water
1 tsp clear honey
½ tbsp kaolin powder
1 tbsp bentonite powder
1 drop rose absolute essential oil

METHOD
1 Combine the aloe vera, rose water, and honey. Add the clay powders by sprinkling them gradually over the mixed liquids while stirring continually. Press the mixture through a sieve. Add the essential oil and stir again to mix well.
2 Apply to freshly cleansed skin (avoiding the area directly around the eyes and mouth). Leave for 10 minutes. Rinse with warm water and pat dry with a towel.

Golden banana facial mask

 CONDITIONS SKIN

Makes enough for 1 treatment

This rich, nourishing treatment revitalizes dry skin. Fresh banana is richly moisturizing and smoothing, while golden calendula oil contains carotenoids, a precursor to skin-nurturing vitamin A. The oil also has excellent healing and anti-inflammatory properties. As it uses fresh fruit ingredients, this recipe is for immediate use.

INGREDIENTS
1 ripe banana
1 egg yolk
2 tsp calendula macerated oil

METHOD
1 Peel the banana, place in a bowl, and mash with a fork. Add the egg yolk and calendula oil and mix all the ingredients together.
2 Apply to freshly cleansed skin (avoiding the area directly around the eyes and mouth). Leave for 10 minutes. Rinse with cool water and pat dry with a towel.

Avocado and aloe vera facial mask

 CONDITIONS SKIN

Makes enough for 1 treatment

A deeply nourishing and soothing facial mask suitable for all skin types. Avocado is vitamin- and mineral-rich, as well as being high in fatty acids, lecithin, and phytosterols, which makes it an excellent moisturizer for dry skin. As it uses fresh fruit and dairy ingredients, this recipe is for immediate use.

INGREDIENTS

1 ripe avocado
1 tsp clear honey
1 tsp lemon juice
1 tsp natural yoghurt
1 tsp aloe vera juice

METHOD

1 Split the avocado in two and scoop the flesh out into a bowl. Mash with a fork to make a paste, then add the other ingredients and mix.
2 Apply to freshly cleansed skin (avoiding the area directly around the eyes and mouth). Leave for 10 minutes. Rinse with cool water and pat dry with a towel.

Apple and cinnamon facial mask

 NOURISHES SKIN

Makes enough for 1 treatment

This cleansing mask is ideally suited to oily or problem skin, as it gently regulates and cleanses the skin. Apples contain natural fruit acids, which help to gently exfoliate the skin, while moisturizing honey and ground oats help to smooth and polish it. As it uses fresh fruit and dairy ingredients, this recipe is for immediate use.

INGREDIENTS

1 ripe apple, peeled and grated
½ tsp single cream
1 tsp clear honey
1 tbsp ground oats
½ tsp ground cinnamon

METHOD

1 Mix all the ingredients together well in a bowl with a fork to form a paste.
2 Apply to freshly cleansed skin (avoiding the area directly around the eyes and mouth). Leave for 10 minutes. Rinse with cool water and pat dry with a towel.

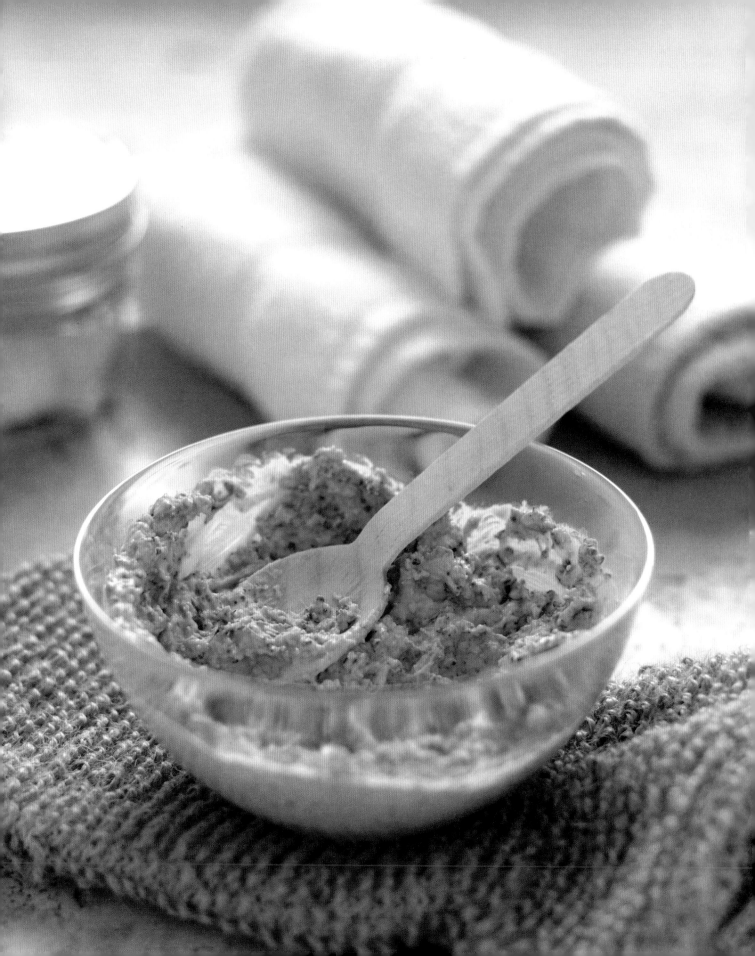

MAKING BODY SCRUBS

Scrubs boost circulation and smooth the skin, leaving it feeling radiant with a healthy glow. If you have sensitive skin or eczema, this may be exacerbated by scrubbing; the best treatment is a moisturizer or anti-inflammatory cream.

Aloe and elderflower body scrub

 EXFOLIATES

Makes enough for 1 application

Aloe vera is an extremely soothing and cooling plant extract, and is rich in nourishing vitamins, amino acids, enzymes, and proteins. This body scrub combines fresh, thick, mucilaginous aloe vera juice with elderflowers, which have anti-inflammatory qualities, and ground rice to create an exfoliating paste that refreshes and smoothes the skin.

INGREDIENTS
20g (¾oz) dried elderflowers
2 tbsp aloe vera juice
25g (scant 1oz) ground rice
3 drops benzoin tincture
4 tsp organic, plain yoghurt
4 drops lavender essential oil

METHOD
1 Cover the elderflowers with the aloe vera juice and leave for 15 minutes.
2 Add the ground rice and mix thoroughly.
3 Add the benzoin, yoghurt, and lavender essential oil. Apply to the skin using firm, circular hand movements.

Strawberries and cream exfoliating facial mask

 CONDITIONS SKIN

Makes enough for 1 treatment

This fruity mask refreshes and brightens skin. Strawberries, which are rich in natural fruit acids that help to exfoliate the skin, are combined with ground oats to give texture and extra polish, unclog pores, and smooth the skin. As it uses fresh fruit and dairy ingredients, this recipe is for immediate use.

INGREDIENTS
2 tbsp ground oats
3 large ripe strawberries
1 tsp single cream

METHOD
1 Using a pestle and mortar, grind the oats to a fine powder. Mash the strawberries with a fork and combine with the oats. Add the cream and mix to a thick paste (add a little more cream if needed to create the right consistency).
2 Apply the paste to freshly cleansed skin (avoiding the area directly around the eyes and mouth) and leave for 10 minutes.
3 Remove the paste by applying a little water in the palms of your hands to loosen it, then gently rub it away in gentle circular movements. Rinse with cool water and pat dry with a towel.

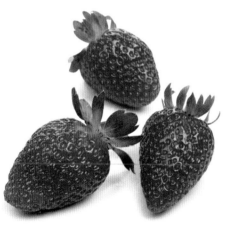

Strawberry (*Fragaria x ananassa*)
These fresh berries are highly nutritious and full of vitamins. Antioxidant anthocyanins give them their red colour.

Lavender clay mask

 CONDITIONS SKIN

Makes enough for 1–2 treatments

Natural clay minerals draw impurities from the skin and deeply cleanse it. With moisturizing honey and antioxidant-rich aloe vera, and reviving, balancing lavender water and essential oil, this soothing, purifying mask leaves skin feeling fresh and smooth. Store in a sterilized dark glass jar (p.370) with a tight-fitting lid and use within 2 months.

INGREDIENTS
2 tbsp aloe vera juice
1 tsp lavender water
1 tsp clear honey
½ tbsp kaolin powder
1 tbsp bentonite powder
1 drop lavender essential oil

METHOD
1 Combine the aloe vera, lavender water, and honey. Add the clay powders by sprinkling them gradually over the mixed liquids while stirring continually. Press the mixture through a sieve. Add the essential oil and stir again to mix well.
2 Apply to freshly cleansed skin (avoiding the area directly around the eyes and mouth). Leave for 10 minutes. Rinse with warm water and pat dry with a towel.

Grapefruit clay mask

 CONDITIONS SKIN

Makes approx 50ml (1¾fl oz)

This variation on a clay mask is more suited to oilier skin types. Grapefruit is naturally rich in fruit acids, and combined with cleansing clay minerals, mildly astringent and toning witch hazel, and soothing, nutrient-rich aloe vera, it leaves skin cleansed, refreshed, and revitalized. Store in a sterilized dark glass jar (p.370) with a tight-fitting lid and use within 2 months.

INGREDIENTS
2 tbsp aloe vera juice
1 tsp witch hazel
1 tsp fresh grapefruit juice
1½ tsp kaolin powder
½ tbsp bentonite powder
1 drop lemon essential oil

METHOD
1 Combine the aloe vera juice, witch hazel, and grapefruit juice. Add the clay powders by sprinkling them gradually over the mixed liquids while stirring continually. Press the mixture through a sieve. Add the essential oil and stir again to mix well.
2 Apply to freshly cleansed skin (avoiding the area directly around the eyes and mouth). Leave for 10 minutes. Rinse with warm water and pat dry with a towel.

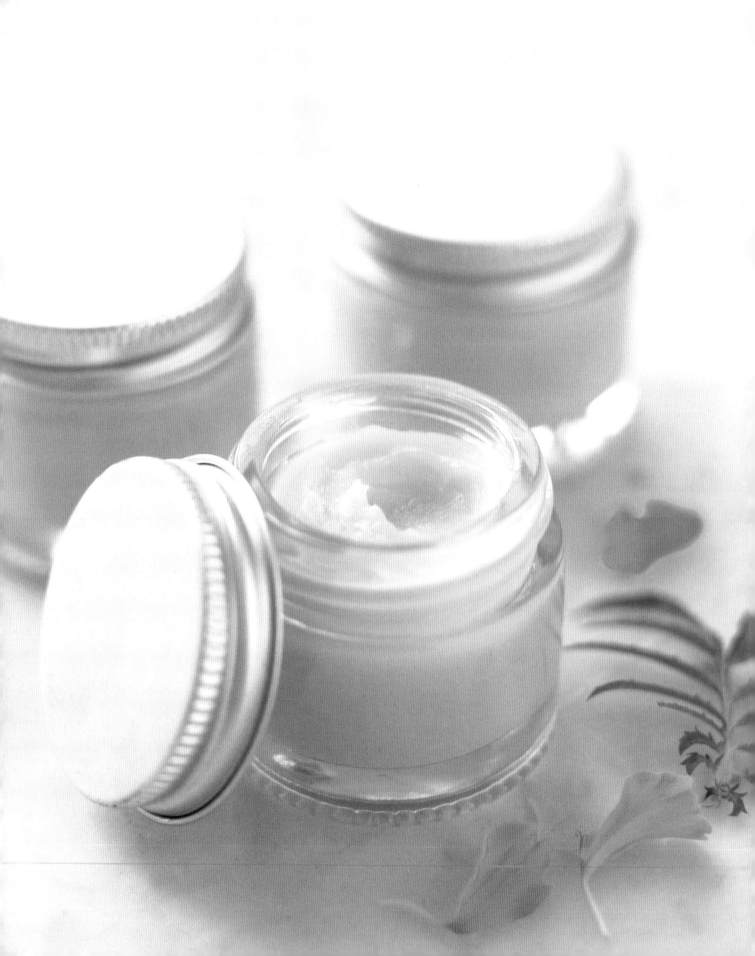

MAKING BALMS

Balms are a simple way to nourish skin and protect it from moisture loss. Make sure that the containers you use to store your home-made balms are sterilized (p.370). If you have very sensitive skin, test any skincare product on a small area of skin first to check that it does not provoke a reaction.

Calendula and mandarin lip balm

 MOISTURIZES SKIN　　**HELPS PREVENT COLD SORES**

INGREDIENTS
1 tsp beeswax
70g (2¼ oz) cocoa butter
1 tsp coconut oil
5 drops lemon balm tincture
5 drops calendula tincture
10 drops mandarin essential oil

Makes 80g (2¾oz)

Mandarin essential oil, expressed from the fresh peel of the fruit, is gently antiseptic and cleansing. Lemon balm is active against the herpes virus, so this balm will also help to prevent or treat cold sores. Cocoa butter helps to condition, soothe, and protect lips.

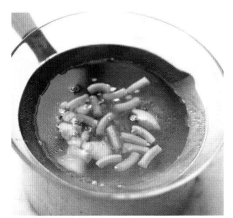

1 *Melt the beeswax*, cocoa butter, and coconut oil over a saucepan of hot water (bain-marie).

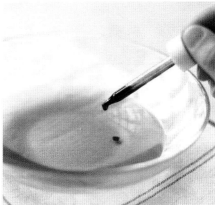

2 *Add the tinctures* and essential oil to the mixture, then stir.

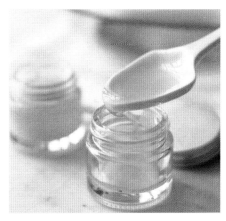

3 *Divide between* two small sterilized jars (p.370) and allow to set. It will keep for about 3 months.

Glossary

Absolute Concentrated aromatic oils extracted from a single plant source by solvent extraction. None of the solvent remains after the process. Absolutes can be used like essential oils.

Adaptogen A substance that can relax or stimulate to help balance body systems, especially in times of stress.

Adaptogenic A restorative herb which helps increase the body's resistance to fatigue or stress.

Adrenaline *See epinephrine*

Alterative Normalizes or re-establishes healthy nutritive processes.

Analgesic A substance that reduces or eliminates pain.

Analgesic A substance that relieves pain.

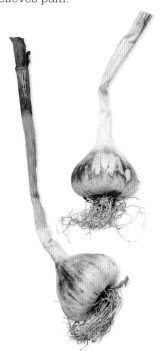

Anaphrodisiac A substance that represses sexual desire.

Anodyne A substance that allays pain.

Antacid Helps neutralize stomach acid.

Anthelmintic Treats infections by parasitic worms.

Anti-allergenic Alleviates allergic reactions.

Antibacterial A substance that inhibits bacterial growth.

Antibiotic With properties that can destroy or inhibit the growth of microorganisms.

Anticatarrhal A substance that is efficacious against catarrh.

Anticoagulant Hinders blood clotting.

Antidepressant A medication or compound that alleviates depression.

Antidiarrhoeal Helps treat diarrhoea.

Anti-emetic Helps reduce vomiting.

Antifungal Inhibits the growth of mould and fungi.

Antihidrotic A substance that reduces sweating.

Antihistamine A substance or medication that counters allergic reactions. Commonly used in the treatment of hay fever, hives, itching, and insect bites and stings.

Anti-inflammatory A substance that prevents or reduces inflammation.

Antimicrobial A substance that reduces or resists microbes, commonly used to refer to substances that are active against a wide range of bacteria, viruses, and fungi.

Antioxidant Substances that inhibit the oxidation of other molecules. Oxidation is a chemical reaction that can produce free radicals, which damage body tissues. It is also a process that can cause oils and fats to become rancid.

Antiparasitic Kills or inhibits the growth or reproduction of parasites.

Antirheumatic A substance that provides relief from the symptoms of rheumatism.

Antiscorbutic Helps prevent scurvy (a condition caused by lack of vitamin C).

Antispasmodic A substance that provides relief from muscle spasms and cramps.

Antithrombotic Preventing or interfering with the formation of a thrombus or blood clotting.

Antitussive Helps alleviate coughing.

Antiviral Capable of killing some viruses.

Aphrodisiac Something that arouses or increases sexual desire.

Aromatherapy The therapeutic use of essential oils. Aromatherapy can involve inhalation or application of essential oil blends to the skin.

Aromatic Refers to the unique aroma emitted by a plant or substance.

Astringent A substance that produces a localized tightening effect on body tissues. Used in preparations to tone the skin and close pores, or to reduce secretions and bleeding from abrasions. Astringents also help to close wounds and ulcers.

Base oil An oil used to dilute essential oils before a massage.

Bitter A digestive tonic, alterative or appetizer.

Bronchodilator Opens up the bronchial tubes (air passages) of the lungs.

Carminative The quality of reducing flatulence and gastric discomfort.

Carrier oil *See Base oil*

Choleretic Increases secretion of bile by the liver.

Cholagogue A substance that stimulates the flow of bile.

Compound A substance formed when two or more chemical elements bond together.

Compress A wet cotton pad or flannel pressed onto the body to relieve pain, inflammation, or to stop bleeding. Can be used hot or cold.

Concentrated Essential oils are concentrated because they are the essence of a large volume of plants distilled into a small amount of oil. For example, it takes around 136kg (300lb) rose petals to produce 30ml (1oz) rose essential oil.

Concrete The first products of solvent extraction; a concrete is a semi-solid mix of plant waxes and essential oils that are used to make solid perfumes.

Decongestant A substance or process that reduces congestion in the nasal passages or lungs.

Demulcent Softens and soothes inflamed surfaces.

Detoxifying Aids the body in eliminating waste and impurities.

Diaphoretic A substance that promotes sweating.

Diffusion/diffuser In aromatherapy, the process by which concentrated essential oil molecules are dispersed/diluted into the air. This can be via a device, such as an electronic diffuser, or a process, such as using a room spray, which releases fragrance molecules into the air.

Dilution The process of making something less concentrated.

Diuretic Increases urine production and output.

Dopamine A neurotransmitter that helps control the brain's reward and pleasure centres.

Elixir In aromatherapy, a blend of essential oils in a base oil. Usually refers to a mixture used on the face for the purposes of improving skin tone.

Emmenagogue Stimulates blood flow to the pelvis and uterine area, may stimulate menstruation.

Emollient Any substance that prevents water loss from the skin. Most natural oils perform this function.

Emulsifier A substance that holds oil and water together, necessary for the production of lotions and creams.

Epinephrine A hormone, commonly called adrenaline, released by the body when a person feels a strong emotion, such as excitement, fear, or anger. It causes the heart to beat faster and prepares the body for a "fight or flight" response.

Esters Chemical compounds derived from an acid. One of a number of constituents of essential oils. Most esters have fruity aromas.

Exfoliate To remove surface layers of the skin, especially dead skin cells, by using an abrasive agent.

Expectorant Encourages mucus to be expelled from the lungs.

Expression The "cold press" method by which essential oils are extracted from citrus peels.

Extraction In aromatherapy, any one of a number of methods by which essential oils are obtained from plant materials. *See also Expression, Steam-distillation, and Solvent extraction*

Febrifuge Something that helps to reduce a fever.

Haemostatic Capable of stopping haemorrhaging or bleeding.

Hepatic restorative Supportive of the liver.

Holistic Treatment of the whole person, taking into account both mental and social factors, rather than just the symptoms of a particular disease.

Hypoglycaemic Lowers the concentration of glucose in the blood.

Hypolipidaemic Regulates cholesterol levels.

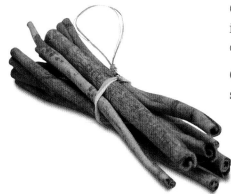

Hypotensive Having low blood pressure.

Infusion When the active constituents of a plant are extracted into a solvent such as water, alcohol, or oil. The process can be aided by heat and/or time. *See also Macerate.*

Irritant A substance that can irritate the skin or mucous membranes.

Laxative A substance that encourages bowel movements.

Macerate A type of infusion made by steeping chopped-up parts of a plant in a base oil to extract the plant's therapeutic properties.

Nervine Affects the nervous system (can be either stimulating or relaxing).

Neurotransmitter Chemicals released by the brain that act like messengers, carrying information and instructions to other parts of the body.

Nutritive Something that is beneficially nutritious.

Oestrogenic Promotes or mimics the action of female hormones.

Ointment An oily substance that is rubbed on the skin for medicinal or cosmetic purposes.

Olfactory Refers to the sense of smell. The olfactory system collects aromatic compounds from the environment and translates these into neural signals that help our brains identify individual aromas.

Organic A method of farming and growing using practices that strive to work with nature and seasonal cycles, promote ecological balance, and conserve biodiversity. Organic farmers and growers, for instance, do not use synthetic pesticides and fertilizers.

Oxytocic Stimulates the smooth muscle of the uterus to contract, hastening or facilitating childbirth.

Peripheral vasodilator Improves blood flow, especially to hands and feet, used to treat conditions of poor circulation.

Photo-allergy A skin reaction, often slow to develop (1–3 days), caused when the sun's UV rays change a substance such as an essential oil into one that the immune system considers foreign. The reaction can spread beyond the sun-exposed area.

Photo-sensitive Referring to any substance that can increase skin damage on exposure to UV rays. *See also Photo-allergy and Photo-toxicity.*

Photo-toxicity A skin reaction, often immediate, caused by the interaction of a substance with UV rays, which produces free radicals that damage skin. This is the most common type of photo-sensitive reaction; rashes tend to be limited to the sun-exposed area.

Progesterogenic
Having or stimulating
a progesterone-like activity.

Purgative A strong
laxative.

Regenerative
Supports healing and the
regeneration of cells and
tissues.

Relaxant Tending to relax or
to relieve tension.

Rubefacient Stimulates the
flow of blood to the skin, causing
localized reddening.

Sedative A substance that has a
tranquillizing effect, reducing
irritability and over-excitement.

Sensitizer Something that causes
an allergic reaction. Often an initial
application will not produce an
effect, but used over time it may
induce a severe inflammatory
response.

Solvent extraction This is a
method of extracting essential oils
from delicate plant materials that
cannot withstand heat treatment.
With this method, the essential oil
is infused in a solvent. The solvent
is then removed leaving behind a
waxy substance called a "concrete"
from which a thick essential oil
known as an absolute is then
extracted. *See also Concrete*
and *Absolute*.

Soporific This describes the
quality of inducing or tending to
induce sleep.

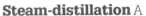

Steam-distillation A
process by which steam is
used to extract an essential
oil from plant material. Steam
flows into a container that
holds the raw plant material.
The heat encourages the
release of the oil into the
steam, which passes into
another container where the
steam is condensed back into water.
The essential oil is then separated
out from the water.

Steam inhalation The process
of inhaling steam deep into the
lungs. Adding essential oils to hot
water creates an aromatic steam
which, once in the lungs, has a
range of medicinal effects.

Stomachic Beneficial to or
stimulating digestion in the
stomach.

Sustainability Refers to the
way we produce and use goods,
specifically to systems that are
regenerative and that work to
conserve the natural balance of
ecosystems.

Styptic Stops external bleeding.

Synergy This describes the action
when several elements work
together to produce an effect that
is greater than the sum of each
part. Synergy usually refers to
compounds in a single essential oil,
but the way an oil blends with other
oils to produce a therapeutic or
aromatic effect is also sometimes
referred to as synergy.

Terpenes These are one of the
naturally occurring constituents
of essential oils. Terpenes are a
large and diverse class of organic
compounds, which are often
strong-smelling and are produced
by a variety of plants, particularly
conifers.

Therapeutic Having a healing
effect on the body and/or mind.

Toxic Something that can cause
damage to living organisms.

Vaporizer A device used to
disperse an essential oil mist into
the air. *See also Diffusion.*

Vasodilator Increases diameter
of blood vessels.

Volatile In aromatherapy, refers to
volatile aromatic compounds: the
molecules that make up individual
essential oils. They are very light
and mobile and quickly disperse
into the air, even at room
temperature.

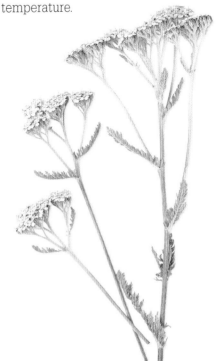

Index

Resources

Neal's Yard Remedies
www.nealsyardremedies.com
Supplier of essential oils and essential oil products. Also provides treatment rooms for consultations with qualified aromatherapists.

For courses in herbal medicine and aromatherapy, call 020 3119 5904, or email: courses@nealsyardremedies.com

National Institute of Medical Herbalists
www.nimh.org.uk

British Association for Nutritional Therapy
www.bant.org.uk

Garden Organic
www.gardenorganic.org.uk

Arne Herbs
www.arneherbs.co.uk

G. Baldwin & Co
www.baldwins.co.uk
Supplier of essential oils and complementary products.

Jekka's Herb Farm
www.jekkasherbfarm.com

Poyntzfield Herb Nursery
www.poyntzfieldherbs.co.uk

Petersham Nurseries
www.petershamnurseries.com

Aromatherapy Trade Council (ATC)
www.a-t-c.org

Provides information and news on essential oils.

International Federation of Professional Aromatherapists (IFPA)
www.ifparoma.org
Has a register of qualified aromatherapy practitioners.

Essential Oil Safety

Tisserand and Young
Comprehensive reference book for aromatherapy practitioners.

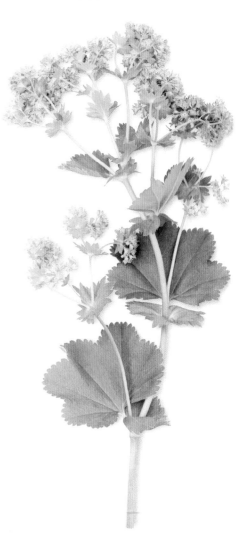

Disclaimer

Essential oils and herbs contain natural therapeutic and medicinal properties and should be treated with respect. This book is not intended as a medical reference book, but as a source of information. Do not use essential oils or herbal remedies for conditions if you are undergoing any other course of medical treatment without seeking professional advice. The reader is advised not to attempt self-treatment for serious or long-term problems, during pregnancy, or for children without consulting a qualified aromatherapist or herbalist. Neither the authors nor the publisher can be held responsible for any adverse reactions to the recipes or remedies, recommendations, and instructions contained herein, and the use of any essential oil or herbal remedy is entirely at the reader's own risk.

Acknowledgments

The authors at Neal's Yard Remedies would like to thank:
Julie Wood, Elly Phillips, Dr Pauline Hili and the NY technical team past and present, Dr Merlin Wilcox, and our great editor, Claire Cross, from DK. Our wonderful essential oil suppliers and experts who work so hard to get fairly traded, organic, and amazing quality oils, and share their expertise freely, especially Patrick Collin, Walter De Boeck, Denzil Phillips and Ulli Wentzler. Also the inspiring and dedicated tutors on our aromatherapy courses, especially Victoria Plum and Elaine Tomkins.

Dorling Kindersley would like to thank
the great team at Neal's Yard Remedies for their expertise and guidance throughout. Peacemarsh, for the use of the organic physic garden in July and August 2010 for many of the herb photographs in this book. We would also like to thank Philip Robbshow at Sheepdrove Organic Farm for his help.

Thanks to the following for supplying plants for photoraphy: Arne Herbs, Jekka's Herb Farm, Petersham Nurseries, Poyntzfield Herb Nursery, and South Devon Chilli Farm.

The publisher would like to thank the following for their kind permission to use their photographs:
(Key: a-above; b-below/bottom; c-centre; f-far; l-left; r-right; t-top)

Beniculturali (bc). 173 SuperStock: Eye Ubiquitous (bc). 176 Dorling Kindersley: Barnabas Kindersley (ca). 178 Science Photo Library: Eye of science (c). 198-99 123RF. com: Elena Lifantseva. Paperbark Co., Fragonia p201, 203 Alamy Stock Photo: Blickwinkel (l). 205 Alamy Stock Photo: Valery Voennyy (r). 207 Alamy Stock Photo: imageBROKER. 213 123RF.com: Arcticphotoworks (r). 215 123RF.com: Igor Dolgov. 220-21 123RF.com: Varaporn Chaisin. 223 123RF.com: Vitaly Suprun / suprunvitaly (r). 225 Dorling Kindersley: Mockford and Bonetti / Villa Giulia and Beniculturali (r). 226 SuperStock: Eye Ubiquitous. 233 123RF.com: Arthit Buarapa (crb). 236-37 123RF.com: Joemat (c). 241 Alamy Stock Photo: Tim Gainey. 247 Alamy Stock Photo: Yooniq Images (crb). 253 Alamy Stock Photo: Stephanie Jackson - Aust wildflower collection (tr). Alan Buckingham, Peppermint p257, Parsley p264, 119 Alamy Stock Photo: imageBROKER (l). Alan Buckingham, Tuberose p270 272 Alamy Stock Photo: Steffen Hauser / botanikfoto. 283 Dorling Kindersley: John Glover / Unwins (tr). 291 123RF.com: Anna Bogush. 292 123RF.com: Pittawut Junmee (crb). 302 Getty Images: Image Source (cla). 303 123RF.com: Mohammed Anwarul Kabir Choudhury (cla). 346 Dorling Kindersley: Alan Buckingham (br). Getty Images: Image Source (tr). 314 Getty Images: felipedupouy.com / Photodisc (bc)

All other images © Dorling Kindersley
For further information see: www.dkimages.com

Recipe and ingredient photography
William Reavell

Recipe styling
Jane Lawrie

Photoshoot prop styling and art direction
Isabel de Cordova, Luis Peral, Nicky Collings

Design/illustration help
Steve Marsden, Debbie Maizels, Dunaya Bunnag, Emma Forge

Food styling Jane Lawrie

Recipe testing Katy Greenwood

Editorial assistance
Roxanne Benson-Mackey, Kajal Mistry

DK Picture Library
Lucy Claxton, Romaine Werblow

Prop styling
Wei Tang

Proofreading
Anna Davidson, Jennifer Latham

Indexing
Hilary Bird

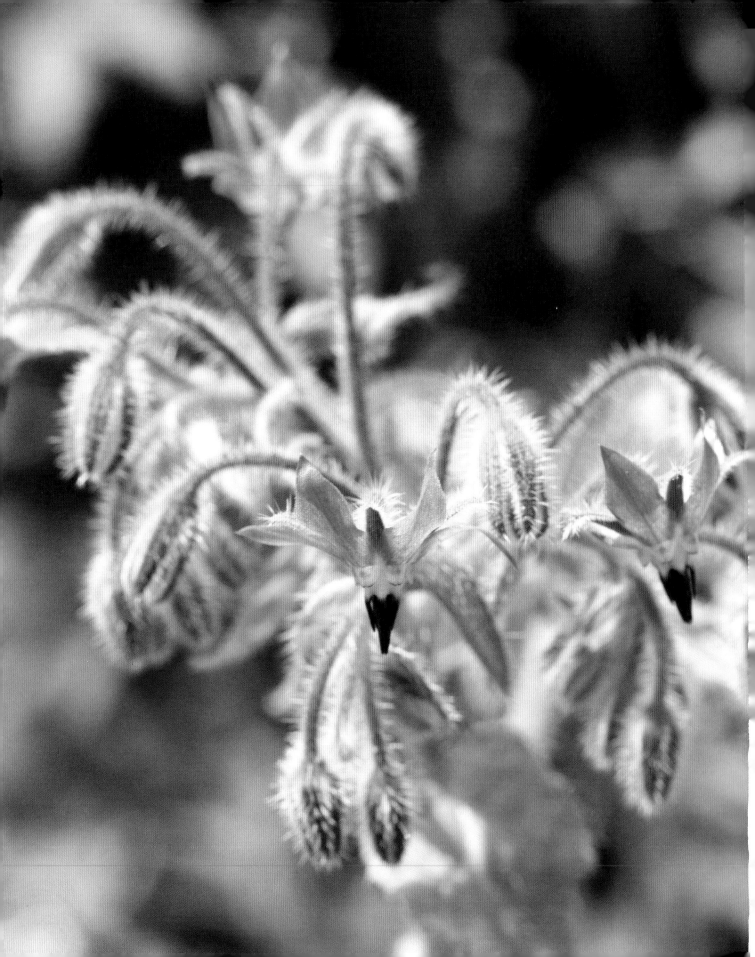